The Juicing Bible Second Edition

Pat Crocker

Robert
ROSE

Design and Production: Joseph Gisini/PageWave Graphics Inc.
Editors: Carol Sherman and Sue Sumeraj
Proofreader: Karen Campbell-Sheviak
Indexer: Gillian Watts
Photography: Colin Erricson
Photograph of Tomato Juice Cocktail: Mark T. Shapiro
Photograph on chapter openers: istockphoto.com/arsat
Food Styling: Kathryn Robertson and Kate Bush
Prop Styling: Charlene Erricson
Illustrations: Kveta/Three In A Box

Cover image: Strawberry Sparkle, see page 204.

We acknowledge the financial support of the Government of Canada through the Book Publishing Industry Development Program (BPIDP) for our publishing activities.

Published by Robert Rose Inc.
120 Eglinton Avenue East, Suite 800, Toronto, Ontario, Canada M4P 1E2
Tel: (416) 322-6552 Fax: (416) 322-6936
www.robertrose.ca

Printed and bound in Canada

11 12 13 TCP 18 17 16 15 14 13 12

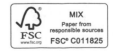

Contents

This book is for Shannon McLaughlin.

In Taoist philosophy, shen, *one of the Three Treasures means "spirit" or "mood."*
It refers to the radiance that comes from someone who is truly healthy.
May you always show bright shen *and vibrate with the*
salubrious energy that comes from healthy living.

Acknowledgments

Thanks go to Susan Eagles, a member of the National Institute of Medical Herbalists. Susan contributed the Health Conditions information. Paulina Zettel, ND, is a health specialist and founder of Continuum Wellness (www.continuumwellness.ca). Ms. Zettel provided body systems information for this book.

I have designed, made and tasted a lot of juices — literally hundreds of different combinations — most of them using the powerful Breville Juice Fountain. Beautifully designed for ease of use and cleaning and able to handle a continuous flow of fruit or vegetables, I can say without reservation that the Breville juice machines are among the best on the market today. (For more information visit www.breville.com.)

Carol Sherman and Sue Sumeraj really take their work as editors seriously and that makes my job easier. They and the Robert Rose team make and market great books.

Introduction

With juice bars and "elixir cafés" springing up in cities throughout North America, it might be tempting to think that juicing is a new trend. But it's really just the latest manifestation of a centuries-old health practice. And in this new age of genetically modified, over-refined, chemical-laden non-food, this "rediscovery" of juicing has never been more appropriate.

Research consistently shows that people who eat the greatest quantity of fruits and vegetables are about half as likely to develop cancer as those who eat little or no fresh fruits and vegetables. So it's not surprising that the United States Cancer Institute recommends eating 5 servings of fresh vegetables and 3 servings of fresh fruit each day. In fact, the phytochemicals in fruit and vegetables hold the keys to preventing many other modern diseases, such as heart disease, as well as debilitating conditions such as asthma, arthritis and allergies.

Still, even the most disciplined person can find it difficult to eat all those fruits and vegetables every day. So why not drink them? Raw fresh juices, blended drinks and homemade frozen treats are an easy and a tasty way to ensure that adults and children get their "daily 8."

Benefits of Juicing

Juicing requires that fruit or vegetables be squeezed or shredded and spun using a machine to separate the liquid from solids. Usually the solids are discarded or recycled into soups or stews.

Easy assimilation • In whole fruits and vegetables (or even in drinks that contain pulp), some enzymes, phytochemicals, vitamins A, C and E — along with minerals like iron, copper, potassium, sodium, iodine and magnesium — are trapped in the indigestible fiber and cannot be assimilated by the body. But once "liberated" from the cellulose in the pulp, those nutrients can be taken into the cells of the body within 15 minutes (as compared to the hour or more it takes for nutrients to be assimilated from food or drinks with the pulp intact). This saves the energy required for digestion and allows the body to rest while detoxifying or cleansing, before or after physical activity, or while recovering from an illness.

Water supply • Our cells consist mostly of water, which is essential to their proper function. That's why we require at least 8 glasses of water a day. Raw juice — unlike coffee, soft drinks and alcohol (which take water from the body in order to metabolize) — supplies the water you need to replenish lost fluid, while providing all the necessary vitamins, minerals, enzymes and phytochemicals. In addition, juices promote the alkalinity of body fluids, which is vital for proper immune and metabolic function.

Cleansing action • Because the fiber is removed by extraction, raw juice has a laxative effect (more evident in fruit juices), which helps to rid the body of toxins. Detoxifying the system and cleansing the digestive tract and colon helps clear the mind and balance your moods. Cleansing also causes your metabolism to become more efficient and, if a whole-food diet is followed, the body will revert to its natural weight.

The spark of life • The living "green power" that is present in all living plants is available to the body when raw fresh juices are consumed. This "life force" is a natural, vital quality that is lost in processing and when fruit and vegetables are stored.

Antioxidants • Herbs, fruits and vegetables are high in antioxidants, which counteract the free radicals that can cause cellular damage, aging and susceptibility to cancers. See pages 110 and 122 for a list of the top antioxidant fruits and vegetables.

Natural sugars • The sugars in fruits and vegetables come bundled with the goodness of vitamins, minerals, enzymes and other phytochemicals that aren't found in refined sugar. They deliver the same energy as pastries, candy and soft drinks, but without the chemicals and fat.

Chlorophyll • Found only in plants, chlorophyll has a unique structure that allows it to enhance the body's ability to produce hemoglobin, which in turn enhances the delivery of oxygen to cells.

Benefits of Pulping

Pulping or blending requires a food processor or blender. The whole fruit or vegetable is pitted, peeled and cut into smaller pieces before being combined with other ingredients for pulping. The blender blades chop the flesh of fruits and vegetables, and then liquify the solids, making them drinkable.

Full of fiber • Fruit and vegetables contain fiber in the form of cellulose, pectin, lignin and hemicellulose — all of which are essential to health. Combined, these types of fiber slow absorption of food (increasing absorption of nutrients); help lower cholesterol; reduce the risk of heart disease; help eliminate toxins and carcinogens; prevent hemorrhoids, varicose veins, constipation, colitis (and possibly colon cancer); and help prevent gallstones. When fruits and vegetables are blended or pulped, their fiber is retained, along with all the vitamins, minerals, enzymes and phytochemicals.

Keeping you satisfied • Pulping different fruit and vegetable combinations and combining them with herbs, nuts, seeds and whole grains nourishes the body. The bulk in the fiber gives a sense of satisfaction that lasts longer than what you get from fast food snacks, soft drinks or coffee.

Water supply • See page 6.

More cleansing action • Fiber in pulped juices cleanses the body in a manner different from that of extracted juices. Insoluble fiber adds bulk to fecal matter, facilitating its rapid elimination through the colon. As a result, there is no undue multiplication of bacteria with production of toxins.

The spark of life • See page 7.

Antioxidants • See page 7.

Natural sugars • See page 7.

Chlorophyll • See page 7.

Juice Machines

Juice is simply the water (up to 90%) and nutrients that have been separated from the indigestible fiber contained in fruits, vegetables and herbs. For this process, a juice machine is essential. Juicing produces a lot of pulp that can be used in other recipes (see Roughies, pages 290 to 297).

Types of Juice Machines

There are two basic types of machines that extract juice. They are as follows:

Masticating • With this type of machine, fruits and vegetables are squeezed through gears that crush them and force them through a fine stainless steel strainer. The pulp is continuously extracted. This type generally extracts more nutrients in the juice; also, because it generates less heat and friction, more enzymes are preserved.

Centrifugal • This type of juicer uses a spinning basket that shreds the fruit and vegetables and forces the juice through a fine stainless steel strainer by centrifugal force. Depending on the make of juicer, pulp can be continuously extracted or collected in the basket. Centrifugal juicers cause slight oxidation of the nutrients by introducing air into the juice.

Criteria for Choosing a Juice Machine

Ease of use • If a juice machine is easy to use and clean, it will be used more often.

Size of opening • Most new juicing machines have an opening large enough to hold a whole apple. The larger the opening, the less preparation required.

Yield • The goal is to extract the most juice from the fruit or vegetable as possible. Juicers that eject the pulp outside the machine yield less juice than juicers that keep the pulp in the basket. However, with continual extraction, a larger quantity of juice may be made without stopping to clean out the basket.

Type • See page 8 for information on masticating versus centrifugal juicers.

Reliability • Look for a 5- to 10-year warranty on motor and parts. Look for companies that supply replacement parts at reasonable cost.

Pulping Machines

Most people use a blender, Vita-Mix or food processor to blend foods in addition to a juice machine because there are some fruits and vegetables that do not juice well. Also there are some ingredients — such as flax seeds, dry herbs and wheat germ — that are easier to add to blended drinks than juices.

To make more than half the recipes in this book, you do not need to use a juice machine. To process the flesh of fruits and vegetables — alone or with herbs, nuts, seeds, whole grains or other ingredients — a blender, liquifier or food processor will suffice. This process is referred to in this book as pulping. Retaining and drinking the pulp has the added boost of all the nutrients, fiber, pith and flesh along with the juice.

Even the best juice machine will leave some nutrients in the pulp. Pulping machines cut the food into tiny pieces, making it possible to drink the pulp along with the juice.

Types of Pulping Machines

Blenders are better at pulping than food processors. The Vita-Mix is the best machine to use for smoothies and blended drinks since it reduces foods (even seeds) to microscopic particles. Most blended drinks or smoothies call for some juice, and it is best if fresh, raw fruits or vegetables are first juiced using a juice extractor then added to a pulping machine to complete the recipe.

Both extracted juices and blended (or pulped) drinks have their place in a whole-food diet.

Citrus Press

Citrus presses are powerful machines that extract the juice from oranges, grapefruit, limes, lemons and pomegranates quickly and with ease. The fruit is cut in half and placed on a molded form. When the handle controlling the cup-shaped press is brought down, the form spins and the cup presses the maximum amount of juice from the fruit.

Citrus presses are a convenient method of juicing oranges, grapefruit, lemons, limes and pomegranates. They make it easy to have a large quantity of fresh citrus and pomegranate juice on hand for drinking and using in recipes.

Note: Citrus fruits may be peeled and juiced using a juicing machine; the result is a creamy juice that contains the nutrients of the outer white pith.

Cleaning Juicers and Blenders

Use a stiff brush and hot running water to clean equipment immediately after making juice or smoothies. Thoroughly clean blades and sieves, ensuring that all bits of vegetable matter are removed. Over time, the strong natural pigments of raw foods will stain the plastic parts of most juicing and pulping equipment. To remove stains, soak in a sink full of warm water to which 2 tbsp (25 mL) of bleach has been added. (Note that some manufacturers recommend that bleach not be used with their products; check your user's manual.) Most parts are safe in the top shelf of an automatic dishwasher, and the bleach in dishwasher detergent will remove most stains.

Healthy Body Systems

Healthy Living

Today, the big killers in Western societies are the cancers, cardiovascular disease, diabetes and hypertension, most of which are preventable by diet. Immunity and obesity play a role in either reducing or elevating disease, and they in turn are both affected by the foods we eat.

Doctors, scientists, naturopaths, nutritionists and medical herbalists all agree: to be healthy and prevent disease, a healthy lifestyle is essential. Following these guidelines will maintain and help to restore good health:

Guidelines to Good Health

- Limit alcohol consumption — use of alcohol is clearly linked to a slightly increased risk of getting breast cancer. Post-menopausal women who take less than one drink per day can increase the risk of dying from breast cancer by up to 30%.
- Exercise — moderate daily physical activity can lower cancer risk, boost the immune system, help prevent obesity, decrease estrogen and insulin growth factor (IGF), improve overall health and emotional well-being.
- Do not smoke — smoking is related to one-third of all cancers and 80% of all lung cancer.
- Eat well — a healthy diet is the best defense against disease.

Guidelines to Eating Well

- Eat a minimum of five servings of fruit and vegetables every day.
- Focus on the most colorful fruit and vegetables, such as red peppers, dark leafy greens, oranges, carrots, apricots, blueberries.
- Choose whole grains over processed grains and white flours.
- Limit refined carbohydrates, such as pastries, sweetened cereals, soft drinks, candy, salty snacks.
- Cook with olive or organic canola oil.
- Avoid trans fats, found in many margarines and baked and convenience products.
- Limit intake of saturated fats and cholesterol found in meats and dairy products.
- Add avocados, natural nuts, seeds, cold water fish (cod, sardines, salmon) to the diet.
- Control portion sizes.

Juicing as Part of a Healthy Diet

Juicing plays a major role in ensuring a healthy diet by making it easier to consume the recommended five to eight daily servings of fruits and vegetables. One large glass of pure, raw, fresh juice per day will help improve the immune system, increase energy, strengthen bones, clear skin and lower the risk of disease. For maximum benefit, it is wise to consume a wide variety of juices from different types of organic herbs, fruits and vegetables.

Be sure to incorporate juices into a well-balanced, high-fiber, whole food diet. Extracted juices should not completely replace whole fruits and vegetables since their fiber is important for eliminating toxins and preventing some forms of cancer.

Healthy Bodies

The body may be characterized by seven major systems: Cardiovascular (the heart and its components), Nervous (the brain, spinal cord and nerves), Endocrine (glands and hormones), Digestive (mucous membranes, stomach, pancreas, bladder, bowel), Musculoskeletal (muscles, bones, joints, connective tissue), Respiratory (nose, trachea, bronchial tubes, lungs) and Immune (protective cells). Each system has a role to play in keeping the body disease-free. And each system responds positively to specific whole foods.

In the following pages, you will find information on each system including its importance to our health, what kinds of problems we develop when the systems break down, and the diet and lifestyle changes we need to make to keep each system working as well as it can. As always, check with a health-care specialist if you are experiencing health problems.

Cardiovascular System

Healthy Cardiovascular System

The cardiovascular system consists of the heart, the arteries and veins, and the blood that runs through them. The heart is a muscular organ responsible for pumping oxygenated blood that has just come from the lungs, and for delivering it via the arteries to all body tissues and organs. The body's tissues and organs depend on this oxygen and other nutrients to function. The heart is also responsible for bringing de-oxygenated blood back from the body via the veins to the heart so this blood can be sent to the lungs to get more oxygen.

See details on the following Cardiovascular Health Conditions:

- Anemia, page 30
- High Cholesterol, High Blood Pressure, Cardiovascular Disease, Heart Failure and Stroke, page 55

See also:

- Heart-Healthy Tonics, page 200

Cardiovascular Problems

Atherosclerosis, high cholesterol, high blood pressure

Cardiovascular disease — or heart disease, as it is most commonly called — is an illness that pertains to the heart and the blood vessels. Atherosclerosis is the most common precursor to heart disease.

Atherosclerosis occurs when fatty deposits build up on the inside of the arteries, restricting blood flow to the organs supplied by the arteries. If this narrowing and decreased blood flow happens in the coronary arteries, the arteries that supply the heart muscle itself, coronary heart disease occurs. Coronary heart disease has few signs or symptoms, until the arteries become severely occluded, resulting in tissue death and a heart attack.

Digestive System

Healthy Digestive System

The digestive system is responsible for mixing the food we eat and breaking it down into smaller molecules that our body can absorb and use. Digestion starts at the mouth with chewing and breaking carbohydrate molecules down with the aid of enzymes found in saliva. Food then travels down the esophagus into the stomach, where hydrochloric acid, also known as HCl, and digestive enzymes break down proteins and allow for the absorption of some substances. Most digestion and absorption of nutrients takes place in the small intestine, with the help of the liver and gall bladder, which provide bile, and the pancreas, which provides digestive enzymes. Food molecules, such as monosaccharides (carbohydrate units), amino acids (protein units) and fatty acids, as well as vitamins, minerals and water are absorbed into the bloodstream and lymphatic system, while indigestible foods (mostly fiber) continue down to the large intestine and eventually get eliminated.

The entire digestive system is lined with mucous membranes. Mucous membranes act as a barrier and are responsible for mucous secretions that aid in the digestive process. A smooth muscle layer also exists in the entire digestive tract, and is responsible for mixing and breaking food down, as well as propelling food downwards through the digestive tract.

Food Combining

Food combining is a disciplined method of eating foods in a specific order or combination. It is used as a short-term aid to digestive problems and, in simple terms, requires eating protein foods, carbohydrate foods and fruit at different times, thus allowing for complete and efficient digestion of these foods.

Protein foods — meat, poultry, fish, eggs, nuts, seeds, dairy products, soy products — require the most time and energy for the body to digest.

Carbohydrates are the starches and sugars found in foods that furnish most of the energy needed for the body's activities. Squash, legumes, grains (wheat, oats, rice, rye, etc.), pasta, beets, parsnips, carrots, sweet potato and pumpkin are starchy carbohydrate foods that break down faster than protein but not as quickly as fruit. Fruits are the high-sugar carbohydrate foods that are digested very quickly, and are thus considered separately in food combining

Fruit requires the least time and energy for digestion and should be eaten before a meal or at least 2 hours after a meal. When taken this way, fruit acts as a digestive cleanser, promoting digestive function. Fruit taken with a meal causes digestive problems. Melons and bananas should be eaten separately from other fruit.

Health conditions that may benefit from food combining are food allergies and intolerances, indigestion, inflammatory bowel, flatulence, fatigue and peptic ulcer.

The best food combination meals

- Fruit alone. This is best taken as a variety of fruits at breakfast.
- Proteins with non-starchy vegetables: leafy green vegetables, asparagus, broccoli, cabbage, celery, cucumber, onion, peppers, sea vegetables, tomatoes, zucchini.
- Grains with non-starchy vegetables.

Digestive Problems

Heartburn, constipation, IBS and IBD, colon cancer

Heartburn is one of the most common digestive complaints. It can be a symptom of gastric reflux, a hiatal hernia or a gastric or duodenal ulcer. Determining the cause of heartburn is important because these conditions can be easily treated but can become serious if not attended to.

Constipation occurs when bowel movements are infrequent or difficult, causing bloating, headaches or hemorrhoids, to name a few symptoms. Constipation can be caused by a lack of fiber or water in the diet, stress, or perhaps disease.

Constipation can be an indicator of other digestive system diseases. For example, constipation alternating with diarrhea can be one of the symptoms of irritable bowel syndrome (IBS). Other symptoms of IBS include abdominal pain and cramps, excess gas and bloating. IBS can be caused by sensitivity to foods and is often associated with emotional stress — and it can be extremely disabling.

Inflammatory bowel disease (IBD) includes two conditions with chronic inflammation of the bowels: Crohn's disease and ulcerative colitis. In these conditions, inflammation of the bowel can result in such symptoms as diarrhea, bleeding, cramping and a feeling of urgency. The cause of these conditions is not known. Consult a physician if you are suffering from any of the above symptoms.

The digestive system is also susceptible to cancer. Colon cancer is the second most common form of cancer, and one that can be easily prevented with a healthy lifestyle and regular bowel movements. Colon cancer is treatable, but early detection and treatment are crucial. If you experience a change in bowel habits, blood in the stool, unexplained weight loss or fatigue, consult your physician.

Endocrine System

Healthy Endocrine System

The endocrine system consists of the endocrine glands and the hormones produced by these glands, which work together to serve as one of the body's main control systems. Hormones are chemicals that carry messages through the blood. To do this, hormones travel from the endocrine glands in which they are produced to the target cells where they will perform their function. For example, the thyroid gland produces and secretes thyroid hormones (thyroxine or T4, and triiodothyronine or T3), which control the body's metabolic rate. The pancreas, which secretes digestive enzymes as part of the digestive system, also performs an endocrine function by releasing the insulin and glucagon responsible for balancing blood sugar.

The reproductive organs are also part of the endocrine system. In females, the ovaries manage the functioning, growth and development of the female reproductive system, including the breasts, via hormones such as estrogen and progesterone. In males, the testes produce testosterone, which is responsible for the functioning, growth and development of the male reproductive system.

Many other glands and organs are part of the endocrine system, including the hypothalamus in the brain and the pituitary gland just below it. Both control many glands through the hormones they secrete. Hormonal feedback can signal to these glands to produce more or less hormones that help keep the body's functions in balance.

Endocrine Disorders

Hormone imbalance, hyperthyroidism, hypothyroidism, diabetes

Most endocrine disorders occur when too much or too little of a hormone is produced by an endocrine gland, when the target cell exerts a reduced response, or in some cases when our body cannot properly eliminate excess hormones.

See details on the following Endocrine Conditions:

• Diabetes, page 43

• Hypoglycemia, page 59

• Menopause, page 74

• Menstrual Disorders, page 75

See also

• Endocrine Elixirs, page 220

Immune System

Healthy Immune System

The immune system consists of a complex collection of cells found throughout the body. These cells are responsible for protecting the body against infection, as well as for constant surveillance and destruction of the cancer cells.

The skin and mucous membranes, along with chemical substances like mucous, tears and stomach acid, are also an important part of the immune system, acting as front-line barriers that prevent foreign materials and pathogenic organisms from entering and harming the body.

When the immune system does not work optimally, we see an increased risk for infections and cancers, as well as the development of allergies and inflammatory disease.

Support and enhancement of the immune system through consumption of whole foods, proper intake of water, regular moderate exercise and mental relaxation can increase the body's resistance to colds, influenza and cancers and keep allergies and inflammation in check.

See details on the following Immune Conditions:

• AIDS + HIV, page 24

• Allergies, page 26

• Cancer Prevention, page 37

• Chronic Fatigue Syndrome, page 39

• Common Cold, page 40

• Herpes Simplex, page 57

• Immune Deficiency, page 59

• Influenza, page 67

• Lupus, page 73

Immune System Disorders

Frequent and chronic infections, cancer, inflammation, allergies

See also
- Immune Boosters, page 226
- The Power of Garlic, page 226

Frequent and chronic infections may include anything from a common cold, flu, ear infections and urinary tract infections to more serious illnesses, such as herpes virus infections, bronchitis and pneumonia. Viruses, bacteria, fungi and parasites can all cause infections, especially when they do not meet adequate resistance from a weakened immune system.

Similarly, cancer risk increases when there is damage to a cell's DNA and the immune system's DNA repair or cancer surveillance systems are not functioning at an optimal level. DNA can be damaged by free radicals produced inside the body or by elements from the external environment, such as chemicals, radiation or viruses.

Musculoskeletal System

Healthy Musculoskeletal System

Muscles, bones, joints and connective tissue make up the musculoskeletal system, responsible for the movement of the human body and its individual parts. The musculoskeletal system also gives structure to the body and physically protects the internal organs.

Nutrition is very important in the management of this system; for example, muscle contraction and relaxation depend on minerals like calcium and magnesium to perform movements and maintain an upright posture and balance. Bones also need minerals to maintain their density and withstand the pulling forces created by the muscles and the impact of accidents and falls.

Another important part of the musculoskeletal system is the joints, such as the hip, knees and elbows. Within the joints, the ends of the bones are covered with cartilage and are surrounded by synovial fluid, a lubricating fluid, which allows smooth and frictionless motion where two bones meet.

Musculoskeletal Disorders

Arthritis, osteoporosis, low back pain, muscle spasms and cramps, sprains and strains

Muscle cramping and spasms can occur with dehydration and if minerals such as calcium, sodium, potassium and magnesium are not in the proper balance. This can cause simple cramping of the calf muscle or more aggravate existing conditions, such as low back pain. Low back pain can also be due to misalignment of the spine or other parts of the skeleton, nerve impingement, injury and chronic inflammation.

Inflammation also occurs during arthritis. There are many types of arthritis, some with more inflammation than others. For example, osteoarthritis, the most common type, is characterized by wear and tear at the joints, wearing down of the joint cartilage, and causing changes in the bone. Although minimal, osteoarthritis consists of some inflammation at the joint and in surrounding tissues. Symptoms can be stiffness and pain at the joint and eventually restricted joint function. On the other hand, rheumatoid arthritis is an autoimmune condition characterized by chronic inflammation that can affect the joints as well as other areas of the body. Rheumatoid arthritis can give symptoms of inflammation at the joint, such as pain, redness, swelling and eventually deformity, but also generalized symptoms of fatigue, weakness and low-grade fever. Regardless of the cause and the differing symptoms and location, nutrition is essential to repair and build cartilage and decrease inflammation.

Unlike arthritis, osteoporosis is mostly symptom-free, which is why people at increased risk must get regular bone-density checks. In osteoporosis, the bone density is diminished and the bones become brittle and susceptible to fractures. The density of the bone depends on many nutrients, such as calcium, magnesium and zinc, for the strength to withstand trauma, perform movement and provide support.

See details on the following Musculoskeletal Conditions:

• Arthritis, page 32

• Osteoporosis, page 79

See also

• Muscle Powers, page 240

Nervous System

Healthy Nervous System

The nervous system is a highly complex system made up of two main parts, the central and the peripheral nervous systems, which together allow us to respond to our internal and external environments. The central nervous system consists of the brain and the spinal cord, while the peripheral nervous system is made up of nerves (sensory and motor) and connects the central nervous system with other parts of the body.

The peripheral nervous system is responsible for receiving information, such as taste, sound or hormone levels, from the internal and external environments and for relaying that information to the central nervous system via peripheral sensory nerves. The spinal cord and brain integrate this information in the central nervous system and generate a response, which is then sent to other parts of the body via the peripheral motor nerves. For example, the peripheral sensory nerves might relay information about a song on the radio to the spinal cord and the brain. A response would then be sent through the peripheral motor nerves to make a movement to turn up the radio.

Of course, not all responses are conscious. The peripheral nervous system also consists of the autonomic nervous system, which controls internal organs and glands, such as the heart, or the thyroid gland, which is responsible for the body's metabolism. Through this system, consisting of sympathetic and parasympathetic responses, the body can maintain an internal balance and react to different stimuli based on the needed responses. For example a sympathetic or "fight or flight" response is created when you are frightened or stressed. This response causes your heart rate to increase. In contrast, a parasympathetic response allows you to perform such functions as relaxing and digesting your food after a meal. These two parts of the autonomic nervous system act on the same organs and glands, but have opposing effects, helping maintain balance in the body.

Nervous System Disorders

Anxiety, depression, seasonal affective disorder, memory loss and decreased cognitive function

Depression is a condition that occurs when there is an imbalance of neurotransmitters in the brain. It can be characterized by a loss of interest or pleasure in usual activities and a lack of energy. It can also affect appetite, with either a decrease or increase, and subsequent changes in body weight. Depression can be quite debilitating and can trigger feelings of worthlessness or even thoughts of death or suicide.

Seasonal affective disorder (SAD) is a form of depression that occurs with diminished exposure to sunlight in the winter months. This disorder may result in the general symptoms of depression, and also an increase in sleep, appetite and perhaps body weight.

Anxiety is a devastating psychiatric disorder that can consist of feelings of agitation, nervousness, fearfulness, irritability or shyness. Other symptoms may include heart palpitations, flushing of the face, sweating, shallow breathing or even fainting. Both anxiety and depression can be caused by psychological factors; a physical cause, such as trauma or illness; nutrient deficiencies; or the side effects of medications.

As a result of normal living and aging, the nervous system suffers from oxidation of its cells, improper nutrient status and a decrease in blood circulation. These and other factors can lead to a decline in neurotransmitter levels, a decrease in the number of connections between neurons and an actual decrease in brain size, leading to a decrease in cognitive function and memory loss.

See details on the following Nervous System Conditions:

- Anxiety States, page 31
- Depression, page 42
- Parkinson's Disease, page 82

See also

- Nerve Nourishers, page 248
- Stress Busters, page 259

Respiratory System

Healthy Respiratory System

The respiratory system is responsible for the exchange of oxygen and carbon dioxide between the external environment and the blood. The air that we breathe travels in through the nose, past the pharynx and larynx, down the trachea, into the bronchi and bronchioles and eventually reaches its destination: the lungs. In the lungs, the exchange of gases occurs in tiny air sacs called alveoli, where oxygen from the air enters the bloodstream and carbon dioxide from the bloodstream enters the air to be expelled. Through the actions of inspiration and expiration, the air flows in and out of the lungs providing all body cells with the fresh supply of oxygen essential to them for survival.

The respiratory system is also responsible for protecting the body against microbes, toxic chemicals and foreign matter. This is achieved with the help of cilia, tiny hair-like structures that sweep mucous and foreign materials out of the system. The cilia also work with the immune system to produce mucous and perform phagocytosis (engulfing pathogens and debris).

Respiratory Disorders

Asthma and allergies, respiratory tract infections, lung cancer

Asthma is the most common illness associated with the respiratory system. It is an inflammatory condition of the lungs and airways in which swelling, smooth muscle contraction and excess mucous production create acute breathing difficulties. Someone who suffers from asthma might experience a feeling of tightness and constriction of the chest, with shortness of breath, wheezing and coughing. It is believed that asthma, like allergies, is a hypersensitivity disorder and therefore greatly linked to the immune system.

The respiratory system is the most susceptible to infection, because it is directly exposed to the external environment. Therefore, respiratory infections, such as colds, sinusitis, bronchitis and pneumonia, also greatly depend on the immune system. Here, the immune system is responsible for protecting the respiratory system by producing mucous, attacking foreign invaders and developing a proper response to fight pathogens once they enter the body.

The respiratory system is also susceptible to cancer. Lung cancer is the most prevalent form of cancer today and can affect one or both lungs. Smoking is the biggest risk factor for lung cancer, so quitting smoking is a valuable method in its prevention. Other methods include eating a vitamin-rich diet, which can help reduce the risk of cancer but also the chance that cancer will come back once treated.

See details on the following Respiratory System Conditions:

• Allergies, page 26
• Bronchitis, page 36
• Cancer Prevention, page 37

See also

• Respiratory Juices, page 255

Health Conditions

The combined wisdom of common sense, human observation and scientific study all point to the importance of our diet in preventing and controlling disease. General dietary principles are set out on page 12. In this section you will find recommendations for specific health conditions.

These recommendations are not intended to take the place of consultation with a medical practitioner. For best results, and especially if faced with a serious condition, contact a doctor, medical herbalist or natural health specialist who can provide you with a diet and lifestyle program suited to your needs. For each condition, the best fruits, vegetables, herbs and other foods are recommended.

AIDS & HIV
Acquired Immunodeficiency Syndrome & Human Immunodeficiency Virus

There is no known cure for AIDS, and anyone with HIV should be under a doctor's care. However, dietary therapy can improve immune function, promote resistance to infections associated with AIDS and reduce symptoms associated with HIV and AIDS.

Healing Foods

Fruits and vegetables
citrus fruits, peaches, pears, strawberries, asparagus, avocados, broccoli, carrots, cauliflower, leafy greens, onions, squash

Herbs
aloe vera, astragalus, burdock (leaf, root and seeds), evening primrose oil, garlic, ginseng, licorice*, turmeric

Other
cereal grasses, flax seeds, kelp, pumpkin seeds, sprouted seeds, soy yogurt, sunflower seeds, tofu, whole grains

* Avoid licorice if you have high blood pressure. The prolonged use of licorice is not recommended under any circumstances.

What to Do

Maximize
- Organic fruits and vegetables, which are free of chemicals
- Shiitake mushrooms, which studies have shown to strongly support the immune system
- Garlic — an antibacterial, antiviral and antifungal — which guards against opportunistic infections

Minimize
- Sweet foods, including honey and fruit juices, which encourage the growth of molds and yeast

Eliminate
- Refined flour
- Animal fats in meat and dairy products, as they decrease immunity
- Alcohol, which increases susceptibility to infection
- Food allergies and intolerances (see Appendix A: Food Allergies, page 359)
- Sugar

Other Recommendations
- Exercise daily, according to your fitness level. This helps improve circulation and eliminates toxins through sweating.
- Practice stress-reduction techniques, such as yoga, tai chi and meditation to strengthen the immune system by decreasing stress.

Healing Drinks

(see also Immune Boosters, page 226; Top Common Antioxidant Fruits and Vegetables, pages 110 and 122)

Add 1 tsp (5 mL) herbs and up to 2 tbsp (25 mL) other ingredients recommended (see page 24) for this condition to the following:

Juices
- Allium Antioxidant, page 227
- Brocco-Carrot, page 181
- Cauliflower Cocktail, page 312
- C-Green, page 184
- Leafy Greens, page 191
- Green Magic (use a recommended herb in place of ginkgo, see page 24), page 190
- Moist & Juicy (use a recommended herb in place of ginkgo, see page 24), page 192

Smoothies
- Green Energy (use a recommended herb in place of ginkgo, see page 24), page 303

Teas
- Antioxi-T, page 229

Coffee Substitutes
- Immune Regulator Tea, page 234
- Immune Tea Blend, page 235
- Root Coffee Blend, page 338

Aging

Several scientific studies show that eating a diet high in nutrients but low in calories helps reduce signs of aging and increases life span. Recent studies also show that oxidation is one of the most important factors that contributes to aging. Oxidation occurs when cells are damaged by free radicals, by-products produced when the body converts oxygen to energy. The progression of Parkinson's disease and Alzheimer's disease have been linked to oxidative stress. Heart disease, cancer, arthritis and wrinkles are also signs of cell damage, often caused by free radicals. Antioxidants, which are found in many fruits and vegetables, protect the body from free-radical damage.

Healing Foods

Fruits and vegetables
apples, blueberries, grapefruit, oranges, pears, raspberries, strawberries, beets, broccoli, cabbage, carrots, celery, leafy greens, onions, pumpkin, sweet potatoes, tomatoes

Herbs
cayenne, German chamomile, garlic, ginger, ginkgo, green tea, lemon balm, milk thistle, oregano, parsley*, peppermint, rosemary, sage, spearmint, thyme, turmeric

* If you are pregnant, limit your intake of parsley to ½ tsp (2 mL) dried or one sprig fresh per day. Do not take parsley if you are suffering from kidney inflammation.

What to Do

Maximize
- Antioxidant-rich fruits and vegetables
- Antioxidant herbal teas (any combination of oregano, rosemary, lemon balm, sage, thyme and peppermint)
- Effective digestion. Remedying digestive problems (see Indigestion, page 62) will improve your body's ability to absorb nutrients

Minimize
- Animal fats in meat and dairy products. Replace some meat meals with fish and vegetable protein

Eliminate
- Unnecessary calories

Other
cereal grasses, flax seeds, nuts, extra-virgin olive oil, pumpkin seeds, sea herbs, sesame seeds, soy products, sunflower seeds, yogurt with active bacterial cultures

Healing Drinks

(see also Immune Boosters, page 226; Top Common Antioxidant Fruits and Vegetables, pages 110 and 122)

Add 1 tsp (5 mL) herbs and up to 2 tbsp (25 mL) other ingredients recommended (see page 25 and left) for this condition to the following:

Juices
- Allium Antioxidant, page 227
- Black Pineapple, page 164
- Blueberry, page 165
- Brocco-Carrot, page 181
- Grape Heart, page 202

- Green Magic, page 190
- Moist & Juicy, page 192
- Rust Proofer #1, page 238
- Rust Proofer #2, page 238

Smoothies
- Beta Boost, page 299
- Smart Smoothie, page 306
- Spa Special, page 307

Teas
- Antioxi-T, page 229
- Green Giant Tea Blend, page 281
- Raspberry Tea, page 265

Coffee Substitutes
- Seed Power Coffee, page 339

Allergies
Hay Fever, Eczema & Asthma

Healing Foods

Fruits and vegetables
apples, blueberries, grapes, mangoes, oranges, raspberries, strawberries, asparagus, beets, carrots, onions, red and green bell peppers, spinach, watercress

The symptoms of allergic reactions evidenced in hay fever, eczema and asthma are caused by inflammation, which is the body's normal healing response to injury. Allergies are an example of chronic inflammation, in which factors such as food intolerance, stress and poor digestion allow a toxin to activate the immune system. This causes inappropriate inflammatory responses on the skin or in the eyes, nose or airways. Proper nutrition and the use of appropriate herbs can reduce the severity of the inflammation.

What to Do

Maximize
- Fruits and vegetables that provide flavonoids and antioxidants, which support appropriate immune response
- Essential fatty acids (found in oily fish, flax seeds and sunflower seeds, among other foods), which are anti-inflammatory and reduce the severity of allergies

- Herbs that optimize digestion (dandelion root, as required), boost immunity (astragalus, garlic) and nourish the nervous system (oat straw, skullcap)

Healing Foods

Herbs

astragalus, burdock root*, calendula*, cinnamon, dandelion leaf and root*, elderflower, garlic, ginger, licorice**, parsley***, stinging nettle, thyme, turmeric, yarrow*

Other

flax seeds, nuts (except peanuts), pumpkin seeds, rice, soy products, yogurt with active bacterial cultures, whole grains

* People who are allergic to ragweed may also be allergic to herbs in the same botanical family (the *Compositae*, or daisy, family). The herbs in this family include burdock, calendula, chamomile, chicory, dandelion, echinacea, feverfew, milk thistle and yarrow (avoid yarrow if you are pregnant).

** Avoid licorice if you have high blood pressure. The prolonged use of licorice is not recommended under any circumstances.

*** If you are pregnant, limit your intake of parsley to ½ tsp (2 mL) dried or one sprig fresh per day. Do not take parsley if you are suffering from kidney inflammation.

Eliminate

- Food allergies and intolerances (see Appendix A: Food Allergies, page 359)
- Sugar, including honey and fruit sugars. Studies have shown that sugars decrease immune function by impairing white-blood-cell activity. Excess sugar also promotes yeast infections, which increase allergic reactions
- Alcohol, which depresses immune function
- Mucus-forming foods (dairy products, bananas)

Other Recommendations

- Reduce stress. Stress and high emotion are factors in lowered immunity, which increases susceptibility to allergies. Sleep and relaxation help to produce immunity-enhancing compounds.
- Improve digestion. Poor digestion keeps the body from eliminating toxins and limits the absorption of nutrients. When food is completely digested, allergic reactions are often eliminated.
- Get adequate protein. Protein is essential for optimum immune function. The best sources of protein are fish, such as tuna, salmon, sardines, trout, cod and herring.

Healing Drinks

(see also Immune Boosters, page 226; Top Common Antioxidant Fruits and Vegetables, pages 110 and 122)

Add 1 tsp (5 mL) herbs and up to 2 tbsp (25 mL) other ingredients recommended (see left) for this condition to the following:

Juices

- Beet, page 180
- Berry Fine Cocktail, page 310
- Blueberry, page 165
- C-Green, page 184
- Citrus Cocktail, page 313
- Grape Power (use a recommended herb in place of rosemary, see left), page 170
- Spring Celebration, page 195

Smoothies

- Green Energy (use a recommended herb from list in place of ginkgo, see left), page 303
- Mango Madness (substitute ¼ cup/50 mL yogurt for banana), page 304

Teas

- Aller-free Tea, page 227
- Immune Regulator Tea, page 234
- Nettle Tea, page 284

Alopecia

Alopecia is a partial or complete loss of hair. It can be caused by severe stress; skin diseases; excessive sunlight; thyroid imbalances; excessive sex hormones; or strong chemicals, such as those used for cancer treatment or on the hair, that interfere with the nutrition of the hair follicles.

Hair consists largely of protein, which is made from amino acids and minerals, and is greatly affected by nutrition. Rosemary is traditionally used to treat hair problems. A rosemary tea can be used both internally and externally to stimulate blood flow to the scalp.

What to Do

Include in Your Diet

- High-protein foods (meat, fish, poultry, eggs, cheese, brown rice, nuts, seeds, soybeans)
- Foods that contain sulfur (egg yolks, cauliflower, cabbage, turnips, onions, garlic)
- Calcium-rich foods (dairy products, leafy greens, sea herbs)

Maximize

- Antioxidant-rich fruits and vegetables, especially broccoli, cabbage, garlic, onions and spinach

Minimize

- Stress. Relaxation techniques, such as meditation and yoga, can help alleviate the stresses and tensions of life

Healing Drinks

Add 1 tsp (5 mL) herbs and up to 2 tbsp (25 mL) other ingredients recommended (see left) for this condition to the following:

Juices

- Allium Antioxidant, page 227
- Cabbage Cocktail, page 311
- Cabbage Rose, page 181
- Nip of Goodness, page 192

Smoothies

- Green Energy, page 303

Teas

- Circulation Tea, page 249

Alzheimer's Disease & Dementia

Dementia is characterized by impairment of memory, judgment and abstract thinking. It may be caused by stress, by impaired circulation caused by a buildup of fatty deposits in the blood vessels of the brain or by a degenerative disease, such as Alzheimer's disease. Recognized risk factors for Alzheimer's disease include acetylcholine deficiency, free-radical damage and inflammation of brain tissue. Diet can play

Healing Foods

Fruits and vegetables
blueberries, citrus fruits, grapes, asparagus, broccoli, beets and beet greens, carrots, green bell peppers, kale, okra, onions, spinach, sweet potatoes, watercress, yams

Herbs
basil, garlic, German chamomile, ginger, ginkgo, ginseng, dandelion leaves and flowers, lemon balm, licorice*, stinging nettle, parsley**, red clover flowers, rosemary, sage, skullcap, turmeric

Other
Brazil nuts, brown rice, cider vinegar, egg yolks, flax seeds, lecithin, legumes, lentils, nuts, oats, extra-virgin olive oil, pumpkin seeds, sea herbs, soy products, wheat germ

* Avoid licorice if you have high blood pressure. The prolonged use of licorice is not recommended under any circumstance.

** If you are pregnant, limit your intake of parsley to ½ tsp (2 mL) dried or one sprig fresh per day. Do not take parsley if you are suffering from kidney inflammation.

a role in the prevention of Alzheimer's by nourishing the brain; by lowering cholesterol, which causes fatty deposits to form in the blood vessels of the brain; and by providing antioxidants to protect against free radicals that cause brain-cell damage. Foods that contain choline, a building block of acetylcholine (a chemical that plays a key role in cognition and reasoning) may help prevent Alzheimer's disease.

What to Do

Maximize

- Fresh fruits and vegetables, which provide vitamins and minerals to feed brain tissue and antioxidants to eliminate free radicals
- Foods that contain choline, a building block of acetylcholine (Brazil nuts, lecithin, dandelion flowers, mung beans, lentils, fava beans)
- Nuts and seeds, which provide essential fatty acids to nourish the brain

Minimize

- Meat and dairy products
- Environmental toxins

Eliminate

- Refined and processed foods
- Alcohol
- Fatty foods, fried foods and oils (except extra-virgin olive oil)
- Aluminum in cookware, foil, deodorants and antacids. There is a suspected relationship between aluminum and Alzheimer's disease. Avoid preparing foods in aluminum cooking utensils. Although no direct link has been established between Alzheimer's and aluminum, high concentrations of aluminum have been found when autopsies were performed on Alzheimer's patients. It is probably wise

to err on the side of caution. Don't prepare foods in aluminum cooking utensils, and avoid products that contain aluminum, such as most deodorants and some processed foods.

Other Recommendations

- Eat oily fish (salmon, sardines, mackerel, herring), which provide essential fatty acids to nourish brain and nerve tissue.
- Rosemary and sage traditionally have been used to improve memory. Both herbs are rich in antioxidants. Studies also show that they contain substances that conserve acetylcholine.
- Ginkgo biloba improves blood flow to the brain, which is helpful in cases in which a doctor has diagnosed that insufficient blood flow to the brain is causing dementia. If dementia is not caused by insufficient cerebral blood flow, do not use ginkgo biloba, as it may cause other problems.
- Take anti-inflammatory herbs (German chamomile, ginseng, licorice, turmeric) to reduce the inflammation of brain tissue associated with Alzheimer's disease.

Healing Drinks

(see also Immune Boosters, page 226; Top Common Antioxidant Fruits and Vegetables, pages 110 and 122)

Add 1 tsp (5 mL) herbs and up to 2 tbsp (25 mL) other ingredients recommended (see page 29) for this condition to the following:

Juices
- Beet, page 180
- Black Pineapple, page 164
- Blueberry, page 165
- Brocco-Carrot, page 181
- C-Blend, page 166
- Grape Power, page 170
- Leafy Greens, page 191
- Sea Herb Surprise, page 194
- Spring Celebration, page 195

Smoothies
- Sea-Straw Smoothie, page 306
- Smart Smoothie, page 306

Teas
- Memory Booster Tea Blend, page 282

Anemia

Anemia is a deficiency of hemoglobin in the blood, which results in fatigue and facial pallor. Other symptoms depend on the type of anemia, which can be determined by a blood test. Iron-deficiency anemia is the most common type and may be precipitated by heavy menstrual flow, internal bleeding, dietary deficiency of iron, pregnancy or rheumatoid arthritis. To treat anemia, you must determine the type, then work to alleviate the underlying cause. For all types of anemia, increasing the body's ability to absorb nutrients is helpful.

Healing Foods

Fruits and vegetables
apples, citrus fruits, grapes, peaches, strawberries, beets and beet greens, broccoli, carrots, fennel, green peas, Jerusalem artichokes, leafy greens, watercress

Herbs
burdock root, dandelion leaf and root, stinging nettle, parsley*

Other
almonds, dried apricots, figs, prunes, raisins, blackstrap molasses, kelp

* If you are pregnant, limit your intake of parsley to ½ tsp (2 mL) dried or one sprig fresh per day. Do not take parsley if you are suffering from kidney inflammation.

What to Do

Maximize
- Iron-rich foods and herbs (sea herbs, beets, dried fruits, almonds, spinach, stinging nettle, parsley*, watercress)
- Foods rich in vitamin C
- Herbal bitters, such as dandelion root, to improve iron absorption

Minimize
- Whole wheat bread, which limits iron absorption

Eliminate
- Foods that limit iron absorption (coffee, tea, chocolate, wheat bran)

Healing Drinks

Add 1 tsp (5 mL) herbs and up to 2 tbsp (25 mL) other ingredients recommended (see page 30) for this condition to the following:

Juices
- Apple Beet Pear, page 162
- Apricot Peach, page 163
- Beet, page 180
- Brocco-Artichoke, page 181
- Green Beet, page 188
- Peas Please, page 193
- Popeye's Power, page 246

Smoothies
- Sea-Straw Smoothie, page 306

Teas
- Iron Builder Tea, page 244
- Nettle Tea, page 284

Coffee Substitutes
- Easy Root Coffee, page 335

Anxiety States
Anxiety, Stress & Panic Attacks

Anxiety is characterized by a mood of fear and is often associated with insomnia. Panic disorders are recurrent attacks of severe anxiety. Causes may include fatigue, stress, nervous disorders, depression or hormone imbalance.

Healing Foods

Fruits and vegetables
apricots, bananas, broccoli, carrots, celery, fennel, leafy greens, onions, watercress

Herbs
alfalfa, borage, dandelion leaf, garlic, German chamomile, kava kava, lavender, lemon balm, parsley*, St. John's wort, skullcap, valerian**

Other
almond milk, dulse, honey, kelp, nuts (especially almonds), tofu, whole grains (especially oats)

* If you are pregnant, limit your intake of parsley to ½ tsp (2 mL) dried or one sprig fresh per day. Do not take parsley if you are suffering from kidney inflammation.

** Valerian has an adverse effect on some people.

What to Do

Maximize
- Fresh fruits and vegetable fiber to boost general health, which allows you to cope better with stress
- Foods rich in B vitamins (whole grains, leafy greens) to support the nervous system
- Foods that are high in calcium and magnesium (kelp, dulse, soy products, almonds, kale, parsley*), which help ease nervous tension
- Herbs that help you relax and that improve sleep (German chamomile, lavender, skullcap)
- Meditation and relaxation exercises to help release nervous energy, allowing a more balanced emotional state

Eliminate
- Caffeine (found in coffee, black and green tea, chocolate and soft drinks)
- Alcohol
- Refined flour and sugar
- Artificial food additives
- Food allergies and intolerances (see Appendix A: Food Allergies, page 359)

(see also Stress Busters, page 259; Nerve Nourishers, page 248)

Add 1 tsp (5 mL) herbs and up to 2 tbsp (25 mL) other ingredients recommended (see page 31) for this condition to the following:

Juices
- C-Green, page 184
- Leafy Greens, page 191
- Popeye's Power, page 246

Smoothies
- Almond-Banana Milk, page 298

Teas
- Adrenal Support Tea, page 220
- Calming Cuppa Tea, page 261
- Lavender Tea, page 282

Coffee Substitutes
- Anxiety Antidote, page 335

Milk Substitutes
- Banana Frappé, page 329

Arthritis
Rheumatoid Arthritis & Osteoarthritis

Healing Foods

Fruits and vegetables
apples, cherries, grapes, mangoes, papayas, asparagus, beets, broccoli, cauliflower, cabbage, carrots, celery, Jerusalem artichokes, turnips, onions, watercress

Rheumatoid arthritis is the most common chronic inflammatory joint disease. It can usually be diagnosed by the presence of antibodies (called rheumatoid factor) in the blood. Since it is blood-related rather than the result of wear and tear, rheumatoid arthritis is a disease that affects the whole body, often resulting in symptoms such as fever, weight loss, fatigue and a general decline in health. The joints (commonly the wrists, elbows, ankles, knees, hips, and hand and foot joints) become swollen and inflamed and are usually affected symmetrically. Neck pain and stiffness result from spinal inflammation. Joints can eventually become deformed due to a buildup of fluid that impairs the healing process in the joint tissue. Pain and stiffness is usually worst in the morning and may wear off during the day.

Osteoarthritis is a wear-and-tear disorder that usually starts after age 50. It is characterized by cartilage degeneration in weight-bearing joints, such as the hips, knees and spine, as well as joints in the hand. As the cartilage degenerates, new bone, cartilage and connective tissues are formed, which remodel the joint, leading to wasted muscle around the joint and limited movement. Inflammation is secondary to the degeneration of cartilage. Pain is usually provoked by movement and disappears with rest, so it typically gets worse as the day progresses. Because osteoarthritis pain is caused by placing weight on the joints, in overweight people it improves with weight loss. It is often related to a mineral imbalance in the diet and/or a defect that limits the body's ability to absorb minerals. As a result, it may improve with dietary changes and/or support for the digestive system.

Arthritis sufferers often have poor circulation (signified by constantly cold hands and feet), don't perspire, get constipated easily and are overweight. These factors contribute to the retention of waste products and must be addressed first by using some of the herbs listed below (see also Constipation, page 41, and Overweight, page 80). Visit a medical herbalist or other natural-health practitioner for additional advice for your individual situation.

What to Do

Maximize

- Fresh fruits and vegetables
- Fluid intake (drink at least eight large glasses of water, juice and/or herbal tea daily) to dilute and wash out toxins
- Oily fish (salmon, tuna, herring, sardines, trout, cod, mackerel), which are anti-inflammatory
- Herbs that support the digestive system (lemon balm, peppermint, chamomile) to improve nutrient absorption
- Herbal analgesics (German chamomile, meadowsweet) for pain relief
- Anti-inflammatory herbs (German chamomile, ginger, licorice*, meadowsweet) to reduce pain and joint deterioration
- Herbal diuretics (dandelion leaf) and lymphatics (red clover flower) to encourage the elimination of waste products
- Herbs that support the liver (dandelion root, licorice*) to help eliminate toxins
- Herbal circulatory stimulants (ginger, stinging nettle) to improve blood supply to the affected joints

Minimize

- Refined foods
- Tea, coffee and soft drinks
- Salt and salty foods
- Acidic fruits and vegetables (rhubarb, cranberries, plums, spinach, Swiss chard, beet greens)

Eliminate

- Junk food
- Food allergies and intolerances (see Appendix A: Food Allergies, page 359). Problem foods are often corn, dairy products, wheat, eggs, chocolate, peanuts and varieties of the nightshade family, which includes peppers, tomatoes, potatoes and eggplant
- Meat, especially red meat (beef, pork, lamb) and processed meat products (ham, hamburgers, sausages, cold cuts), which can stimulate inflammation
- Margarine, shortening and heat-processed oils (replace with extra-virgin olive oil)
- Shellfish. When protein from shellfish is digested, toxins (urea, uric acid, purines) in it are deposited in the fat and at the ends of the long bones (joints), where they lead to slow, chronic inflammation. Toxins created when shellfish are digested seem to cause more problems than other proteins
- Processed and refined foods

Eliminate

- Sugar and artificial sweeteners (replace with honey, maple syrup or stevia, page 148)
- Citrus fruits, which often cause allergic reactions in people with rheumatoid arthritis
- Vinegar and vinegared foods (pickles), which leach minerals from the body (except apple cider vinegar and brown rice vinegar)
- Alcohol
- Artificial food additives
- Food contaminants from pesticides (eat as much organically produced food as possible)

Healing Drinks

Add 1 tsp (5 mL) herbs and up to 2 tbsp (25 mL) other ingredients recommended (see page 33) for this condition to the following:

Juices
- Allium Antioxidant, page 227
- Apple Spice Cocktail, page 310
- Breakfast Cocktail, page 311
- Brocco-Artichoke, page 181
- Brocco-Carrot, page 181
- Cabbage Cocktail, page 311
- Carrot Apple, page 183
- Cauli-Slaw, page 184
- Cell Support Juice, page 274
- Crimson Cleanser Juice, page 275
- Sea Herb Surprise, page 194

Smoothies
- Almond-Banana Milk, page 298
- Calming Chamomile Smoothie, page 301

Teas
- Chamomile-Licorice-Ginger Tea, page 261
- Ginger Tea, page 279
- Gout Buster Tea, page 280

ADD & ADHD
Attention Deficit Disorder & Attention Deficit Hyperactivity Disorder

Healing Foods

Fruits and vegetables
apples, pears, carrots, beets, broccoli, spinach

A child may be diagnosed with ADD if he or she is easily distracted, has a short attention span, has difficulty concentrating and impulsively moves from one activity to another. In ADHD, there are also signs of hyperactivity. Studies have shown that increasing a child's intake of whole, nutrient-rich foods increases the supply of nutrients to the brain and improves mental performance. Other studies show that iron deficiency can cause attention deficits.

Introducing fresh juice and smoothies into a child's diet is an easy way to help him or her eat more raw fruits and vegetables. Certain herbs can also help calm a child's nerves while the process of diet detoxification takes place.

Healing Foods

Herbs
catnip, cinnamon, German chamomile, lemon balm, parsley*, St. John's wort, stinging nettle

Other
almonds, kelp, sunflower seeds, pumpkin seeds, oats

* If you are pregnant, limit your intake of parsley to ½ tsp (2 mL) dried or one sprig fresh per day. Do not take parsley if you are suffering from kidney inflammation.

What to Do

Maximize
- Whole foods
- Antioxidant-rich fruits and vegetables
- Iron-rich foods (beets; leafy greens; almonds; sea herbs; watercress; and dried fruits, such as figs, raisins and apricots)
- Nuts and seeds to provide zinc, which is necessary for brain function

Minimize
- Foods that limit iron absorption (coffee, tea, chocolate, egg yolks, wheat bran)

Eliminate
- Artificial food additives, colorings, preservatives and sweeteners, which can be toxic to a child

- Sugar and sweet foods and drinks, which deplete the B vitamins necessary for nerve-cell function
- Refined foods, including white flour and white sugar products, which deplete the body's zinc supply
- Food allergies (see Appendix A: Food Allergies, page 359). They are often implicated in ADD, and some of the most common allergens are dairy products (see pages 327–28 for information on milk substitutes), eggs, wheat and oranges

Healing Drinks

(see also Top Common Antioxidant Fruits and Vegetables, pages 110 and 122)

Add 1 tsp (5 mL) herbs and up to 2 tbsp (25 mL) other ingredients recommended (see left) for this condition to the following:

Juices
- Autumn Refresher, page 163
- Brocco-Carrot, page 181
- Leafy Greens, page 191
- Pear Pineapple, page 173

Smoothies
- Almond-Banana Milk, page 298
- Green Energy (omit ginkgo), page 303

Teas
- Lavender Tea, page 282

Milk Substitutes
- Banana Frappé, page 329
- Chocolate Shake, page 331
- Date and Nut Shake, page 331

Breastfeeding

A nourishing diet that's rich in minerals is essential for the health of a nursing mother and her baby. Adding fennel, dill or anise to the mother's food or tea helps prevent infant colic. While weaning, drink sage tea to reduce breast milk production.

Healing Foods

Fruits and vegetables
bananas, avocados, carrots, green beans, leafy greens, sweet potatoes, watercress

Herbs
alfalfa, borage leaves and flowers, dandelion leaf and root, fennel seeds, German chamomile, parsley*, red raspberry leaves, stinging nettle

Other
almonds, blackstrap molasses, legumes, sunflower seeds, pumpkin seeds, sea herbs, wheat germ, whole grains, yogurt with active bacterial cultures

* If you are pregnant, limit your intake of parsley to ½ tsp (2 mL) dried or one sprig fresh per day. Do not take parsley if you are suffering from kidney inflammation.

What to Do

Maximize
- Whole foods
- Foods that contain B vitamins (whole grains, leafy greens, sea herbs), which encourage a rich supply of breast milk
- Foods that contain calcium (leafy greens, sea herbs) to support baby's bone development
- Mineral-rich herbal teas (stinging nettle, red raspberry leaf, alfalfa, red clover flower, dandelion)

Minimize
- Garlic, onions and hot peppers, which can create gas in the baby
- Refined foods (white flour, white sugar)

Eliminate
- Artificial food additives, colorings and sweeteners, which can be toxic to a child

Healing Drinks

Add 1 tsp (5 mL) herbs and up to 2 tbsp (25 mL) other ingredients recommended (see left) for this condition to the following:

Juices
- Folic Plus, page 187
- Kelp, page 190
- Leafy Greens, page 191
- Sea Herb Surprise, page 194

Smoothies
- Avocado Pineapple, page 299

Teas
- Mother's Own, page 284
- Raspberry Tea, page 265

Other
- Digestive (Gripe) Water, page 211

Bronchitis

Bronchitis is an inflammation of the bronchial tubes that is usually characterized by chest congestion and a persistent cough. Typical causes include bacteria, virus, or exposure to smoke or chemicals. Without treatment, the condition can become chronic.

Healing Foods

Fruits and vegetables
apricots, citrus fruits, cranberries, pears, broccoli, cabbage, carrots, leafy greens, onions, red and green bell peppers, turnips, watercress

Healing Foods

Herbs
cayenne, cinnamon, elderberries, fenugreek seeds, garlic, ginger, hyssop, licorice*, marshmallow, stinging nettle, parsley**, plantain, thyme

Other
legumes, sesame seeds, sunflower seeds, pumpkin seeds, soy products, soy yogurt

* Avoid licorice if you have high blood pressure. The prolonged use of licorice is not recommended under any circumstances.

** If you are pregnant, limit your intake of parsley to ½ tsp (2 mL) dried or one sprig fresh per day. Do not take parsley if you are suffering from kidney inflammation.

What to Do

Maximize
- Fruits and vegetables, especially those high in vitamin C and beta carotene
- Raw garlic for its antibiotic effect on the lungs

Minimize
- Meat
- Salt and salty foods

Eliminate
- Dairy products
- Sugar
- Refined flour
- Alcohol
- Food allergies and intolerances (see Appendix A: Food Allergies, page 359)

Healing Drinks

(see also Respiratory Juices, page 255)

Add 1 tsp (5 mL) herbs and up to 2 tbsp (25 mL) other ingredients (see left) for this condition to the following:

Juices
- Allium Antioxidant, page 227
- Carrot Allium, page 183
- C-Blitz, page 166
- Gingered Broccoli, page 187
- Tomato Juice Cocktail, page 315

Teas
- Lung Relief Tea, page 257

Cancer Prevention

Risk factors for cancer include the use of tobacco and alcohol, exposure to toxins in food and the environment, and family history of cancer. Factors that protect against cancer include eating a diet that consists primarily of fresh fruits, vegetables and other whole foods; a healthy, active lifestyle; and avoiding foods and toxins that have been linked to cancer (see Eliminate, below).

Healing Foods

Fruits and vegetables
apples, apricots, blueberries, cherries, citrus fruits, cranberries, figs, grapes, kiwis, mangoes, papayas, peaches, raspberries, strawberries, watermelon, asparagus, beets, broccoli, cabbage, carrots, leafy greens, onions, parsnips, squash, sweet potatoes, tomatoes, watercress

Herbs
astragalus, burdock root, calendula, cayenne, echinacea, garlic, green tea, licorice*, parsley**, red clover flower, rosemary, sage, turmeric

What to Do

Maximize
- Organic foods
- Soy products
- Antioxidant-rich fruits and vegetables
- Nuts and seeds

Minimize
- Animal protein in meat and dairy products

Other Recommendations
- Exercise daily, according to your fitness level.

Eliminate
- Margarine, shortening and cooking oils (except extra-virgin olive oil)
- Alcohol
- Sugar
- Coffee
- Salt; pickled and salt-cured foods
- Fried foods
- Fried, grilled or barbecued meat, fish and poultry

Healing Foods

Other
extra-virgin olive oil, fish oil, flax seeds, legumes, nuts (except peanuts), pumpkin seeds, shiitake mushrooms, soy products, spirulina, sunflower seeds, yogurt with active bacterial cultures, wheat grass, whole grains

What to Do

Eliminate
- Smoked or cured meats (ham, bacon, hot dogs, cold cuts)
- Artificial food additives
- Refined food

Healing Drinks

(see also Immune Boosters, page 226; Top Common Antioxidant Fruits and Vegetables, pages 110 and 122)

Add 1 tsp (5 mL) herbs and up to 2 tbsp (25 mL) other ingredients recommended (see page 37 and left) for this condition to the following:

Juices
- Allium Antioxidant, page 227
- Brocco-Carrot, page 181
- Cabbage Cocktail, page 311
- Cauliflower Cocktail, page 312
- Citrus Cocktail, page 313
- Immunity, page 190
- Rust Proofer #1, page 238
- Rust Proofer #2, page 238
- Tomato Juice Cocktail, page 315

Teas
- Antioxi-T, page 229
- Ginger Tea, page 279

Candida

Candida is a yeast infection that typically occurs on the external genitalia. It appears as a discharge in women and a rash in men. It may occur in the mouth, causing a burning sensation, or in the digestive system, causing bloating. General symptoms include fatigue, mood changes, depression, poor memory, headaches, cravings for sweets, bowel irregularities, muscle and joint problems, and skin problems.

Low thyroid function, diabetes, pregnancy, antibiotics, steroids, poor diet and sexual transmission can cause candida. Vaginal deodorants and scented soaps aggravate the condition by irritating the protective mucosa of the vagina. Stress, oral contraceptives, hormones and preservatives in food can encourage chronic candida. Reduce stress by using nerve-nourishing herbs, such as skullcap and oats.

Healing Foods

Fruits and vegetables
cranberries, broccoli, cabbage, carrots, cauliflower, celery, leafy greens, onions, squash, sweet potatoes, red bell peppers

Herbs
calendula, cloves, dandelion leaf and root, echinacea, garlic, ginger, lemon balm, stinging nettle, parsley*, peppermint, rosemary, thyme

* If you are pregnant, limit your intake of parsley to ½ tsp (2 mL) dried or one sprig fresh per day. Do not take parsley if you are suffering from kidney inflammation.

What to Do

Maximize
- Antioxidant-rich vegetables
- Vegetable protein (soy products, legumes with rice)
- Raw garlic (several cloves a day) to kill the yeast fungus
- Yogurt with active bacterial cultures to control yeast growth

Minimize
- Fruits and fruit juices to reduce excess fruit sugars that encourage yeast growth
- High-carbohydrate vegetables (potatoes, corn, parsnips)

Other
caprylic acid, dulse, kelp, legumes, nuts, extra-virgin olive oil, seeds, soy products, whole grains, unsweetened yogurt with active bacterial cultures

Eliminate

- Food allergies and intolerances (see Appendix A: Food Allergies, page 359)
- Bananas, citrus fruits, dried fruits and mushrooms
- Alcohol, coffee, chocolate and tea
- Dairy products, which contain sugars that encourage candida growth (except unsweetened yogurt with active bacterial cultures)
- Honey, molasses, soy sauce, sugar and sweeteners
- Meat
- Refined foods
- Vinegared foods (pickles, mustard, ketchup, salad dressings)
- Yeast (including bakery products made with yeast)

Healing Drinks

(see also Top Common Antioxidant Vegetables, page 122)

Add 1 tsp (5 mL) herbs and up to 2 tbsp (25 mL) other ingredients recommended (see page 38 and left) for this condition to the following:

Juices

- C-Blend, page 166
- C-Green, page 184
- Digestive Cocktail Juice, page 210
- Green Goddess, page 188
- Popeye's Power, page 246
- Rust Proofer #1, page 238
- Squash Special, page 196

Teas

- Ginseng, page 280
- St. John's Wort, page 148

Tonics

- Antibiotic Toddy, page 228
- Dandelion Tonic, page 186

Chronic Fatigue Syndrome

Chronic fatigue syndrome is not well understood. It is characterized by overwhelming fatigue, lack of energy, sleep disturbances and depression, and often features headaches, sore throats or swollen glands. It often follows a viral infection that has weakened the immune system. Other possible causes are food allergies, poor digestion or nutrient absorption, antibiotic use and long-term stress.

Healing Foods

Fruits and vegetables
apples, bananas, citrus fruits, broccoli, carrots, green beans, green and red bell peppers, leafy greens, squash, sweet potatoes, tomatoes, watercress

What to Do

Maximize

- Immunity and proper digestion (see Immune Deficiency, page 59, and Indigestion, page 62)
- Antioxidant-rich fruits and vegetables
- Nuts and seeds

Healing Foods

Herbs

alfalfa, cayenne, dandelion leaf and root, echinacea, evening primrose oil, garlic, ginger, ginseng*, lemon balm, licorice**, milk thistle, parsley***, St. John's wort, stinging nettle

Other

brown rice, cereal grasses, dulse, fish oils, flax seeds, kelp, legumes, maitake mushrooms, oats, extra-virgin olive oil, pumpkin seeds, sesame seeds, shiitake mushrooms, sunflower seeds, whole grains, yogurt with active bacterial cultures

* Do not take ginseng if you have high blood pressure or if you drink coffee. Never take ginseng daily for longer than four weeks.

** Avoid licorice if you have high blood pressure. The prolonged use of licorice is not recommended under any circumstances.

*** If you are pregnant, limit your intake of parsley to ½ tsp (2 mL) dried or one sprig fresh per day. Do not take parsley if you are suffering from kidney inflammation.

**** Do not take sage if you have high blood pressure or are pregnant or breastfeeding.

What to Do

Minimize
- Animal protein in meat and dairy products

Other Recommendations
- Get regular daily exercise, according to your fitness level.

Eliminate
- Processed and refined foods
- Caffeine (found in coffee, black and green tea, chocolate and soft drinks)
- Sugar, alcohol, yeast (or foods made with yeast), which can encourage candida infection (see Candida, page 38), often a factor in the illness
- Foods allergies and intolerances (see Appendix A: Food Allergies, page 359). Common triggers are dairy products, wheat and corn
- Artificial food additives

Healing Drinks

(see also Immune Boosters, page 226; Top Common Antioxidant Fruits and Vegetables, pages 110 and 122)

Add 1 tsp (5 mL) herbs and up to 2 tbsp (25 mL) other ingredients recommended (see left) for this condition to the following:

Juices
- C-Blend, page 166
- C-Green, page 184
- Digestive Cocktail Juice, page 210
- Green Goddess, page 188
- Lemon Lime, page 171
- Orange Zinger, page 173
- Popeye's Power, page 246
- Rust Proofer #1, page 238
- Squash Special, page 196

Teas
- Digestive Stress Soother, page 262
- Immune Regulator Tea, page 234

Common Cold

The common cold is a viral infection of the airways. During cold season, consuming a diet high in fresh fruits, vegetables and garlic is an excellent preventive measure. The severity and duration of any cold can be diminished by promoting elimination through the skin (by sweating) and the bowel (by consuming an abundance of fresh fruit and avoiding slow-digesting meat and dairy products).

> ### Help for Common Cold
> - Nausea: tea made from peppermint, chamomile, ginger or cinnamon
> - Sore throat: gargle or tea made from sage****
> - Cough: tea made from thyme, licorice**, hyssop, plantain or marshmallow root

Healing Foods

Fruits and vegetables
lemons, citrus fruits, carrots, onions

Herbs
astragalus, cayenne, echinacea, elderflowers and elderberries, garlic, ginger, licorice*, peppermint

Other
honey**

* Avoid licorice if you have high blood pressure. The prolonged use of licorice is not recommended under any circumstances.

** Do not feed honey to children under one year of age.

What to Do

Maximize

- Fresh fruits and vegetables and their juices
- Hot herbs (cayenne, ginger) to promote body heat and discourage the virus
- Fluid intake (drink at least eight large glasses of water, juice and/or herbal tea daily)

Eliminate

- Animal protein. The large amount of energy required to digest meat and dairy products is better used as healing energy

Healing Drinks

(see also Immune Boosters, page 226; Top Common Antioxidant Fruits and Vegetables, pages 110 and 122)

Add 1 tsp (5 mL) herbs and up to 2 tbsp (25 mL) other ingredients recommended (see left) for this condition to the following:

Juices

- Allium Antioxidant, page 227
- Carrot-Allium, page 183

- C-Blend, page 166
- C-Blitz, page 166
- Flaming Antibiotic, page 186
- Immunity, page 190
- Lemon Lime, page 171
- Tomato Juice Cocktail, page 315

Teas

- Flu Fighter, page 278
- Throat Saver Tea Blend, page 287

Constipation

Constipation may be caused by diseases, such as diverticulitis (see Diverticular Disease, page 45) or anemia (see Anemia, page 30), both of which require treatment. Less-serious causes include stress, lack of exercise, insufficient dietary fiber or the overuse of laxatives, which make the bowel lazy.

Constipation can often be relieved by increasing the amount of fiber in the diet, getting regular exercise and drinking an adequate amount of water (eight or more large glasses a day).

Constipation may be a result of either excessive relaxation or tension of the bowel muscles. Stimulation with cayenne or ginger can benefit a person who is too relaxed. A calming tea of German chamomile, lavender or lemon balm can relax a tense, overstimulated person. Dairy products cause constipation, especially in children. Replacing dairy products with soy or rice-based dairy substitutes often relieves constipation in a child.

Healing Foods

Fruits and vegetables
apples, pears, prunes, rhubarb, beets, leafy greens, leeks, onions

Herbs
burdock root, German chamomile, cinnamon, dandelion root, fennel seeds, garlic, ginger, lavender, lemon balm, licorice*, peppermint, yellow dock

Other
dried fruit, flax seeds, legumes, molasses, nuts, psyllium seeds, pumpkin seeds, sesame seeds, yogurt with active bacterial cultures

* Avoid licorice if you have high blood pressure. The prolonged use of licorice is not recommended under any circumstances.

What to Do

Maximize
- Whole foods
- Fiber (found in fresh, raw fruits and vegetables; legumes; nuts; seeds; and whole grains)
- Fluid intake (drink at least eight large glasses of water, juice and/or herbal tea daily)

- Bitter herbs (dandelion root; German chamomile; burdock leaf, root or seeds; ginger; fennel; yellow dock) to stimulate the bowel

Eliminate
- Refined foods

Healing Drinks

(see also Aperitifs and Digestives, page 206, and Bitters, page 217)

Add 1 tsp (5 mL) herbs and up to 2 tbsp (25 mL) other ingredients recommended (see left) for this condition to the following:

Juices
- Cabbage Head, page 209
- Fennel Fantasy, page 207
- Papaya Punch, page 208
- Pear Fennel, page 173
- Rhubarb, page 175
- Roo-Berry Pie, page 175

Smoothies
- Prune Smoothie, page 305

Teas
- Calming Cuppa Tea, page 261
- Chamomile-Licorice-Ginger Tea, page 261
- Digestive Seed Tea, page 211
- Ginger Tea, page 279

Other
- Applesauce, page 291
- Dandelion Delight, page 219

Depression

Depression, a persistently low mood, is often accompanied by headaches, insomnia or constant drowsiness, inability to concentrate and low immunity. Although a long-term cure may require counseling, good nutrition promotes healing by helping to restore nervous-system function.

Healing Foods

Fruits and vegetables
black beans, broccoli, carrots, mangoes, soybeans, spinach, watercress

Herbs
borage, burdock root, cardamom, cayenne, cinnamon, cloves, dandelion root, garlic, German chamomile, ginger, ginkgo, lemon balm, oat seeds, parsley**, rosemary, skullcap, St. John's wort

What to Do

Maximize
- A healthy diet
- Foods rich in B vitamins (whole grains, leafy greens) to improve nerve function
- Herbs that encourage relaxation and sleep and that counter stress and anxiety (borage, skullcap, St. John's wort, German chamomile, lemon balm)
- Herbs that support liver function (dandelion root, burdock root, rosemary)
- Nuts and seeds

Eliminate
- Artificial food additives, which can contribute to depression

Other
cereal grasses, evening primrose oil, flax seeds, kelp, nuts, oats (including bran), pumpkin seeds, sunflower seeds, whole grains

** If you are pregnant, limit your intake of parsley to ½ tsp (2 mL) dried or one sprig fresh per day. Do not take parsley if you are suffering from kidney inflammation.

Healing Drinks

(see also Nerve Nourishers, page 248; Stress Busters, page 259)

Add 1 tsp (5 mL) herbs and up to 2 tbsp (25 mL) other ingredients recommended (see page 42 and left) for this condition to the following:

Juices
• Brocco-Carrot, page 181
• C-Green, page 184
• Leafy Greens, page 191

Smoothies
• Green Energy, page 303
• Smart Smoothie, page 306

Teas
• Memory Booster Tea Blend, page 282
• Spirit Raising Tea, page 253

Coffee Substitutes
• Seed Power Coffee, page 339

Diabetes

Diabetes mellitus is an insulin deficiency that results in a high blood-sugar level. This deficiency affects the body's ability to metabolize carbohydrates, protein and fat, which often leads to an increase in the incidence of infections. It is important that a health-care practitioner monitor a patient with diabetes. If diabetes is not controlled, changes in the blood vessels can lead to high blood pressure and deterioration of circulation, causing kidney, nerve and eye problems.

Type I diabetes begins in childhood. The pancreas is unable to produce an adequate supply of insulin, so the disease is controlled with daily insulin injections.

Type II diabetes usually occurs in adulthood, and obesity is a major risk factor. The pancreas often produces sufficient insulin, but the body is unable to use it efficiently. High blood sugar can be reversed by diet and weight loss. In type II diabetes, diet and herbs can help regulate blood sugar, improve digestion and intestinal absorption of nutrients, support blood circulation and improve immunity.

Healing Foods

Fruits and vegetables
apples, avocados, blueberries, grapefruit, lemons, limes, pears, broccoli, Jerusalem artichokes, leafy greens, onions

Herbs
cinnamon, cloves, coriander, dandelion root and leaf, evening primrose oil, fenugreek seeds, garlic, ginger, ginkgo, linden flower, stevia, turmeric, yarrow*

* Avoid yarrow if you are pregnant.

What to Do

Maximize
• A mainly vegetarian diet of fresh organic fruits, vegetables, legumes and unrefined grains, which helps regulate blood sugar and boosts the immune system's ability to resist infection
• Omega-3 fatty acids (found in oily fish and fish oils, hemp oil, flax seeds, pumpkin seeds and soybean products), which are beneficial to blood circulation

Minimize
• Animal fats in meat and dairy products (replace some meat meals with fish and vegetable protein; replace dairy products with soy alternatives)

Eliminate
- Food allergies and intolerances (see Appendix A: Food Allergies, page 359)
- Dairy products
- Potatoes
- Dried fruits, sugar and sweeteners (except stevia and small amounts of raw honey)
- Fats and oils (except extra-virgin olive oil)
- Processed foods
- Refined foods
- Caffeine (found in coffee, black and green tea, and soft drinks)

Other Recommendations
- Chronic stress affects sugar levels. Skullcap and oats can help calm nervous stress.
- Daily exercise makes an important contribution to regulating blood sugar levels.

Healing Drinks

(see also Endocrine Elixirs, page 220)

Add 1 tsp (5 mL) herbs and up to 2 tbsp (25 mL) other ingredients recommended (see page 43 and left) for this condition to the following:

Juices
- Allium Antioxidant, page 227
- Apple Beet Pear, page 162
- Beta Blast, page 164
- Brocco-Artichoke, page 181

Smoothies
- Blue Cherry, page 300
- Green Energy, page 303
- Spa Special, page 307

Teas
- Circulation Tea, page 249
- Immune Regulator Tea, page 234

Coffee Substitutes
- Easy Root Coffee, page 335
- Seed Power Coffee, page 339

Diarrhea

Diarrhea is an inflammation of the bowel caused by bacterial or viral infection, food allergies or intolerances, or malfunctions of the digestive system. Consult a health-care practitioner if diarrhea lasts longer than one week. Diarrhea causes dehydration, which can be life threatening for small children. In such cases, consult your health-care practitioner immediately.

What to Do

Maximize
- Water intake (to be safe, boil all water to eliminate any bacteria, then cool to drinking temperature)
- Herbal teas
- Starchy foods (potatoes, carrots, rice)

Minimize
- Raw fruits (except bananas), which can promote diarrhea
- Raw vegetables, as the fiber may irritate an inflamed bowel
- Dried fruits

Healing Foods

Other
evening primrose oil, flax seeds, pumpkin seeds, rice, sunflower seeds, whole grains, yogurt with active bacterial cultures

Eliminate
- Alcohol, caffeine (found in coffee, black and green tea, chocolate and soft drinks), soft drinks

- Dairy products (except yogurt with active bacterial cultures)
- Sugar and sweeteners
- Food allergies and intolerances (see Appendix A: Food Allergies, page 359)

Healing Drinks

Add 1 tsp (5 mL) herbs and up to 2 tbsp (25 mL) other ingredients recommended (see page 44 and left) for this condition to the following:

Smoothies
- Best Berries (use blueberries), page 299

Teas
- Raspberry Ginger, page 285

Milk Substitutes
- Banana Frappé, page 329

Other
- Apple Rice Pudding, page 291
- Applesauce, page 291

Diverticular Disease
Diverticulitis & Diverticulosis

Healing Foods

Fruits and vegetables
apples, bananas, grapes, mangoes, pears, prunes, broccoli, cabbage, carrots, celery, leafy greens, watercress

Herbs
cinnamon, fenugreek seeds, garlic, German chamomile, ginger, licorice*, marshmallow leaf and root, peppermint, psyllium seeds, slippery elm bark powder, valerian**

* Avoid licorice if you have high blood pressure. The prolonged use of licorice is not recommended under any circumstances.

** Valerian has an adverse effect on some people.

Diverticulosis is characterized by the presence of multiple small pouches (diverticula) on the large intestine. Diverticulitis occurs when these pouches become inflamed. It is usually associated with constipation and caused by a low-fiber diet. Symptoms typically include continuous pain on the left side of the abdomen, flatulence and, sometimes, diarrhea.

What to Do

Maximize
- Fruits and vegetables
- Whole grains and legumes
- Water intake (drink at least eight large glasses daily)

Minimize
- Animal protein in meat and dairy products

Eliminate
- Caffeine (found in coffee, black and green tea, chocolate and soft drinks)

- Alcohol
- Fried foods
- Pickled foods
- Ham, bacon and fatty meats
- Refined and processed foods
- Spicy foods
- Sugar
- Dairy products (except yogurt with active bacterial cultures)
- Constipation, if present (see Constipation, page 41)

Other
flax seeds, legumes, oats, spirulina, wheat bran, whole grains, yogurt with active bacterial cultures

Other Recommendations

- Gradually introduce a high-fiber diet to avoid digestive problems.
- During periods of inflammation, avoid high-fiber foods (raw vegetables, bran), which can irritate the bowel.
- Drink plenty of healing vegetable juices (spinach, cabbage, beet, garlic, carrot) with the addition of soothing slippery elm bark powder

Healing Drinks

Add 1 tsp (5 mL) herbs and up to 2 tbsp (25 mL) other ingredients recommended (see page 45 and left) for this condition to the following:

Juices

- Apple Pear, page 162
- Cabbage Cocktail, page 311
- Gingered Broccoli, page 187
- Leafy Greens, page 191
- Popeye's Power, page 246
- Slippery Beet, page 194

Smoothies

- Mango Madness, page 304
- Prune Smoothie, page 305

Teas

- Digestive Seed Tea, page 211
- Digestive Stress Soother, page 262

Endometriosis

Endometriosis is a condition in which tissue that is normally found in the uterus wall, or endometrium, is found in places outside the uterus, such as the bladder, bowel or fallopian tubes. This tissue responds to a woman's monthly hormonal cycle, shedding blood at these sites. Symptoms can include pain, irregular bleeding, depression and bowel problems.

Healing Foods

Fruits and vegetables
apples, apricots, cherries, grapefruit, strawberries, beets, broccoli, cabbage, leafy greens, peas, red and green bell peppers, squash, sweet potatoes

Herbs
calendula, chasteberry, dandelion leaf and root, evening primrose oil, German chamomile, meadowsweet, passionflower, rosemary, turmeric, valerian*

* Valerian has an adverse effect on some people.

What to Do

Maximize

- Antioxidants (preferably from vegetable sources) to support the immune system in eliminating imperfect or misplaced tissues
- Essential fatty acids (found in nuts, seeds and grains), which have a healing effect

Minimize

- Animal protein in meat and dairy products. Use organic meats, which are sure to be hormone-free, if possible
- Fruits, which may contribute to blood-sugar problems. Candida (see page 38) is often associated with endometriosis

Eliminate

- Sugar and sweeteners
- Yeast and foods made with yeast (bread)
- Coffee
- Alcohol
- Junk food
- Food allergies and intolerances (see Appendix A: Food Allergies, page 359). Dairy and wheat products are common culprits

Healing Foods

Other

barley, fish oils, legumes, nuts, oats, extra-virgin olive oil, seeds, tofu, whole grains, soy yogurt with active bacterial cultures

Other Recommendations

- Balance hormones with chasteberry (*Vitex agnus-castus*).
- Take analgesic herbs (German chamomile, meadowsweet, passionflower, rosemary, valerian) for pain.
- Take nervous-system tonics (passionflower, valerian).

- Use turmeric for its antimicrobial/antiseptic/anti-inflammatory properties.
- Consume herbs that support the liver (calendula, dandelion root, rosemary).
- Evening primrose oil is an antidepressant and helps to support the immune system in eliminating imperfect or misplaced tissues.

Healing Drinks

(see also Endocrine Elixirs, page 220; Top Common Antioxidant Fruits and Vegetables, pages 110 and 122)

Add 1 tsp (5 mL) herbs and up to 2 tbsp (25 mL) other ingredients recommended (see page 46 and left) for this condition to the following:

Juices

- Beet, page 180
- Cabbage Cocktail, page 311

- Cherry Sunrise, page 167
- Peas Please, page 193
- Peppers Please, page 193
- Squash Special, page 196

Teas

- Hormone Balancing Tea, page 222
- Lavender Tea, page 282

Coffee Substitutes

- Easy Root Coffee, page 335
- Seed Power Coffee, page 339

Eye Problems
Cataracts, Glaucoma & Macular Degeneration

Healing Foods

Fruits and vegetables

apricots, blackberries, blueberries, citrus fruits, cranberries, grapes, mangoes, peaches, raspberries, strawberries, watermelon, asparagus, avocados, broccoli, cabbage, carrots, green and red bell peppers, leafy greens, pumpkin, squash, sweet potatoes, tomatoes, watercress

Research shows that your risk of cataracts, glaucoma and macular degeneration decreases if you eat a diet rich in antioxidants.

What to Do

Maximize

- Antioxidant-rich fruits and vegetables (see pages 110 and 122) to protect the eyes from free-radical damage. Carrot juice, spinach and blueberries are especially effective
- Fresh garlic, which is a strong antioxidant

Minimize

- Fat in meat and dairy products

Eliminate

- Refined foods
- Fried foods
- Sugar and sweeteners

Herbs
dandelion leaf, garlic, ginger, ginkgo, parsley*, rosemary, turmeric

Other
extra-virgin olive oil, nuts, pumpkin seeds, wheat germ, yogurt with active bacterial cultures

* If you are pregnant, limit your intake of parsley to ½ tsp (2 mL) dried or one sprig fresh per day. Do not take parsley if you are suffering from kidney inflammation.

Healing Drinks

Add 1 tsp (5 mL) herbs and up to 2 tbsp (25 mL) other ingredients recommended (see left) for this condition to the following:

Juices
- Beta-Carro, page 164
- Black Pineapple, page 164
- Blueberry, page 165
- Blue Water, page 165
- Cabbage Cocktail, page 311
- C-Blend, page 166
- C-Blitz, page 166

- Citrus Cocktail, page 313
- Grape Power, page 170
- Squash Special, page 196
- Sunrise Supreme, page 177
- Tomato Juice Cocktail, page 315

Smoothies
- Liquid Gold, page 304
- Mango Madness, page 304

Teas
- Antioxi-T, page 229
- The Green Diablo, page 232

Fatigue

Fatigue is a symptom of many diseases — including anemia, diabetes, hepatitis, hypoglycemia and thyroid disease — and can be determined by blood tests and diagnosed by your doctor. Common nondisease factors often come from a lack of lifestyle balance, which includes diet, exercise, work and social life. A balanced diet provides the digestive enzymes the body requires for processing nutrients and converting food into energy.

Healing Foods

Fruits and vegetables
bananas, grapes, limes, mangoes, oranges, pineapple, strawberries, broccoli, carrots, leafy greens, onions, spinach, watercress

Herbs
alfalfa, burdock root, cardamom, cayenne, cinnamon, cloves, dandelion leaf and root, garlic, ginger, ginseng*, licorice**, parsley***, peppermint, red raspberry leaf, rose hips, stinging nettle, yellow dock

* Do not take ginseng if you have high blood pressure or if you drink coffee. Never take ginseng daily for longer than four weeks.

** Avoid licorice if you have high blood pressure. The prolonged use of licorice is not recommended under any circumstances.

*** If you are pregnant, limit your intake of parsley to ½ tsp (2 mL) dried or one sprig fresh per day. Do not take parsley if you are suffering from kidney inflammation.

What to Do

Maximize
- Fresh fruits and vegetables
- Whole grains
- Nuts and seeds
- Essential fatty acids

Minimize
- Fat in meat and dairy products
- Fried foods

Eliminate
- Caffeine and sugar, which can cause fatigue
- Refined flour products, which rob the body of nutrients
- Processed foods, which are often low in nutrients and high in chemical additives

- Margarine, shortening and salad oils (except extra-virgin olive oil)
- Alcohol

Other Recommendations
- Exercise daily, according to your fitness level.
- Eat smaller, more-frequent meals to maintain a constant blood-sugar level.
- Practice stress-reduction techniques, such as yoga, tai chi and meditation. Stress depletes vitality.
- Take herbs that support the liver (dandelion root, burdock root) to stimulate metabolism and remove toxins that can cause fatigue.

Healing Foods

Other
almonds, cereal grasses, dates, fish oil, flax seeds, oats, pumpkin seeds, sea herbs, sunflower seeds, whole grains, tofu, wheat germ, yogurt with active bacterial cultures

Healing Drinks

(see also Stress Busters, page 259)

Add 1 tsp (5 mL) herbs and up to 2 tbsp (25 mL) other ingredients recommended (see page 48 and left) for this condition to the following:

Juices
- Apple Fresh, page 162
- Brocco-Carrot, page 181
- Eye Opener, page 169
- Moist & Juicy (use any recommended herb in place of ginkgo, see page 48), page 192
- Spiced Carrot, page 195
- Sunrise Supreme, page 177

Smoothies
- B-Vitamin, page 300
- Green Energy, page 303
- Mango Madness, page 304
- Pineapple-C, page 305
- Taste of the Tropics, page 307

Teas
- Adrenal Support Tea, page 220
- Ginseng, page 280
- Iron Builder Tea, page 244
- Mother's Own, page 284

Fibromyalgia

Fibromyalgia is characterized by tender, aching muscles, joint pain similar to that of rheumatoid arthritis, fatigue and sleep disturbances. The areas typically affected are the neck, shoulders, lower back, chest and thighs. It is considered a form of chronic fatigue syndrome, with pain rather than fatigue as the dominant feature. Depression is often a feature, due to lack of sleep. The cause can be viral or a buildup of toxins. Food, drugs, allergies and nutritional deficiencies can also be involved. Neither the cause nor the cure is well understood, but good nutrition can help recovery.

Healing Foods

Fruits and vegetables
apples, beets, broccoli, cabbage, cauliflower, celery, fennel, green beans, Jerusalem artichokes, onions, squash, sweet potatoes, watercress

Herbs
alfalfa, astragalus, burdock root and seeds, calendula, dandelion leaf and root, echinacea, evening primrose oil, garlic, licorice*, milk thistle, parsley**, passionflower, slippery elm bark powder, St. John's wort, turmeric

* Avoid licorice if you have high blood pressure. The prolonged use of licorice is not recommended under any circumstances.

** If you are pregnant, limit your intake of parsley to ½ tsp (2 mL) dried or one sprig fresh per day. Do not take parsley if you are suffering from kidney inflammation.

What to Do

Maximize
- Antioxidant-rich vegetables
- Vegetable protein
- Nuts and seeds
- Legumes

Minimize
- Fruits, which may contribute to low blood sugar (see Hypoglycemia, page 59)

Other Recommendations
- Eat oily fish (salmon, mackerel, sardines, tuna) two or three times a week.
- Practice stress-reduction techniques, such as tai chi, yoga and meditation.
- Exercise daily, according to your fitness level.

Healing Foods

Other
barley grass, fish oils, flax seeds, legumes, pumpkin seeds, soy products, sunflower seeds, unsweetened yogurt with active bacterial cultures, whole grains (especially brown rice)

Eliminate

- Sugar; products that contain sugar; and high-sugar fruits, such as dried fruit, bananas and watermelon
- Refined flour
- Artificial food additives
- Alcohol
- Food allergies and intolerances (see Appendix A: Food Allergies, page 359). Gluten (in wheat products) and members of the nightshade family (potatoes, tomatoes, eggplant and all peppers) often cause problems
- Caffeine (found in coffee, black and green tea, chocolate and soft drinks), which decreases mineral absorption and contributes to the condition
- Dairy products (replace with soy- or rice-based alternatives)
- Salty and pickled foods
- Fried foods
- Pork, shellfish and fatty meats

Healing Drinks

(see also Immune Boosters, page 226)

Add 1 tsp (5 mL) herbs and up to 2 tbsp (25 mL) other ingredients recommended (see page 49 and left) for this condition to the following:

Juices

- Beet, page 180
- Breakfast Cocktail, page 311
- Brocco-Artichoke, page 181
- Cabbage Cocktail, page 311
- Cauli-Slaw, page 184
- C-Green, page 184
- Rust Proofer #2, page 238

Teas

- Immune Regulator Tea, page 234

Coffee Substitutes

- Easy Root Coffee, page 335
- Root Coffee Blend, page 338

Flatulence

Healing Foods

Fruits and vegetables
apples, kiwis, papayas

Herbs
basil, cardamom, cayenne, German chamomile, cinnamon, cloves, coriander, cumin, dill, fennel seeds, garlic, ginger, mustard seeds, peppermint, thyme

Other
yogurt with active bacterial cultures

Gas is a normal result when food is digested. Foods high in carbohydrates, such as beans, produce more gas because they are not entirely broken down by digestive enzymes. When bacteria ferment the undigested carbohydrates, gas is released. Other foods produce excess gas when the digestive enzyme they require is not available. The most common example is the enzyme needed to digest lactose in dairy products. Artificial sweeteners can also cause gas.

Changing your diet to include more high-fiber foods, such as beans and legumes, may also increase the incidence of gas. Consequently, dietary changes intended to increase the quantity of fiber should be made gradually, over a four- to six-week period.

Tip: To reduce the "gas effect" of legumes, soak them overnight in plenty of water. Discard the soaking water before cooking and rinse the cooked legumes well before adding them to recipes. Cook beans (and other foods) that give you gas with the recommended herbs, which expel gas from the digestive tract.

What to Do

Maximize
- Digestive herbal teas, such as chamomile and fennel, between meals
- Food-combining techniques (see Food Combining, page 15), taking care to eat fruits at least half an hour before or two hours after meals

Eliminate
- Artificial sweeteners and all foods that contain them
- Dairy products

Healing Drinks

(see also Aperitifs and Digestives, page 206, and Bitters, page 217)

Digestives
- Before Dinner Mint, page 207
- Digestive (Gripe) Water, page 211
- Digestive Seed Tea, page 211
- James Duke's Carminatea, page 214
- Rosy Peppermint Tea, page 215
- Spiced Papaya Tea, page 216

Gallstones

Cholesterol from animal fats is a major factor in the formation of gallstones. Symptoms include indigestion, severe pain in the upper right abdomen, constipation, flatulence, nausea and vomiting. If a gallstone remains stuck in the bile duct, causing inflammation, it may need to be surgically removed.

Vegetarians are less likely to develop gallstones than people who eat meat, and dietary changes can reduce the risk of gallstone formation.

Healing Foods

Fruits and vegetables
apples, blackberries, blueberries, cherries, citrus fruits, lemons, pears, raspberries, red grapes, asparagus, beets, broccoli, carrots, celery, leafy greens, radishes, tomatoes, watercress

Herbs
dandelion leaf and root, garlic, ginger, milk thistle, parsley*, turmeric

* If you are pregnant, limit your intake of parsley to ½ tsp (2 mL) dried or one sprig fresh per day. Do not take parsley if you are suffering from kidney inflammation.

What to Do

Maximize
- Vegetable protein
- Fruits, vegetables and whole grains

Minimize
- Fatty meats
- Dairy products

Eliminate
- Sugar
- Refined foods
- Coffee
- Food allergies and intolerances (see Appendix A: Food Allergies, page 359). Often, eggs, pork, onions, coffee, milk, corn, beans and nuts affect gallstone sufferers

Other Recommendations

- Eat oily fish (salmon, mackerel, sardines, tuna) to help lower cholesterol levels.
- Consume bitter foods (dandelion leaf, endive, radicchio, watercress) to increase bile flow, which helps prevent gallstone formation.
- Increase consumption of extra-virgin olive oil to discourage gallstone formation.

Healing Drinks

Add 1 tsp (5 mL) herbs and up to 2 tbsp (25 mL) other ingredients recommended (see page 51 and left) for this condition to the following:

Juices

- Apple Beet Pear, page 162
- Autumn Refresher, page 163
- Brocco-Carrot, page 181
- Carrot-Apple, page 183
- C-Blitz, page 166
- C-Green, page 184
- Dandelion Bitters, page 218
- Gallstone Solvent, page 187
- Lemon Lime (use 1 tsp/5 mL recommended herb in place of licorice, see page 49), page 171
- Spring Celebration, page 195
- Tomato Juice Cocktail, page 315
- Zippy Tomato, page 197

Teas

- Ginger Tea, page 279

Coffee Substitutes

- Easy Root Coffee, page 335
- Root Coffee Blend, page 338

Gout

Gout is an inflammatory joint problem characterized by increased production of uric acid, which is deposited in the joints, especially those of the fingers and toes. It may be hereditary or may be caused by the consumption of excess alcohol, meat or starchy food, which increases the production of uric acid. Decreasing the production of uric acid and increasing its excretion in the urine helps control gout.

What to Do

Maximize
- Water intake (drink at least eight large glasses daily) to assist in the elimination of uric acid
- A vegetarian diet
- Herbal teas that dissolve uric acid (celery seed) and help eliminate uric acid (dandelion leaf, stinging nettle)

Minimize
- Protein (chicken, turkey and whitefish are fine in moderation)
- Fat in meat and dairy products
- Salt and salty foods
- Eggs (those from free-range chickens are preferable)
- Wheat, which is acid forming (use brown rice and buckwheat, which produce less acid)

Healing Foods

Herbs
burdock root and seeds, celery seeds, dandelion leaf, fennel seeds, garlic, ginger, licorice*, parsley**, stinging nettle, turmeric, yarrow***, yellow dock

Other
flax seeds

* Avoid licorice if you have high blood pressure. The prolonged use of licorice is not recommended under any circumstances.

** If you are pregnant, limit your intake of parsley to ½ tsp (2 mL) dried or one sprig fresh per day. Do not take parsley if you are suffering from kidney inflammation.

*** Avoid yarrow if you are pregnant.

Eliminate
- *Foods and substances that form acid in the body, including:*
- pork and beef;
- preserved meats, such as salami;
- tomatoes and spinach;
- vinegar (except apple cider vinegar);
- refined sugar and flour;
- coffee and tea;
- cheese;
- artificial food additives; and
- alcohol.
- *Foods that are high in purines, including:*
- organ meats (kidney, liver);
- shellfish, herring, sardines, anchovies and mackerel;
- peanuts;
- asparagus;
- mushrooms; and
- legumes (peas, beans, lentils).

Healing Drinks

Add 1 tsp (5 mL) herbs and up to 2 tbsp (25 mL) other ingredients recommended (see left) for this condition to the following:

Juices
- Berry Best, page 163
- Celery, page 184
- Gout Buster Juice, page 188
- Immunity, page 190

Teas
- Gout Buster Tea, page 280

Coffee Substitutes
- Root Coffee Blend, page 338

Hangover

Drinking too much alcohol can result in headache, fatigue, nausea, dizziness and depression, which together are called hangover. Hangovers occur because alcohol dehydrates the body, increases acidity in the digestive system, causes the loss of potassium and vitamins, and affects the liver and nervous system. You may get faster relief from hangover symptoms if you follow these recommendations, preferably before retiring.

Healing Foods

Fruits and vegetables
apples, bananas, lemons, limes

Herbs
cumin, evening primrose oil, ginger, German chamomile, lavender, meadowsweet, slippery elm bark powder

Other
foods that are rich in B vitamins (whole grains, leafy greens)

What to Do

Maximize
- Water to hydrate the body before, during and after drinking
- Juices that are high in vitamin C
- Herbal teas that settle the stomach (chamomile)
- Slippery elm bark powder to protect the stomach from excess acid

Healing Drinks

Add 1 tsp (5 mL) herbs and up to 2 tbsp (25 mL) other ingredients recommended (see page 53) for this condition to the following:

Juices
- Hangover Helper, page 170
- Hangover Remedy, page 170

Smoothies
- Calming Chamomile Smoothie, page 301

Teas
- Hangover Rescue Tea, page 281

Headaches
(Non-Migraine)

Healing Foods

Fruits and vegetables
apples, bananas, broccoli, leafy greens, watercress

Herbs
cayenne, evening primrose oil, German chamomile, lavender, lemon balm, linden flower, passionflower, rosemary, skullcap, thyme, valerian*

Other
almonds, legumes, oats, sunflower seeds, tofu, walnuts, wheat germ, whole grains, yogurt with active bacterial cultures

* Valerian has an adverse effect on some people.

Headaches, other than migraines, can be caused by many factors, including muscular and nervous tension, digestive disorders, blood pressure changes, low blood sugar, caffeine, alcohol or drug withdrawal, eye strain, food allergies, a stuffy room, weather changes or poor posture. Avoiding foods that are common headache triggers (see Eliminate, below) may help reduce the incidence of headaches.

What to Do

Maximize
- Foods that are high in magnesium (whole grains, legumes, sea herbs, wheat germ, apples, bananas, nuts, seeds, fish), which relaxes muscles and helps reduce spasms

Minimize
- Salt and salty foods
- Fatty foods

Eliminate
- Artificial food additives, especially monosodium glutamate (MSG)
- Food allergies and intolerances (see Appendix A: Food Allergies, page 359). Dairy products, wheat, corn, oranges and eggs commonly trigger headaches
- Meats preserved with nitrates (bacon, ham, hot dogs)
- Aspartame and foods that are sweetened with aspartame
- Caffeine (found in coffee, black and green tea, chocolate and soft drinks)
- Cheese and red wine

Other Recommendations
- Lemon balm and meadowsweet tea may help relieve headaches caused by digestive disorders.
- Skullcap and valerian* teas can be helpful for stress-related headaches.
- Antispasmodic herbs (cayenne, German chamomile, lemon balm, linden flower, passionflower, skullcap, thyme, valerian*) may help when a headache is caused by muscular tension.

Add 1 tsp (5 mL) herbs and up to 2 tbsp (25 mL) other ingredients recommended (see page 54) for this condition to the following:

Juices
- Brocco-Carrot, page 181
- Cabbage Rose, page 181
- C-Green, page 184
- Leafy Greens, page 191

Smoothies
- Green Energy (substitute skullcap for ginkgo), page 303

Teas
- Lavender Tea, page 282

Heart Problems
High Cholesterol, High Blood Pressure, Cardiovascular Disease, Heart Failure & Stroke

Family history, cigarette smoking, high alcohol consumption and high "bad" cholesterol are major risk factors for high blood pressure, circulation disorders and cardiovascular disease. In most cardiovascular diseases and circulation disorders, cholesterol deposits narrow the arteries, constricting the flow of blood.

Cholesterol is necessary to sustain life. There are two types in human blood: low-density lipoprotein (LDL, or "bad" cholesterol), which increases the risk of high blood pressure, heart disease and gallstones; and high-density lipoprotein (HDL, or "good" cholesterol), which reduces these risks. To improve health, eat a diet that lowers LDL and raises HDL.

Healing Foods

Fruits and vegetables
apples, apricots, blueberries, blackberries, cranberries, grapefruit*, grapes, kiwis, mangoes, melons, oranges, papayas, pineapple, strawberries, asparagus, avocados, broccoli, carrots, celery, leafy greens, lettuce, onions, parsnips, all peppers, peas, squash, watercress

Herbs
cayenne, dandelion leaf and root, fenugreek seeds, garlic, ginger, linden flowers, parsley**, rosemary, stinging nettle, turmeric

* Avoid grapefruit if you are using calcium channel blocker medication.

** If you are pregnant, limit your intake of parsley to ½ tsp (2 mL) dried or one sprig fresh per day. Do not take parsley if you are suffering from kidney inflammation.

What to Do

Maximize
- Fresh fruits and vegetables, whole grains, nuts and seeds, all of which help regulate blood pressure, reduce LDL and raise HDL
- Garlic and onions to reduce blood pressure and cholesterol
- Antioxidant-rich fruits and vegetables to help prevent cholesterol deposits from forming on artery walls
- Red grape juice to prevent blood clotting

Minimize
- Alcohol
- Coffee
- Eggs
- Salt and salty foods (processed foods)
- Sugar and products that contain sugar

Other
almonds, barley, fish oil, kelp, lecithin, legumes, oats, extra-virgin olive oil, seeds (flax, pumpkin, sesame, sunflower), soy products, sprouted seeds and beans, walnuts, whole grains, yogurt with active bacterial cultures

Eliminate

- High-fat meats (such as bacon, pork, beef) and dairy products (except skim milk)
- Margarine and salad oils (except extra-virgin olive oil)
- Fried foods
- Pastries
- Milk chocolate
- Alcohol
- Refined sugar and flour
- Coconut

Other Recommendations

- Supportive therapy for heart problems includes daily exercise (such as walking for 30 minutes a day, depending on your level of fitness) and stress-reduction techniques, such as yoga, tai chi and meditation.
- Eat oily fish (salmon, mackerel, sardines, tuna) two to three times a week.
- Substitute vegetable protein for some meat meals.
- Use herbs (see left) to help lower cholesterol and improve circulation.

Healing Drinks

(see also Immune Boosters, page 226; Top Common Antioxidant Fruits and Vegetables, pages 110 and 122)

Add 1 tsp (5 mL) herbs and up to 2 tbsp (25 mL) other ingredients recommended (see page 55 and left) for this condition to the following:

Juices

- Allium Antioxidant, page 227
- Apple Fresh (use rosemary in place of ginseng), page 162
- Black Pineapple, page 164
- Brocco-Carrot, page 181
- C-Blend, page 166
- C-Blitz, page 166
- Citrus Cocktail, page 313
- Eye Opener, page 169
- Grape Heart, page 202
- Grape Power (use red grapes), page 170
- Melon Morning Cocktail, page 313
- Peas and Carrots, page 192
- Spring Celebration, page 195

Teas

- Circulation Tea, page 249

Coffee Substitutes

- Easy Root Coffee, page 335
- Root Coffee Blend, page 338

Heartburn

Healing Foods

Fruits and vegetables
bananas, papayas, beets, cabbage, carrots, celery, cucumbers, parsnips

Heartburn is a burning sensation in the chest that is related to digestive problems. It may be caused by a hiatal hernia, indigestion or inflammation of the stomach. Check with your health-care practitioner to determine the cause. It is especially important to eliminate the possibility of heart disease. Frequent drinks of therapeutic fruit and vegetable juices, antacid herbs (dandelion root, meadowsweet) and soothing herbs (marshmallow root, slippery elm bark powder) can offer relief.

Herbs
calendula, cardamom, dandelion root, dill, fennel, ginger, German chamomile, licorice*, marshmallow root, meadowsweet, parsley**, slippery elm bark powder

Other
flax seeds

* Avoid licorice if you have high blood pressure. The prolonged use of licorice is not recommended under any circumstances.

** If you are pregnant, limit your intake of parsley to ½ tsp (2 mL) dried or one sprig fresh per day. Do not take parsley if you are suffering from kidney inflammation.

What to Do

Maximize
- Fresh fruits and vegetables
- Water intake (drink at least eight large glasses daily, between meals only)
- Slippery elm bark powder (especially at night) to protect the stomach from excess acid

Eliminate
- Coffee, soft drinks, alcohol and chocolate
- Fried, fatty and spicy foods
- Citrus fruits and tomatoes
- Pickled foods
- Refined flour and sugar
- Cigarette smoking
- Large meals
- Antacid and anti-inflammatory drugs, which can irritate the stomach lining

Minimize
- Acid-forming foods (meat, dairy products)

Healing Drinks

Add 1 tsp (5 mL) herbs recommended (see left) for this condition and up to 2 tbsp (25 mL) flax seeds to the following:

Juices
- Beet, page 180
- Cabbage Cocktail (omit garlic), page 311
- Carrot Apple, page 183

Teas
- Digestive Stress Soother, page 262

Coffee Substitutes
- Root Coffee Blend, page 338

Herpes Simplex
Cold Sores & Genital Herpes

Healing Foods

Fruits and vegetables
apples, apricots, berries, grapes, papayas, pears, asparagus, broccoli, cabbage, carrots, leafy greens, onions, squash, watercress

Herpes simplex virus type 1 can cause cold sores. Genital herpes is caused by herpes simplex virus type 2 and should always be treated by a doctor. Once contracted, the virus remains dormant in the nerve endings and may reactivate when triggered by factors such as lowered immune system function; high stress; alcohol; or certain foods, such as processed foods and foods that are high in arginine (see Eliminate, page 58). Diet can be used to complement therapy prescribed by a qualified health-care practitioner. The most effective therapy is to avoid outbreaks by keeping immunity high, managing stress and avoiding foods that trigger the virus. Herbs can help by supporting the immune system and nourishing the nerves, where the virus resides.

Healing Foods

Herbs

astragalus, burdock (leaf, root and seeds), calendula, cayenne, cloves, dandelion root, echinacea, elderflowers, garlic, ginseng, lemon balm, parsley*, St. John's wort, yarrow**

Other

legumes (except chickpeas), nutritional yeast, sea herbs, sprouted beans, yogurt with active bacterial cultures

* If you are pregnant, limit your intake of parsley to ½ tsp (2 mL) dried or one sprig fresh per day. Do not take parsley if you are suffering from kidney inflammation.

** Avoid yarrow if you are pregnant.

What to Do

Maximize

- Antioxidant-rich vegetables
- Fish (salmon, sardines, tuna, halibut), legumes and nutritional yeast. These foods are high in the amino acid lysine, which appears to inhibit the virus from replicating
- Antiviral herbs (astragalus, calendula, echinacea, garlic, lemon balm, St. John's wort)
- Immunity-boosting herbs (astragalus, echinacea, burdock (leaf, root or seeds)
- Antistress herbs (ginseng, St. John's wort, lemon balm)

Minimize

- Fruits
- Whole grains, seeds and brown rice. While these foods are high in arginine (see Eliminate, below), they can be balanced with vegetables that are high in lysine

Eliminate

- Foods that are high in arginine (nuts, wheat, caffeine, chocolate, carob, bacon, coffee, sugars, tomatoes, eggplants, all peppers, mushrooms). Arginine is an amino acid that encourages the herpes virus to replicate
- Alcohol, processed foods and refined foods, which depress the immune system

Other Recommendations

- Practice stress-reduction techniques, such as meditation, yoga and breathing exercises.

Healing Drinks

(see also Immune Boosters, page 226; Top Common Antioxidant Fruits and Vegetables, pages 110 and 122)

Add 1 tsp (5 mL) herbs and up to 2 tbsp (25 mL) other ingredients recommended (see left) for this condition to the following:

Juices

- Allium Antioxidant, page 227
- Breakfast Cocktail, page 311
- Brocco-Carrot, page 181
- Cabbage Rose (use 2 tsp/ 10 mL lemon balm instead of rosemary), page 181
- C-Green, page 184

Teas

- Cleansing Tea, page 274
- Herp-eze Tea, page 233
- Immune Regulator Tea, page 234
- Nerve Nourisher, page 250
- Nerve Support, page 251

Hypoglycemia

Hypoglycemia, or low blood sugar, is a disorder characterized by an overproduction of insulin. Symptoms can include aches and pains, constant hunger, dizziness, headache, fatigue, insomnia, digestive disorders, palpitations, tremors, sweating, nausea and nervous tension. You may notice some of these symptoms if you miss a regular meal. Attention to diet can help control blood-sugar levels.

Healing Foods

Fruits and vegetables
apples, cherries, grapefruit, plums, raw beets, broccoli, cabbage, cauliflower, raw carrots, Jerusalem artichokes, leafy greens, tomatoes

Herbs
dandelion root, German chamomile, ginseng, licorice*

Other
cereal grasses, flax seeds, kelp, legumes, nuts, seeds, spirulina, whole grains, yogurt with active bacterial cultures

* Avoid licorice if you have high blood pressure. The prolonged use of licorice is not recommended under any circumstances.

What to Do

Maximize
- Whole grains, vegetables and legumes
- Smaller meals, eaten more frequently
- Cruciferous vegetables (broccoli, cabbage, cauliflower) to help control blood sugar
- Protein with each meal

Minimize
- Sweet foods, including fruits (particularly bananas, watermelon and dried fruits)

Eliminate
- Refined flour and sugar
- Black tea, coffee, soft drinks and alcohol
- Cigarette smoking, which interferes with blood-sugar mechanisms

Healing Drinks

(see also Endocrine Elixirs, page 220)

Add 1 tsp (5 mL) herbs and up to 2 tbsp (25 mL) other ingredients recommended (see left) for this condition to the following:

Juices
- Brocco-Artichoke, page 181
- Cabbage Cocktail, page 311
- Cauliflower Cocktail, page 312

- Cherry Sunrise, page 167
- Cruciferous, page 185
- Leafy Greens, page 191

Teas
- Chamomile-Licorice-Ginger Tea, page 261
- Root Decoction, page 275

Coffee Substitutes
- Seed Power Coffee, page 339

Immune Deficiency

Healing Foods

Fruits and vegetables
brightly colored fruits and vegetables, such as apricots, carrots, melons, broccoli, leafy greens

A healthy immune system is the key to resisting infections, allergies and chronic illnesses. The immune system protects and defends the body against viruses, bacteria, parasites and fungi. If it is not in top condition, it won't be able to resist these disease-causing agents. Balance in all areas of life — diet, exercise, mental perspective, social activity and spirituality — helps protect the immune system and keep it functioning well.

Healing Foods

Herbs
astragalus, burdock (leaf, root and seeds), cayenne, cloves, echinacea, elderflower and elderberries, garlic, ginseng, green tea, licorice*, parsley**, red clover, rosemary, sage, St. John's wort, thyme, turmeric, yarrow***

Other
cereal grasses, legumes, nuts, seeds, shiitake mushrooms, whole grains, yogurt with active bacterial cultures

* Avoid licorice if you have high blood pressure. The prolonged use of licorice is not recommended under any circumstances.

** If you are pregnant, limit your intake of parsley to ½ tsp (2 mL) dried or one sprig fresh per day. Do not take parsley if you are suffering from kidney inflammation.

*** Do not take yarrow if you are pregnant.

What to Do

Maximize
- Whole foods
- Fresh, raw, organic fruits and vegetables to provide the vitamins, minerals, digestive enzymes and antioxidants necessary for a healthy immune system
- Whole grains
- Essential fatty acids (found in legumes; nuts; seeds; and oily fish, such as salmon, mackerel, sardines and tuna), which is necessary for growth and maintenance of cells
- Fluid intake (drink at least eight large glasses of water, juice and/or herbal tea daily)

Minimize
- Non-organic meat, which is likely to contain antibiotics and steroid hormones, which depress immunity
- Excess animal fat, which suppresses immunity
- Antibiotics and corticosteroids. While these drugs can be lifesaving, overuse can deplete the immune system, causing more-complex health problems

Eliminate
- Sugar, which depletes vitamins and minerals, impairs the immune system and promotes yeast infections
- Refined, processed or preserved foods and soft drinks, which disrupt mineral levels, leading to poor metabolism of essential fatty acids
- Artificial food additives and pesticides likely found in non-organic food
- Alcohol, which depresses immune function
- Margarine, salad dressings and cooking oils (except extra-virgin olive oil and some other cold-pressed oils)
- Nitrates in bacon and sausage, which are converted to toxic substances in the body
- Food allergies and intolerances (see Appendix A: Food Allergies, page 359). Dairy products, gluten, corn products, eggs, oranges, strawberries, pork, tomatoes, coffee, tea, peanuts and chocolate often affect the immune system

Other Recommendations
- Consume sufficient protein, which helps build antibodies and healthy tissue and organs.
- Optimize digestion to improve the absorption of nutrients (see Indigestion, page 62).
- Stress depletes the immune system. Practice stress-reduction techniques, such as yoga, meditation and tai chi.
- Use herbs that are immune-system regulators (astragalus, echinacea, garlic, licorice*, thyme).
- Use antibiotic herbs (burdock leaf, root and seeds; cayenne; cloves; echinacea; garlic; red clover flower; thyme).
- Use antiviral herbs (burdock leaf, root and seeds; elderflower and elderberries; garlic; ginger; lemon balm; licorice*; marjoram; St. John's wort; yarrow***).
- Use antioxidant herbs (astragalus, ginkgo, green tea, hawthorn, milk thistle, rosemary, sage, turmeric).

Healing Drinks

(see also Immune Boosters, page 226; Top Common Antioxidant Fruits and Vegetables, pages 110 and 122)

Add 1 tsp (5 mL) herbs and up to 2 tbsp (25 mL) other ingredients recommended (see page 60) for this condition to the following:

Juices

- Allium Antioxidant, page 227
- Artichoke Carrot, page 179
- Berry Fine Cocktail, page 310
- Black Pineapple, page 164
- Blazing Beets, page 180
- C-Green, page 184
- Eye Opener, page 169
- Flaming Antibiotic, page 186
- Immunity, page 190
- Liquid Lunch, page 191
- Melon Morning Cocktail, page 313
- Rust Proofer #2, page 238

Teas

- Antioxi-T, page 229
- Flu Fighter, page 278
- The Green Diablo, page 232
- Immune Regulator Tea, page 234

Impotence

Impotence, a man's inability to achieve or maintain an erection, may be caused by stress, insufficient blood supply to the penis (from cholesterol deposits in the blood vessels), excess alcohol, drugs, tobacco, diabetes, prostate enlargement or low testosterone.

A whole-food diet helps provide the vitamins and minerals necessary for sexual health. Herbal circulatory stimulants, such as ginger and cayenne, are often helpful for impotence caused by deficient circulation. See Anxiety States, page 31, for suggestions on alleviating emotional stress.

Healing Foods

Fruits and vegetables
all

Herbs
cinnamon, cayenne, dandelion leaf, evening primrose oil, garlic, ginger, ginkgo, ginseng, nutmeg, saw palmetto, stinging nettle

Other
legumes, fish oil, flax seeds, kelp, nuts, oats, sunflower seeds, pumpkin seeds, soy products, wheat germ

What to Do

Maximize

- Fresh fruits and vegetables, whole grains, nuts and seeds
- Foods that contain vitamin E (whole-grain cereals, brown rice, nuts, seeds, wheat germ, soy products, kelp, dandelion leaf, extra-virgin olive oil) to protect the arteries that go to the penis from free-radical damage. Recent studies indicate better antioxidant effects occur when vitamin E comes from food rather than supplements

Minimize

- Animal protein (except for that in fish and chicken)

Eliminate

- Fried foods and junk foods
- Sugar
- Caffeine (found in coffee, black and green tea, chocolate and soft drinks)
- Refined flour
- Alcohol

Add 1 tsp (5 mL) herbs and up to 2 tbsp (25 mL) other ingredients recommended (see page 61) for this condition to the following:

Juices
- Blazing Beets, page 180
- Cajun Cocktail, page 312
- Flaming Antibiotic, page 186
- Immunity, page 190

Smoothies
- B-Vitamin, page 300
- Green Energy, page 303

Teas
- Adrenal Support Tea, page 220
- Circulation Tea, page 249
- Ginseng, page 280

Coffee Substitutes
- Seed Power Coffee, page 339

Indigestion

Overeating, irregular eating, excess alcohol or nervous tension may cause occasional indigestion. Symptoms can include abdominal discomfort, nausea or gastric reflux (flowing of stomach and small-intestine contents backward into the esophagus). Chronic indigestion can be caused by irritable bowel syndrome, food intolerances, ulcer or gallbladder disorder. Symptoms of chronic indigestion can include bloating, fatigue, diarrhea and constipation.

Healing Foods

Fruits and vegetables
apricots, bananas, lemons, mangoes, melons, papayas, pineapple, Jerusalem artichokes, leafy greens, squash, sweet potatoes

Herbs
cardamom, cayenne, coriander seeds, dandelion root, dill, cinnamon, cumin, fennel, German chamomile, ginger, lemon balm, meadowsweet, peppermint, slippery elm bark powder, turmeric

Other
almonds, barley, apple cider vinegar, flax seeds, rice, yogurt with active bacterial cultures

To avoid indigestion, be sure to wait at least one hour after a meal before drinking fruit smoothies. If fruit is eaten immediately after a meal, digestive problems may result (see Food Combining, page 15).

What to Do

Maximize
- Relaxed, unhurried meals
- Daily intake of yogurt with active bacterial cultures
- Antioxidant-rich fruits and vegetables
- Digestive herbal teas, such as chamomile, fennel, ginger, lemon balm or peppermint, taken regularly between meals

Minimize
- Alcohol
- Tea
- Eggs and meat

Eliminate
- Food allergies and intolerances (see Appendix A: Food Allergies, page 359)
- Sugar and artificial sweeteners
- Cold drinks, especially during or after meals
- Fruit juices
- High-fat and fried foods
- Dairy products (except yogurt with active bacterial cultures)
- Salty and spicy foods
- Refined foods
- Heavy meals
- Coffee

Natural Aids to Digestion

- Acidophilus (see Yogurt, page 156). Lactobacillus acidophilus is "friendly" bacteria used to ferment milk into yogurt. This bacteria can replace intestinal bacteria necessary for digestion when it has been destroyed by antibiotics.
- Calendula (*Calendula officinalis*), page 126. Because it stimulates bile production, calendula aids digestion. Calendula may be included in smoothies (use 1 tbsp/15 mL fresh petals) and makes an attractive garnish for drinks.
- Cinnamon (*Cinnamomum zeylanicum*), page 128. A warming carminative used to promote digestion, cinnamon adds a pleasant taste to smoothies.
- Dandelion root (*Taraxacum officinale*), page 130. An easily obtained, fairly mild but bitter laxative. Dandelion stimulates the liver and gallbladder and increases the flow of bile to aid digestion. Dandelion leaf acts as a diuretic.
- Fennel (*Foeniculum vulgare*), pages 116 and 132. Add a chopped fresh fennel bulb or an infusion of fennel seeds to smoothies to aid digestion and soothe discomfort from heartburn and indigestion.
- Fiber, page 363. Insoluble fiber in fruits, vegetables and whole grains helps prevent constipation and digestive diseases, such as diverticulosis and colon cancer.
- German chamomile (*Matricaria recutita*), page 133. As Peter Rabbit's mother knew, chamomile soothes upset tummies and inflammations and reduces flatulence and gas pains.
- Ginger (*Zingiber officinale*), page 134. Ginger is used to stimulate blood flow to the digestive system and to increase the absorption of nutrients. It increases the action of the gallbladder while protecting the liver against toxins.
- Kiwifruits (*Actinidia chinensis*), page 103. The enzymes in kiwis help digestion.
- Licorice (*Glycyrrhiza glabra*), page 139. Soothes gastric mucous membranes and eases spasms of the large intestine. Avoid licorice if you have high blood pressure.
- Papayas (*Carica papaya*), page 105. Papaya is a traditional remedy for indigestion. It contains an enzyme called papain, which is similar to pepsin, an enzyme that helps digest protein in the body.
- Peppermint (*Mentha piperita*), page 143. Because it contains flavonoids that stimulate the liver and gallbladder, peppermint increases the flow of bile. It has an antispasmodic effect on the smooth muscles of the digestive tract, making peppermint tea a good choice as an after-dinner drink.
- Pineapples (*Ananas comosus*), page 106. Pineapple is rich in the antibacterial enzyme bromelain. It is also anti-inflammatory and helps in the digestive process. Due to its digestive properties, raw pineapple prevents gelatin from setting and cannot be used in molded salads.
- Turmeric (*Curcuma longa*), page 149. Increases bile production and bile flow, which improves digestion.

Healing Drinks

Add 1 tsp (5 mL) herbs and up to 2 tbsp (25 mL) other ingredients recommended (see page 62) for this condition to the following:

Juices
- Breakfast Cocktail, page 311
- Leafy Greens, page 191
- Pineapple-Kiwi Cocktail, page 315
- Squash Special, page 196

Smoothies
- B-Vitamin, page 300

- Mango Madness, page 304

Digestives
- Digestive (Gripe) Water, page 211
- Digestive Seed Tea, page 211
- James Duke's Carminatea, page 214
- Rosy Peppermint Tea, page 215
- Spiced Papaya Tea, page 216

Infertility — Female

Healing Foods

Fruits and vegetables
apricots, oranges, peaches, raspberries, asparagus, avocados, beets, broccoli, carrots, leafy greens, sweet potatoes

Herbs
dandelion leaf and root, evening primrose oil, red clover flower, red raspberry leaf, rosemary, stinging nettle

Other
almonds, adzuki beans, Brazil nuts, bulgur, kidney beans, sea herbs, seeds (sunflower, pumpkin, flax, sesame), soy products, wheat germ, yogurt with active bacterial cultures

Factors that affect female fertility include age, vaginal infections, artificial lubricants, surgical scarring, ovarian cysts, endometriosis, uterine fibroids, low thyroid function and diets deficient in the nutrients required for healthy pregnancy, stress relief and hormone balance.

The most important factor in ensuring a healthy pregnancy and birth is the mother's health before and during pregnancy. Whole, fresh, natural foods provide the vitamins and minerals necessary for good health. To help ensure the baby's good health, it is worth taking a few months to improve the mother's health before pregnancy.

An irregular menstrual cycle is a sign of hormonal imbalance. The herb chasteberry, also known as *Vitex agnus-castus* (see page 150), and herbs that support the liver, such as dandelion root (see page 130), may be used to regulate hormone production.

What to Do

Maximize
- Whole foods
- Antioxidant-rich fruits and vegetables
- Nuts and seeds
- Foods that contain folic acid (bulgur, orange juice, spinach, beans, sunflower seeds, wheat germ)

Minimize
- Acid-forming foods (meat, fish, grains, cheese, eggs, tea, coffee, alcohol, cranberries, plums, prunes, lentils, chickpeas, peanuts, walnuts), which can make cervical mucus acidic, which will destroy sperm

Eliminate
- Refined flour
- Cigarette smoking
- Sugar
- Artificial food additives

Other Recommendations
- Drink tea made from nerve-nourishing herbs (German chamomile, skullcap, oat straw) and regularly include relaxing activities, such as walking, meditation, yoga and tai chi, to reduce stress.
- Balance your intake of meat and fish protein (organic if possible) with vegetable protein, such as that in soybean products or beans with rice.

Healing Drinks

Add 1 tsp (5 mL) herbs and up to 2 tbsp (25 mL) other ingredients recommended (see page 64) for this condition to the following:

Juices
- Apricot Peach, page 163
- Beet, page 180
- Brocco-Carrot, page 181
- Raspberry Juice, page 174
- Rust Proofer #2, page 238

Smoothies
- Beta Blast, page 164
- B-Vitamin, page 300

Teas
- Hormone Balancing Tea, page 222
- Raspberry Tea, page 265

Infertility — Male

Male infertility is characterized by low sperm count and low sperm motility (a situation in which the semen is too thick to allow proper sperm mobility). Causes can be related to a deficiency in dietary nutrients, hormone imbalance or stress. There is some evidence that suggests that the estrogens in pesticides and other chemical pollutants may be a cause of declining sperm counts over the past 50 years.

Healing Foods

Fruits and vegetables
berries, cantaloupe, grapefruit, kiwis, oranges, strawberries, asparagus, avocados, broccoli, cabbage, cauliflower, leafy greens (especially spinach), red and green bell peppers

Herbs
astragalus, cayenne, ginger, ginkgo, ginseng, red raspberry leaf

Other
bran, fish oils, legumes, nuts, oats, seeds (especially sunflower and pumpkin), soybean products, whole grains

What to Do

Maximize
- Antioxidant-rich fruits and vegetables, especially those that contain vitamin C. Studies have shown that high sperm motility requires a sufficient intake of vitamin C
- Foods that contain zinc (seafood, legumes, whole grains, sunflower seeds, pumpkin seeds), which is required for sperm motility
- Herbs that improve circulation (cayenne, ginger) of all body fluids, including semen

Minimize
- Iodized salt. Excess iodine lowers sperm count
- Refined foods (white rice, white flour, white sugar)
- Animal fats in meat and dairy products

Eliminate

- Alcohol, coffee, tea and soft drinks, which decrease sperm health

Other Recommendations

- Drink tea made from nerve-nourishing herbs (German chamomile, skullcap, oat straw) and regularly include relaxing activities, such as walking, meditation, yoga and tai chi, to reduce stress.

Healing Drinks

Add 1 tsp (5 mL) herbs and up to 2 tbsp (25 mL) other ingredients recommended (see page 65) for this condition to the following:

Juices

- Berry Fine Cocktail, page 310
- Cauli-Slaw, page 184
- C-Blitz, page 166
- C-Green, page 184
- Citrus Cocktail, page 313

Teas

- Circulation Tea, page 249
- Ginseng, page 280
- Raspberry Tea, page 265

Inflammatory Bowel Disease

Crohn's disease and ulcerative colitis are serious diseases. Read all reference information on these diseases and consult with an experienced medical practitioner.

Healing Foods

Fruits and vegetables
juice of beets and beet tops, carrot juice and boiled carrots, spinach juice

Herbs
garlic, German chamomile, marshmallow root, slippery elm bark powder, valerian*

Other
ground flax seeds, kelp, psyllium seed, rice

* Valerian has an adverse effect on some people.

What to Do

Maximize

- Rice and cooked root vegetables
- Beet juice, which provides nutrition, cleanses the blood and supports detoxification in the liver
- Raw garlic daily, to cleanse the bowel of toxins
- Food combining (see page 15) to optimize nutrition and absorption of nutrients
- Water and herbal teas between meals

Eliminate

- Red meat, which contributes to inflammation. Substitute with oily fish (salmon, sardines, tuna) and a little white chicken meat
- All foods that commonly cause bowel irritation: coffee, chocolate, mushrooms, alcohol, soft drinks, all junk food, all artificial coloring and flavoring, fried foods, salt

Eliminate

- Foods that trigger allergies and intolerances, commonly dairy products, wheat, rye, oats and corn products, citrus fruits, eggs, cruciferous vegetables (broccoli, cabbage, cauliflower, Brussels sprouts), tomatoes, yeast (see Appendix A: Food Allergies, page 359)
- Sugar and sugar products
- Cigarettes

Healing Drinks

Add 1 tsp (5 mL) herbs and up to 2 tbsp (25 mL) other ingredients (see page 66) recommended for this condition to the following:

Juices
- Beet, page 180
- Leafy Greens, page 191
- Popeye's Power, page 246

Teas
- Digestive Stress Soother, page 262

Influenza

Healing Foods

Fruits and vegetables
lemons, oranges, pineapple, strawberries, broccoli, carrots, Jerusalem artichokes, spinach, watercress

Herbs
cayenne, cinnamon, echinacea, elderflower and elderberries, garlic, ginger, licorice*, parsley**, peppermint, thyme, yarrow***

* Avoid licorice if you have high blood pressure. The prolonged use of licorice is not recommended under any circumstances.

** If you are pregnant, limit your intake of parsley to ½ tsp (2 mL) dried or one sprig fresh per day. Do not take parsley if you are suffering from kidney inflammation.

*** Do not take yarrow if you are pregnant.

Influenza (flu) is a viral infection of the respiratory tract. Symptoms include chills, fever, cough, headache, aches, fatigue and lack of appetite. Treating the flu early can shorten recovery time and help prevent more-serious disease. Top priorities are getting rest to allow the body's energies to focus on healing and drinking plenty of fluids to encourage the elimination of toxins.

Eating small meals, mainly of vegetable juices, reduces the energy required for digestion, allowing more energy to be focused on healing. "Hot" herbs, such as ginger and cayenne, increase body temperature, which discourages the influenza virus from multiplying.

What to Do

Maximize
- Fresh fruits and vegetables
- Fluid intake (drink at least eight large glasses of water, juice and/or herbal tea daily)

Eliminate
- Alcohol, sugar and sugar products, which decrease immunity

Other
kelp, psyllium seed, well-cooked (mushy) rice

Healing Drinks

(see also Immune Boosters, page 266; Top Common Antioxidant Fruits and Vegetables, pages 110 and 122)

Add 1 tsp (5 mL) herbs and up to 2 tbsp (25 mL) other ingredients recommended (see page 67 and left) for this condition to the following:

Juices
• Brocco-Artichoke, page 181
• Brocco-Carrot, page 181

• Carrot Allium, page 183
• Flaming Antibiotic, page 186
• Immunity, page 190
• Pineapple Citrus, page 174
• Spring Celebration, page 195

Teas
• Antioxi-T, page 229
• Flu Fighter, page 278

Mulled Juices
• Antibiotic Toddy, page 228

Insomnia

Healing Foods

Fruits and vegetables
apples, bananas, lettuce, leafy greens

Herbs
German chamomile, hops*, lavender, lemon balm, passionflower, skullcap, St. John's wort, valerian**, wild lettuce

Other
honey, nuts, oats, sunflower seeds, brown rice, yogurt with active bacterial cultures

* Do not take hops if you are suffering from depression.

** Valerian has an adverse effect on some people.

Insomnia, or the inability to sleep, may be caused by low blood-sugar levels (see Hypoglycemia, page 59), anxiety, depression, temperature (too hot or too cold) or caffeine ingestion. Foods high in B vitamins, calcium and magnesium supply nutrients that calm the nervous tension that can prevent sleep (see Anxiety States, page 31, and Depression, page 42).

What to Do

Maximize
• Calming, caffeine-free drinks
• Foods that are high in B vitamins (whole grains, leafy greens, broccoli, wheat germ), calcium (yogurt, tofu, broccoli) and magnesium (apples, avocados, dark grapes, nuts, brown rice)

Eliminate
• Alcohol
• Caffeine (found in coffee, black and green tea, chocolate and soft drinks)
• Artificial food additives

Healing Drinks

(see also Stress Busters, page 259)

Add 1 tsp (5 mL) herbs and up to 2 tbsp (25 mL) other ingredients recommended (see left) for this condition to the following:

Juices
• Leafy Greens, page 191

Smoothies
• Almond-Banana Milk, page 298

Teas
• Calming Cuppa Tea, page 261
• Lavender Tea, page 282
• Nerve Support, page 251

Coffee Substitutes
• Anxiety Antidote, page 335

Irritable Bowel Syndrome

Irritable bowel syndrome is a long-standing bowel dysfunction for which no organic cause can be found. It is characterized by bloating, abdominal pain, and diarrhea or constipation. Healing factors include diet, stress management and elimination of allergens. Herbs can be used to soothe the intestines, reduce inflammation, improve digestion, calm the nerves and promote intestinal healing.

What to Do

Maximize

- Fish and vegetable proteins (nuts, seeds, tofu, beans, legumes)
- Raw fruits and vegetables to provide immunity-boosting vitamins C and E, improve bowel function and eliminate toxins
- Flax seeds and flax seed oil, which are soothing and anti-inflammatory and help heal the bowel and improve bowel function

Eliminate

- Alcohol
- Coffee
- Red meat
- Refined sugar and flour
- Artificial sweeteners
- Fats and oils (except extra-virgin olive oil)
- Foods allergies and intolerances (see Appendix A: Food Allergies, page 359). Common culprits are dairy products and citrus fruits
- Caffeine, wheat and corn

Healing Drinks

Add 1 tsp (5 mL) herbs and up to 2 tbsp (25 mL) other ingredients recommended (see left) for this condition to the following:

Juices
- Cabbage Cocktail, page 311
- Cauliflower Cocktail, page 312

Teas
- Digestive Stress Soother, page 262
- Ginger Tea, page 279

Kidney Stones

Healing Foods

Fruits and vegetables
apricots, mangoes, melons, peaches, asparagus, broccoli, celery, corn, fennel, leeks, onions

Herbs
goldenrod, marshmallow leaf and root, plantain, stinging nettle

Other
brown rice, seeds (flax, pumpkin, sesame, sunflower), whole grains

Kidney stones are 60% less common in people who follow vegetarian diets. A high-fiber, high-fluid, low-protein diet is the best preventive medicine. Diets high in animal protein encourage stone formation.

Kidney stones are usually made of calcium and oxalic acid. For this type of stone, limit foods that contain oxalic acid and large amounts of salt (sodium can stimulate calcium excretion). Stones that are made of uric acid and other minerals are less common. Eliminating shellfish can help prevent uric acid stones. Consult your health-care practitioner to determine which type of stone you have and what the possible causes are.

What to Do

Maximize
- Water intake (drink at least two large glasses of water four times a day between meals) to flush out stones and prevent bacterial buildup
- Alkaline-forming foods (oranges, lemons, all vegetables) for uric acid stones

Minimize
- Animal protein in meat and dairy products

Eliminate
- Salt and high-sodium foods (bacon, processed foods)
- Sugar
- High-oxalate foods (leafy greens, rhubarb, coffee, tea, chocolate, grapefruit, parsley, peanuts, strawberries, tomatoes) for oxalic acid stones
- Seafood for uric acid stones
- Alcohol
- Refined flour

Other Recommendations
- Replace animal protein with soy and other vegetable proteins.
- Marshmallow leaf tea, which is soothing to the urinary system, may help break up stones.

Healing Drinks

Add 1 tsp (5 mL) herbs and up to 2 tbsp (25 mL) other ingredients recommended (see left) for this condition to the following:

Juices
- ABC Juice, page 179
- Allium Antioxidant, page 227
- Apricot Peach, page 163

Smoothies
- Mango Madness, page 304

Teas
- Free Flow Tea, page 279

Coffee Substitutes
- Seed Power Coffee, page 339

Laryngitis

Healing Foods

Fruits and vegetables
all fruits, carrot juice

Herbs
garlic, ginger, sage*, thyme

Other
honey**

* Avoid sage if you have high blood pressure or are pregnant or breastfeeding.

** Do not give honey to children under one year of age.

Laryngitis is an inflammation of the vocal cords that may be associated with a cold or other infection, or caused by excessive use of the voice. It is important to rest the voice for a few days. If laryngitis is accompanied by fever and a cough or lasts longer than two days, consult your health-care practitioner.

What to Do

Maximize
• Fruits and fruit juices

• Herbal teas and gargles (thyme and sage)

Healing Drinks

Add 1 tsp (5 mL) herbs and up to 2 tbsp (25 mL) other ingredients recommended (see left) for this condition to the following:

Juices
• Apricot Peach, page 163

• Beta Blast, page 164
• C-Blend, page 166
Teas
• Antioxi-T, page 229
• Throat Saver Tea Blend, page 287

Liver Problems

Healing Foods

Fruits and vegetables
apples, blackberries, dark grapes, plums, raspberries, beets, carrots, celery, leafy greens, onions, tomatoes, watercress

The liver is responsible for removing toxins from the blood that can interfere with the functions of the heart, nervous system, digestive system and circulatory system. Excess fat, chemicals, intoxicants, and refined and processed foods disrupt liver function. Anger, nervous tension, mood swings, depression, skin problems, gallbladder problems, menstrual and menopausal difficulties and candida infections can result from poor liver function. It can be improved by diet, and the following dietary suggestions can complement traditional treatment of liver diseases, such as hepatitis, which must be treated by a physician.

What to Do

Maximize
• Fruits and vegetables
• Legumes and whole grains
• Bitter foods and herbs (asparagus; citrus peel; dandelion leaf, root and flowers; milk thistle seeds; German chamomile flowers) to stimulate liver function

• Water intake (drink at least eight large glasses of water daily)
• Dandelion root tea
Minimize
• Animal protein (replace with small amounts of fish and vegetable protein)

Herbs
alfalfa, astragalus, burdock root, cayenne, dandelion leaf and root, fennel, fenugreek, German chamomile, ginger, lemon balm, licorice*, garlic, milk thistle, parsley**, rosemary, stinging nettle, turmeric, yellow dock

Other
cereal grasses, flax seeds, lecithin, legumes, extra-virgin olive oil, sea herbs, spirulina, whole grains

* Avoid licorice if you have high blood pressure. The prolonged use of licorice is not recommended under any circumstances.

** If you are pregnant, limit your intake of parsley to ½ tsp (2 mL) dried or one sprig fresh per day. Do not take parsley if you are suffering from kidney inflammation.

Eliminate
- Foods that interfere with liver function (animal fats, dairy products, eggs, refined foods, margarine, shortening, oils — except extra-virgin olive oil — alcohol, processed foods)

Healing Drinks

Add 1 tsp (5 mL) herbs and up to 2 tbsp (25 mL) other ingredients recommended (see left) for this condition to the following:

Juices
- Apple Beet Pear, page 162
- Apple Fresh, page 162
- Apple Pear, page 162
- Beet, page 180
- Carrot Apple, page 183
- Cell Support Juice, page 274

- Fried foods
- All tobacco products
- Sugar, sweets and junk foods
- Non-organic foods, which may contain pesticide residues or toxins

- Popeye's Power, page 246
- Sunrise Supreme (use blackberries instead of strawberries), page 177
- Tomato Tang, page 197

Teas
- Cleansing Tea, page 274
- Immune Regulator Tea, page 234

Coffee Substitutes
- Root Coffee Blend, page 338

Low Libido

Healing Foods

Fruits and vegetables
apples, lemons, red grapes, beets, leafy greens, leeks, onions, watercress

Herbs
cayenne, cinnamon, cloves, fennel seeds, garlic, ginger, ginseng, mustard, parsley*, peppermint, rose petals, rosemary, stinging nettle

* If you are pregnant, limit your intake of parsley to ½ tsp (2 mL) dried or one sprig fresh per day. Do not take parsley if you are suffering from kidney inflammation.

You can remedy low libido, a lack of sexual interest or energy, by nourishing the reproductive organs and boosting your overall energy level. A diet that consists of whole foods, which provide basic vitamins and minerals, as well as valuable phytochemicals, will encourage sexual health. Antioxidant-rich fruits and vegetables improve circulation by preventing cholesterol deposits from forming on blood-vessel walls. The essential fatty acids in nuts and seeds are especially important in regulating sexual response. If stress is a factor, use nerve-nourishing oats, lemon balm or skullcap.

What to Do

Maximize
- Antioxidant-rich fruits and vegetables
- Nuts and seeds
- Whole grains
- Herbs that stimulate circulation and energy (cayenne, cinnamon, cloves, garlic, ginger, rosemary)
- Herbs such as ginseng, fennel, parsley*, nutmeg, lavender, mustard and rose, which have been traditionally used as aphrodisiacs

Minimize
- Meat

Other
almonds, Brazil nuts, fish oil, flax seeds, honey, legumes, oats, pumpkin seeds, soy products, cereal grasses, sunflower seeds, walnuts, wheat germ, whole grains

Eliminate
- Alcohol
- Coffee
- Dairy products
- Refined and processed foods
- Sugar

Healing Drinks

Add 1 tsp (5 mL) herbs and up to 2 tbsp (25 mL) other ingredients recommended (see page 72 and left) for this condition to the following:

Juices
- Allium Antioxidant, page 227
- Apple Fresh, page 162
- Beet, page 180
- Blazing Beets, page 180
- Leafy Greens, page 191

Smoothies
- Green Energy, page 303

Teas
- Circulation Tea, page 249
- Ginseng, page 280

Other
- Applesauce, page 291

Lupus

Healing Foods

Fruits and vegetables
apples, apricots, blackberries, black currants, blueberries, cantaloupe, cherries, grapes, pineapple, avocados, broccoli, cabbage, carrots, cauliflower, fennel, leafy greens, onions, squash, watercress

There are two forms of this autoimmune disease: discoid lupus erythematosus (DLE), which affects only the skin, and systemic lupus erythematosus (SLE), which affects the connective tissues throughout the body. In DLE, the skin lesions are red and scaly. Early symptoms of SLE are fatigue, weight loss and fever, which progress to arthritis-like joint pain. In the later stages, SLE may affect the kidneys and heart. Because this disease attacks the body's immune system, it is important to avoid viral infections, stress and fatigue. Nutrition and herbs can help by providing support and nourishment to the immune system and the organs through which detoxification takes place: skin, lungs, kidneys, liver and bowels. Relaxation exercises and plenty of sleep also support the immune system.

What to Do

Maximize
- Antioxidant-rich fruits and vegetables
- Water intake (drink at least eight large glasses of water daily) to eliminate toxins
- Essential fatty acids (found in nuts and seeds, especially freshly ground flax seeds) to strengthen the immune system and improve blood flow

Herbs
burdock root, dandelion root and leaf, echinacea, elderflower, evening primrose oil, fennel, garlic, ginger, lemon balm, licorice*, meadowsweet, parsley**, red clover flower, St. John's wort, stinging nettle, thyme, turmeric

Other
cereal grasses, fish oil, flax seeds, legumes, extra-virgin olive oil, seeds, shiitake mushrooms, soy products, whole grains, soy yogurt

* Avoid licorice if you have high blood pressure. The prolonged use of licorice is not recommended under any circumstances.

** If you are pregnant, limit your intake of parsley to ½ tsp (2 mL) dried or one sprig fresh per day. Do not take parsley if you are suffering from kidney inflammation.

Eliminate

- Animal protein in meat and dairy products, which contributes to the progression of lupus. Substitute vegetable proteins in soy products and legumes with rice
- Food allergies and intolerances (see Appendix A: Food Allergies, page 359). Keep a diet diary to note symptom changes in relation to food eaten
- Salad and cooking oils (except extra-virgin olive oil), which promote inflammation
- Sugar and alcohol, which inhibit immune function
- Alfalfa seeds and sprouts, which can cause inflammation

Healing Drinks

(see also Immune Boosters, page 226; Top Common Antioxidant Fruits and Vegetables, pages 110 and 122)

Add 1 tsp (5 mL) herbs and up to 2 tbsp (25 mL) other ingredients recommended (see left) for this condition to the following:

Juices

- Apricot Peach, page 163
- Black Pineapple, page 164
- Blueberry, page 165

Other Recommendations

- Eat oily fish (salmon, mackerel, sardines and tuna), which provide healing omega-6 oils, three times a week.
- Use anti-inflammatory herbs (German chamomile, elderflower, fennel, ginger, meadowsweet, turmeric).
- Use herbs that help eliminate toxins (burdock leaf, root and seeds; dandelion root and leaf; parsley**).
- Consume herbs and foods that support the immune system (echinacea, garlic, shiitake mushrooms, cereal grasses).
- Exercise daily, according to your fitness level.

- Brocco-Carrot, page 181
- Cauli-Slaw, page 184
- C-Green, page 184
- Cruciferous, page 185
- Pine-Berry, page 174

Teas
- Antioxi-T, page 229
- Immune Regulator Tea, page 234
- Nerve Nourisher, page 250

Coffee Substitutes
- Easy Root Coffee, page 335

Menopause

Healing Foods

Fruits and vegetables
apples, avocados, bananas, berries, grapes, peaches, pears, asparagus, carrots, celery, fennel, green bell peppers, leafy greens, tomatoes, watercress

Menopause occurs when menstruation ceases. Hormonal changes around that transitional time can result in irregular menstruation and other symptoms, such as hot flashes, mood swings and vaginal dryness. Stress magnifies these symptoms.

After menopause, a woman's estrogen level decreases. Decreased estrogen is one of the many factors involved in the development of osteoporosis and heart disease. Daily exercise, relaxation and good diet will help you make a smooth transition and decrease your risk of heart disease and osteoporosis. Nutritional

Herbs
dandelion root, fennel, garlic, ginseng, lemon balm, licorice*, motherwort, red clover flower, rosemary, sage

Other
dried fruits, flax seeds, lentils, sea herbs, soy products, sunflower seeds, extra-virgin olive oil, pumpkin seeds, wheat germ, whole grains, yogurt with active bacterial cultures

* Avoid licorice if you have high blood pressure. The prolonged use of licorice is not recommended under any circumstances.

and herbal support help balance hormone levels, improve blood circulation, eliminate toxins and reduce nervous tension.

In addition to the transition-smoothing herbs listed on the left, use the following herbs for specific conditions and symptoms:
- chasteberry (also known as *Vitex agnus-castus*) to balance hormones;
- ginseng, skullcap or oats for stress and nervous tension;
- valerian for insomnia;
- black cohosh for joint pain, hot flashes or depression; and
- hawthorn berries for women with a family history of heart disease.

What to Do

Maximize
- Antioxidant-rich fruits and vegetables (see pages 110 and 122)
- Nuts and seeds
- Whole grains

Minimize
- Animal fats in meat and dairy products

Eliminate
- Caffeine (found in coffee, black and green tea, chocolate and soft drinks)
- Sugar
- Cigarette smoking
- Alcohol

Healing Drinks

(see also Endocrine Elixirs, page 220)

Add 1 tsp (5 mL) herbs and up to 2 tbsp (25 mL) other ingredients recommended (see left) for this condition to the following:

Juices
- Apple Fresh, page 162
- Bone Builder, page 241
- Grape Power, page 170
- Leafy Greens, page 191
- Pear Fennel, page 173
- Peppery Tomato Cocktail, page 314
- Spring Celebration, page 195

Smoothies
- Best Berries, page 299
- Green Energy (use ginseng in place of ginkgo), page 303

Teas
- Cleansing Tea, page 274
- Woman's Own, page 288

Menstrual Disorders

Fruits and vegetables
apricots, blueberries, blackberries, citrus fruits, grapes, strawberries, beets and beet greens, broccoli, carrots, leafy greens

Amenorrhea (absence of menstruation), dysmenorrhea (painful menstruation) and premenstrual syndrome (PMS) are often caused by a hormone imbalance, which is sometimes related to excess stress, exercise or animal products in the diet. Other factors can include poor circulation and insufficient blood or lymphatic circulation.

The natural approach is to:

- balance hormones;
- support blood (and lymphatic) circulation to the pelvic organs;
- promote relaxation, regular moderate exercise and good nutrition; and
- improve digestion and elimination to improve nutrient absorption and regulate hormones.

What to Do

Maximize
- Fruits and vegetables, especially those on page 75

Minimize
- Salt and salty foods
- Alcohol

Eliminate
- Refined foods, which lack minerals and vitamins and contain potentially harmful additives
- Caffeine which depletes calcium and other minerals
- Sugar and sweeteners
- Non-organic meat and dairy products, which can contain artificial hormones and toxins

Other Recommendations
- Balance your intake of lean meat or fish protein with vegetable protein.
- Get sufficient dietary calcium by eating foods such as yogurt, broccoli and tofu.
- Exercise daily.

Healing Drinks

(see also Endocrine Elixirs, page 220)

Add 1 tsp (5 mL) herbs and up to 2 tbsp (25 mL) other ingredients (see left) for this condition to the following:

Juices
- Beet, page 180
- Brocco-Carrot, page 181
- C-Green, page 184
- Eye Opener (use blueberries, blackberries or strawberries), page 169
- Leafy Greens, page 191
- Popeye's Power, page 246
- Sunrise Supreme, page 177

Smoothies
- Best Berries, page 299
- Pump It Up, page 246

Teas
- Ginger Tea, page 279
- Hormone Balancing Tea, page 222

Migraines

A migraine headache starts with the constriction of blood vessels in the brain, which is then followed by an expansion, which causes pain. Warning symptoms (such as vision changes or mood swings) can come with the blood-vessel constriction. The pain usually starts on one side of the head, but may spread to both sides, and may be accompanied by nausea or dizziness. Migraine triggers can include strong emotions, hormonal changes, food allergies and some medications, including oral contraceptives.

Healing Foods

Fruits and vegetables
blackberries, cantaloupe, beets, broccoli, carrots, celery, leafy greens, onions

Herbs
cayenne, cinnamon, dandelion leaf and root, feverfew, garlic, German chamomile, ginger, lemon balm, parsley*

Other
brown rice and rice bran, flax seeds, legumes, pumpkin seeds, sunflower seeds, whole grains

* If you are pregnant, limit your intake of parsley to ½ tsp (2 mL) dried or one sprig fresh per day. Do not take parsley if you are suffering from kidney inflammation.

What to Do

Maximize
- Vegetable protein
- Fresh fruits and vegetables

Minimize
- Animal fats in meat and dairy products
- Sugar

Eliminate
- Caffeine (found in coffee, black and green tea, chocolate and soft drinks)
- Foods that precipitate migraine attacks by causing constriction of the blood vessels (red wine, cheese, corn, smoked or pickled fish, sausages, hot dogs and all other preserved meats, pork, shellfish, walnuts)
- Artificial food additives
- Alcohol
- Food allergies and intolerances (see Appendix A: Food Allergies, page 359), which are usually the cause of migraine headaches. Migraine sufferers are commonly intolerant of dairy products, wheat, eggs, oranges and/or monosodium glutamate (MSG). When food allergies and intolerances are alleviated, the incidence of migraines is either eliminated or greatly reduced

Other Recommendations
- Eat oily fish (salmon, mackerel, sardines and tuna) two or three times a week to maintain steady blood flow to the brain.
- Eat a leaf or two of fresh feverfew daily.
- Practice food-combining techniques (see Food Combining, page 15).

Healing Drinks

Add 1 tsp (5 mL) herbs and up to 2 tbsp (25 mL) other ingredients recommended (see left) for this condition to the following:

Juices
- Beet, page 180
- Brocco-Carrot, page 181
- C-Green, page 184
- Liquid Lunch, page 191

Smoothies
- Calming Chamomile Smoothie, page 301

Teas
- Ginger Tea, page 279
- Migraine Buster, page 283

Multiple Sclerosis

Multiple sclerosis is the breakdown of the protective myelin sheaths around the brain and spinal cord. Symptoms may include muscular weakness, numbness, blurred vision, light-headedness and urinary incontinence. Although a cure is not known, dietary changes, such as those recommended below, have shown impressive results in slowing the disease's progress by preventing the breakdown of myelin sheaths and returning to health.

What to Do

Maximize
- Foods that are low in saturated fat
- Essential fatty acids (found in evening primrose oil, flax seeds, fish oils)
- Immunity (see Immune Deficiency, page 59)
- Foods that are high in B vitamins (fish, wheat germ, sea herbs) and magnesium (apples, avocados, bananas, leafy greens, fish, nuts, soy products, brown rice, wheat germ) to nourish nerve tissue
- Lifestyle quality. Evaluate and reduce stress in your life by practicing meditation, yoga, tai chi or taking daily long walks in natural surroundings

Minimize
- Animal fats

Eliminate
- Candida infections (see Candida, page 38)
- Food allergies and intolerances (see Appendix A: Food Allergies, page 359)
- Coffee
- Red meat and dark meat of chicken or turkey
- Dairy products and eggs
- Gluten
- Fats and oils (except cold-pressed oils, such as extra-virgin olive oil)

Healing Drinks

Add 1 tsp (5 mL) herbs and up to 2 tbsp (25 mL) other ingredients recommended (see left) for this condition to the following:

Juices
- Beet, page 180
- Cauli-Slaw, page 184
- Green Beet, page 188
- Leafy Greens, page 191
- Sea Herb Surprise, page 194

Smoothies
- Smart Smoothie, page 306

Teas
- Immune Regulator Tea, page 234
- Immune Tea Blend, page 235
- Nerve Nourisher, page 250

Tonics
- Spring Tonic, page 271

Osteoporosis

Osteoporosis is a disease characterized by progressive bone loss and decreased bone density and strength. It is caused when bones lose calcium. Consumption of calcium- and nutrient-rich foods helps keep bones strong. In order for the body to absorb calcium, it requires adequate levels of certain vitamins and minerals, especially vitamin D and magnesium.

Factors in bone loss are:
- age;
- decreased estrogen level (estrogen enhances calcium absorption);
- not doing weight-bearing exercise, which decreases calcium absorption (doing weight-bearing exercise increases it);
- some prescription drugs, such as corticosteroids, anticonvulsants, diuretics and antacids, which contain aluminum, which interferes with calcium absorption;
- chronic stress, which depletes calcium;
- lack of minerals and vitamins in the diet, which inhibits calcium absorption; and
- disease of the thyroid or adrenal glands.

Healing Foods

Fruits and vegetables
all raw fruits, except those that are acid forming (cranberries, plums, prunes). Broccoli, cabbage, leafy greens and watercress are especially good sources of calcium

Herbs
alfalfa, dandelion leaf, German chamomile, oat straw, parsley*, plantain, stinging nettle

Other
blackstrap molasses, dried fruits, fish and fish oil, legumes, nuts, seeds, feta cheese, sardines, salmon, spirulina, tofu, whole grains, yogurt with active bacterial cultures

Sea herbs are especially good sources of calcium

* If you are pregnant, limit your intake of parsley to ½ tsp (2 mL) dried or one sprig fresh per day. Do not take parsley if you are suffering from kidney inflammation.

What to Do

Maximize
- *Foods that promote calcium absorption:*
- raw fruits;
- green vegetables;
- nuts and seeds; and
- legumes.

Minimize
- Foods high in oxalic acid (almonds, Swiss chard, rhubarb, spinach), which inhibits calcium uptake
- Foods that use up calcium while being metabolized by the body (citrus fruits, vinegar, wine)
- Sodium fluoride (found in drinking water, soft drinks, canned food, preserved meats, boxed cereals, and residues of insecticides and fertilizers on commercially grown produce).

Although fluoride is needed in bone formation, an excess inhibits the process.
- Sugar, salt and caffeine, which cause calcium to be excreted through the urine;
- Alcohol;
- High-protein (meat and dairy) diets, which lead to bone loss through calcium excretion in the urine. (This is partly because calcium is used in the process of protein breakdown.) Moderate amounts of fish, poultry, eggs and dairy products can be included in the diet. Note that a lack of protein will also cause weakness in the whole system, including all of the bone-making organs and systems

Minimize

- Phosphorus-rich foods, especially soft drinks, which contribute most to bone loss. Although phosphorous is necessary to bone health, an excess inhibits calcium metabolism
- Refined flour, which is nutrient-depleted, leading to a loss of minerals in the diet
- Vegetables in the nightshade family (tomatoes, potatoes, eggplants, all peppers), which contain the calcium inhibitor solanine
- Commercially prepared foods that contain chemicals, which add toxins and deplete minerals
- Food grown with non-organic fertilizers, which cause depletion of their minerals
- Grains and brans, particularly raw bran, which are high in phytic acid, which binds to calcium, making it unavailable to the body. Soak grains overnight to neutralize the phytic acid and make the vitamins and minerals available to the body

Healing Drinks

(see also Muscle Powers, page 240)

Add 1 tsp (5 mL) herbs and up to 2 tbsp (25 mL) other ingredients recommended (see page 79) for this condition to the following:

Juices
- Black Pineapple, page 164
- Bone Builder, page 241
- Brocco-Carrot, page 181
- Leafy Greens, page 191

Smoothies
- Avocado-Pineapple, page 299
- B-Vitamin, page 300
- Sea-Straw Smoothie, page 306

Teas
- Bone Blend Tea, page 241
- Cleansing Tea, page 274
- Digestive Seed Tea, page 211

Overweight

Healing Foods

Fruits and vegetables
apples, blackberries, cherries, citrus fruits, grapes, pineapple, strawberries, watermelon, asparagus, broccoli, cabbage, celery, cucumber, fennel, leafy greens, lettuce, Jerusalem artichokes, radishes, watercress

Excessive weight is most often caused by insufficient exercise relative to the amount eaten. In a few cases, weight gain can be attributed to hormonal imbalances and some drugs (including corticosteroids and birth control pills). Long-term weight loss is most effectively achieved by adopting a whole-food diet and increasing exercise.

Healing Foods

Herbs
cayenne, chickweed, dandelion leaf and root, evening primrose oil, fennel, garlic, ginger, parsley*, psyllium seeds

Other
cider vinegar, flax seeds, kelp, legumes, soy products, walnuts, whole grains

* If you are pregnant, limit your intake of parsley to ½ tsp (2 mL) dried or one sprig fresh per day. Do not take parsley if you are suffering from kidney inflammation.

What to Do

Maximize
- Fresh fruits and vegetables, which help speed up the metabolism and eliminate toxins
- Water intake (drink at least eight large glasses daily) to reduce appetite and eliminate toxins

Minimize
- Refined flour products, fast foods and junk foods
- Fats in meat, dairy products and salad oils (except extra-virgin olive oil)
- Starchy foods (breads, corn, parsnips, potatoes, squash, sweet potatoes)

Eliminate
- Sugar and artificial sweeteners
- Fried foods
- Artificial food additives
- Food allergies and intolerances (see Appendix A: Food Allergies, page 359). Milk products, eggs, oranges and gluten may affect digestion

Other Recommendations
- Eat oily fish (salmon, sardines, mackerel, tuna) two or three times a week to help the body burn excess fat.
- Eat fruit between meals for optimum digestion and to discourage snacking on inappropriate foods.
- Exercise daily, according to your fitness level.
- Replace empty-calorie drinks and snacks with nutrient-rich smoothies.

Healing Drinks

Add 1 tsp (5 mL) herbs and up to 2 tbsp (25 mL) other ingredients recommended (see left) for this condition to the following:

Juices
- Black Pineapple, page 164
- Brocco-Artichoke, page 181
- C-Green, page 184
- Cherry Sunrise, page 167
- The Chiller, page 185
- Citrus Cocktail, page 313
- Melon Morning Cocktail, page 313
- Popeye's Power, page 246
- Soft Salad, page 195
- Sunrise Supreme, page 177

Smoothies
- B-Vitamin, page 300
- Sea-Straw Smoothie, page 306

Teas
- Cleansing Tea, page 274
- Digestive Seed Tea, page 211
- Ginger Tea, page 279

Parkinson's Disease

Healing Foods

Fruits and vegetables
bananas, blueberries, strawberries, beets, carrots, leafy greens, lettuce, potatoes

Herbs
alfalfa, evening primrose oil, ginger, ginkgo, milk thistle seed, passionflower, St. John's wort

Other
legumes, nuts, oats, extra-virgin olive oil, peanuts, seeds (flax, sesame, sunflower, pumpkin), soy lecithin, spelt flour, whole grains (except wheat)

Symptoms of Parkinson's disease include muscle rigidity, loss of reflexes, slowness of movement, trembling and shaking. It is caused by the degeneration of nerve cells within the brain, which leads to a deficiency of the neurotransmitter dopamine. While there is no cure for Parkinson's disease, dietary therapy can help prevent further degeneration of neurons by neurotoxins. Choose foods that are high in antioxidants and avoid pollutants by choosing fresh, organic foods.

What to Do

Maximize

- Raw antioxidant-rich organic fruits and vegetables to optimize vitamin and mineral intake and provide digestive enzymes (see pages 110 and 122)
- Legumes, nuts and seeds (especially sunflower seeds) to provide vitamin E, which can slow progression of the disease

Minimize

- Animal protein in meat and dairy products, which aggravates symptoms

Eliminate

- Refined and processed foods
- Sugar and artificial sweeteners
- Alcohol
- Wheat and liver, which contain manganese, which may aggravate the disease
- Fatty foods, fried foods, margarine and oils (except extra-virgin olive oil)

Other Recommendations

- Eat fava beans (broad beans), which contain levodopa, a precursor to dopamine. Eating $\frac{1}{2}$ cup (125 mL) a day can decrease the amount of medication required. Discuss this with your doctor to avoid overdosing.
- Passionflower can help reduce tremors.
- Ginkgo improves blood circulation to the brain, bringing it more nutrients, which helps prevent cell damage.
- Avoid antacids, cookware, deodorants and water that contain aluminum, which may have adverse effects on Parkinson's sufferers.
- Ground flax seeds help cure and prevent constipation and provide essential fatty acids to nourish brain and nerve tissue.
- Oily fish (salmon, sardines, mackerel, tuna) provides essential fatty acids that nourish brain and nerve tissue.

Healing Drinks

(see also Nerve Nourishers, page 248)

Add 1 tsp (5 mL) herbs and up to 2 tbsp (25 mL) other ingredients recommended (see page 82) for this condition to the following:

Juices
- Beet, page 180
- C-Green, page 184
- Eye Opener, page 169

Smoothies
- Pump It Up (use flax seeds instead of protein powder), page 246
- Smart Smoothie, page 306
- Spa Special, page 307

Teas
- Antioxi-T, page 229
- Circulation Tea, page 249
- Ginger Tea, page 279

Peptic Ulcers
Gastric & Duodenal Ulcers

Stomach and intestinal ulcers, called peptic ulcers, occur when the protective mucous lining of the stomach or intestine breaks down. Ulcers can be caused by infection from *Heliobacter pylori* bacteria; a breakdown of the protective mucous lining of the intestine caused by steroid medications, such as Aspirin, or nonsteroidal anti-inflammatory medications, which increase acid secretions that break down the lining; stress; and food allergies. Healing involves minimizing the consumption of acids that erode the stomach and intestinal lining, protecting and soothing the intestinal lining, stimulating the immune system and inhibiting the growth of harmful bacteria. Anti-inflammatory, antibacterial, calming and mucous-protective herbs are also helpful in healing ulcers.

Healing Foods

Fruits and vegetables
apples, apricots, bananas, blueberries, cantaloupe, cherries, red grapes (with seeds), mangoes, papayas, pears, avocados, cabbage, carrots, cucumbers, broccoli, leafy greens, onions, watercress

Herbs
calendula, cinnamon, cloves, dandelion root, echinacea, garlic, German chamomile, ginger, green tea, licorice*, marshmallow root, meadowsweet, parsley**, slippery elm bark powder, turmeric

* Avoid licorice if you have high blood pressure. The prolonged use of licorice is not recommended under any circumstances.

** If you are pregnant, limit your intake of parsley to ½ tsp (2 mL) dried or one sprig fresh per day. Do not take parsley if you are suffering from kidney inflammation.

What to Do

Maximize
- Fruits and vegetables, which provide healing vitamins and protection from infection. Fully ripe, sweet fruits are more soothing than sour fruits
- Slippery elm bark powder (especially at bedtime) to form a coating in the intestinal tract that protects against acid
- Fluid intake (drink at least eight large glasses of water, juice and/or herbal tea daily, between meals only, to ensure that your digestive juices are not diluted)

Minimize
- Salt

Other
barley, cereal grasses,
extra-virgin olive oil, honey,
legumes, seeds, oats

Eliminate

- Caffeine (found in black and green tea, coffee, chocolate, soft drinks and decaffeinated coffee), which stimulates secretion of stomach acid
- Dairy products, which lead to increased stomach acidity
- Alcohol, soft drinks and refined grains, which promote ulceration
- Refined flour and sugar
- Ulcer-causing drugs (steroids, such as Aspirin, and nonsteroidal anti-inflammatories)
- Cigarette smoking
- Very hot liquids, which irritate ulcers
- Fried foods and oils (except extra-virgin olive oil)

Other Recommendations

- Eat smaller, more-frequent meals and avoid eating late at night.
- Try stress-reducing techniques, such as meditation, yoga and tai chi.
- Drink raw cabbage juice (1 cup/250 mL taken four times a day on an empty stomach immediately after juicing is effective in healing ulcers).
- Practice food-combining techniques (see Food Combining, page 15).

Healing Drinks

Add 1 tsp (5 mL) herbs and up to 2 tbsp (25 mL) other ingredients recommended (see page 83 and left) for this condition to the following:

Juices

- Berry Best, page 163
- Cabbage Cocktail, page 311
- Pear Fennel, page 173

Smoothies

- Blue Cherry, page 300
- Calming Chamomile Smoothie, page 301
- Mango Madness (use apple juice instead of orange juice), page 304
- Pump It Up, page 246

Teas

- Chamomile-Licorice-Ginger Tea, page 261
- Digestive Stress Soother, page 262
- Immune Regulator Tea, page 234

Coffee Substitutes

- Root Coffee Blend, page 338

Pregnancy

Nutrition is vital to a baby's health, from preconception to birth. Ideally, a mother should get enough nutrients from food rather than supplements. Whole foods provide high-quality, easily digestible nutrients in forms and proportions that your body can use more easily than supplements. Make natural, unprocessed whole grains, beans, fruits, vegetables, nuts and seeds the basis of your diet. Add sufficient protein in the form of lean meat, fish or soy products.

Healing Foods

Fruits and vegetables
bananas, cantaloupe, citrus fruits, strawberries, avocados, carrots, leafy greens, peas, sweet potatoes, watercress

Herbs
alfalfa, dandelion root and leaf, lemon balm, oat straw, red raspberry leaf, rose hips, stinging nettle

Other
dulse, flax seeds, kelp, legumes, blackstrap molasses, nuts (especially almonds), extra-virgin olive oil, soy products, seeds (especially sunflower), wheat germ, whole grains, yogurt with active bacterial cultures

Note: See Appendix C: Herbs to Avoid in Pregnancy, page 361.

What to Do

Maximize
- Fruits and vegetables
- Nuts and seeds
- Folic acid (found in egg yolks, wheat germ, leafy greens, soybeans, asparagus, oranges), which is necessary for normal fetal development
- Foods that are rich in omega-3 fatty acids (found in flax seeds; walnuts; and oily fish, such as salmon, tuna, mackerel and sardines), which are needed to maintain a mother's hormone balance and for proper fetal development

Minimize
- *Foods that increase calcium loss (common in pregnancy), such as:*
- sugar and sweeteners;
- tea, coffee and soft drinks;
- fats;
- refined flour; and
- bran, tomatoes, potatoes, eggplant and all peppers.

Eliminate
- Alcohol
- Artificial food additives
- Non-organic foods, which can contain pesticide residues
- Junk foods

Healing Drinks

Add 1 tsp (5 mL) herbs and up to 2 tbsp (25 mL) other ingredients recommended (see left) for this condition to the following:

Juices
- Beta Blast, page 164
- Citrus Cocktail, page 313
- Folic Plus, page 187

- Kelp, page 190
- Leafy Greens, page 191
- Peas and Carrots, page 192

Smoothies
- Avocado Pineapple, page 299

Teas
- Mother's Own, page 284

Prostate Enlargement, Benign

Prostate enlargement occurs in 50% of men aged 50, 60% of men aged 60 and so on to 100% of men aged 100. The enlarged prostate blocks the urinary tract, obstructing the flow of urine.

What to Do

Maximize
- Antioxidant-rich fruits and vegetables (see pages 110 and 122)
- Tomatoes, which reduce the risk of prostate cancer
- Soy products, which protect the prostate from disease
- Foods that are rich in zinc (shellfish, brown rice, legumes, leafy greens, dried fruits, onions, sunflower seeds, pumpkin seeds, egg yolks) to reduce prostate size
- Foods that contain vitamin C (citrus fruits, berries, leafy greens, parsley, all peppers) to aid zinc absorption
- Foods that are rich in vitamin B6 (bananas, cabbage, egg yolks, leafy greens, legumes, prunes, raisins, soybeans, sunflower seeds) to improve the effectiveness of zinc

Minimize
- Animal fat in meat and dairy products

Eliminate
- Caffeine (found in coffee, black and green tea, chocolate and soft drinks), which limits calcium absorption
- Alcohol, which flushes zinc out of the system
- Foods that contain artificial additives, pesticides or hormones
- Margarine and cooking oils (except extra-virgin olive oil)
- Fried foods
- Sugar and sugar products

Other Recommendations
- Eat oily fish (salmon, mackerel, sardines, tuna) two or three times a week.
- Ensure that you get sufficient dietary protein to help absorb zinc.

Healing Drinks

Add 1 tsp (5 mL) herbs and up to 2 tbsp (25 mL) other ingredients recommended (see left) for this condition to the following:

Juices
- ABC Juice, page 179
- Allium Antioxidant, page 227
- Beet, page 180
- Berry Fine Cocktail, page 310

- C-Blend, page 166
- C-Blitz, page 166
- C-Green, page 184
- Cruciferous, page 185
- Kelp, page 190
- Leafy Greens, page 191
- Raspberry Juice, page 174
- Spring Celebration, page 195

Juices
- Strawberry-Orange Lemonade, page 176
- Tomato Juice Cocktail, page 315

Smoothies
- B-Vitamin, page 300

Teas
- Free Flow Tea, page 279
- Ginger Tea, page 279
- Saw Palmetto, page 285

Sinusitis

Sinusitis is an inflammation of the sinuses, which is caused by colds, influenza, allergies or dental infections. The most effective prevention and treatment strategies are to avoid mucus-producing foods and to identify, then avoid, food allergies (see Appendix A: Food Allergies, page 359).

Healing Foods

Fruits and vegetables
apricots, cantaloupe, citrus fruits, mangoes, pumpkin, strawberries, watermelon, asparagus, broccoli, cabbage, carrots, green beans, leafy greens, papayas, red and green bell peppers

Herbs
cayenne, dandelion leaf and root, elderflowers, ginger, echinacea, garlic, parsley*

Other
legumes, lentils, pumpkin seeds, sea herbs, sunflower seeds, wheat germ

* If you are pregnant, limit your intake of parsley to ½ tsp (2 mL) dried or one sprig fresh per day. Do not take parsley if you are suffering from kidney inflammation.

What to Do

Maximize
- Foods that are rich in vitamin C (citrus fruits, strawberries, parsley*)
- Foods that are rich in vitamin E (wheat germ, nuts, seeds, cabbage, soy lecithin, spinach, asparagus)
- Foods that are rich in beta carotene (carrots, mangoes, cantaloupes, apricots, watermelon, red bell peppers, pumpkin, leafy greens, parsley*, papayas)
- Foods that are rich in zinc (pumpkin seeds, fish, sea herbs)
- Liquid intake (drink at least eight large glasses of water a day)
- Raw garlic to reduce and prevent sinus congestion (take daily)

Minimize
- Starchy foods

Eliminate
- Alcohol
- Bananas
- Dairy products (except yogurt with active bacterial cultures)
- Eggs
- Food allergies and intolerances (see Appendix A: Food Allergies, page 359)
- Refined sugar and flour

Healing Drinks

Add 1 tsp (5 mL) herbs and up to 2 tbsp (25 mL) other ingredients recommended (see left) for this condition to the following:

Juices
- Allium Antioxidant, page 227
- Beta Blast, page 164
- Beta-Carro, page 164
- Brocco-Carrot, page 181
- C-Blitz, page 166

Coffee Substitutes
- Seed Power Coffee, page 339

Skin Conditions
Acne, Dry Skin, Psoriasis & Rosacea

Healing Foods

Fruits and vegetables
apples, apricots, berries, cantaloupe, grapes, mangoes, papayas, pears, carrots, cucumbers, leafy greens, beets and beet greens, pumpkin, squash, watercress

Herbs
burdock root, leaf and seeds; calendula; dandelion root and leaf; echinacea; evening primrose oil; fennel seeds; licorice*; red clover flower; stinging nettle; yellow dock

Other
extra-virgin olive oil, soy products, pumpkin seeds, sesame seeds, sunflower seeds, flax seeds, lentils, oats, sea herbs, spirulina, whole grains, yogurt with active bacterial cultures

* Avoid licorice if you have high blood pressure. The prolonged use of licorice is not recommended under any circumstances.

Acne: This condition, characterized by raised red pimples, usually responds to the dietary changes and cleansing herbs listed on the left. When acne is related to the menstrual cycle, include the hormone-balancing herb chasteberry (*Vitex agnus-castus*).

Dry Skin: Adding essential fatty acids to your diet helps nourish dry skin. Food sources include extra-virgin olive oil, freshly ground flax seeds, fresh walnuts and hazelnuts, and oily fish (mackerel, sardines, salmon, tuna).

Psoriasis: This condition is caused by an increase in the production of skin cells, causing red, scaly plaques. It usually affects the elbows and knees. The cause is unknown, but it is often related to stress and emotional state; herbs such as German chamomile, skullcap and lemon balm can help calm and relax you. Exposing the plaques to sunlight and bathing in the sea are also helpful. Relaxation techniques, such as meditation, yoga and tai chi, can help bring balance to your life. Avoid nuts, citrus fruits and tomatoes, all of which can aggravate psoriasis.

Rosacea: Acne rosacea is a chronic inflammatory skin disease in which too much oil is produced by the glands in the skin. It is often associated with digestive disorders, and the dietary suggestions and cleansing herbs (left) are usually effective in clearing rosacea up.

What to Do

Maximize
- Fresh fruits and vegetables
- Foods that are rich in beta carotene (carrots, broccoli, leafy greens, apricots, papayas)
- Blood-cleansing herbs (dandelion root, burdock root, yellow dock)
- Herbal nerve relaxants (German chamomile, skullcap, lemon balm, oat seeds)
- Seeds (flax, pumpkin, sunflower)

Minimize
- Salt and salty foods
- Animal protein (replace with vegetable protein)

Eliminate
- Red meat and shellfish
- Sugar
- Fried foods
- Oranges
- Chocolate
- Refined flour
- Coffee and black tea
- Dairy products
- Soft drinks
- Artificial food additives, including sweeteners
- Alcohol

Other Recommendations
- Drink at least eight glasses of water, juice and/or herbal tea daily to flush out toxins.
- Eat oily fish (salmon, sardines, mackerel, tuna) two or three times a week.

Healing Drinks

Add 1 tsp (5 mL) herbs and up to 2 tbsp (25 mL) other ingredients recommended (see page 88) for this condition to the following:

Juices
- Beet, page 180
- Beta Blast, page 164
- Breakfast Cocktail, page 311
- Carrot Apple, page 183
- Crimson Cleanser Juice, page 275
- Leafy Greens, page 191
- Pear Fennel, page 173
- Popeye's Power, page 246

Teas
- Cleansing Tea, page 274

Smoking — Quitting

In addition to being a major cause of heart and lung disease and cancer, smoking encourages the loss of calcium (leading to osteoporosis) and is a risk factor for high blood pressure and ulcers. Smoking constricts the blood vessels, decreasing circulation to peripheral parts of the body, and increases the risk of stroke for both men and women, as well as impotence in men. It also causes wrinkles.

Healing Foods

Fruits and vegetables
cantaloupe, citrus fruits, broccoli, carrots, leafy greens

Herbs
German chamomile, red clover (flowering tops), skullcap

Other
oats, oat bran, pumpkin seeds, sunflower seeds, tofu

Reduce Cravings

- Maintain constant blood sugar by eating six meals a day that consist mainly of fresh fruits and vegetables, with a little protein and whole grains.
- Ease withdrawal symptoms with a mainly vegetarian diet, which slows down the removal of nicotine from the body.
- Exercise regularly. Walking and breathing exercises are excellent.
- Snack on sunflower and pumpkin seeds — the zinc content may reduce cravings by blocking taste enzymes.
- Eat plenty of oats. Studies show that oats diminish cravings.
- Drink calming herbal teas to soothe your nerves.

Healing Drinks

(see also Nerve Nourishers, page 248)

Add 1 tsp (5 mL) herbs and up to 2 tbsp (25 mL) other ingredients recommended (see left) for this condition to the following:

Juices
- Beta Blast, page 164
- Brocco-Carrot, page 181
- C-Blend, page 166
- Grapefruit, page 169
- Leafy Greens, page 191
- Orange Zinger, page 173

Smoothies
- Beta Boost, page 299
- Calming Chamomile Smoothie, page 301
- Green Energy, page 303

Healing Drinks

Specialty Drinks
- Melon Cocktail, page 313

Teas
- Calming Cuppa Tea, page 261
- Lavender Tea, page 282
- Nerve Nourisher, page 250

Urinary Tract Infections

Urinary tract infections can be caused by yeast or bacteria. The infection can then pass into the bladder. Cystitis, an inflammation of the bladder, is caused when yeast or bacteria settle into the irritated tissue of the bladder. It is characterized by frequent, painful urination.

Healing Foods

Fruits and vegetables
blueberries, cranberries, lemons, watermelon, carrots, celery, fennel, onions, parsnips, turnips

Herbs
buchu, cinnamon, coriander, cumin, dandelion leaf, echinacea, fennel seeds, garlic, marshmallow root, slippery elm bark powder, stinging nettle, yarrow*

Other
pumpkin seeds, yogurt with active bacterial cultures, barley

* Do not take yarrow if you are pregnant.

What to Do

Maximize
- Liquid intake (drink 8 to 10 cups/2 to 2.5 L water, vegetable juice and/or herbal tea daily) to dilute and wash out bacteria
- Unsweetened cranberry and blueberry juices to prevent bacteria from adhering to the bladder wall
- Onions and garlic, which are antibacterial. Raw garlic is best. Add it to main dishes, sauces, dips and smoothies; add freshly crushed to salads and vegetables; or chop into pieces small enough to swallow
- Antibacterial herbs (buchu, yarrow) to soothe the bladder and herbs that promote urination (marshmallow root, buchu, dandelion leaf)

Minimize
- Meat (replace with vegetable protein, such as that found in tofu, or legumes and rice)
- Alcohol, sugar and artificial food additives, which irritate an inflamed bladder
- Refined sugar and flour
- Dairy products

Eliminate
- Caffeine (found in coffee, black and green tea, chocolate and soft drinks)

Healing Drinks

Add 1 tsp (5 mL) herbs and up to 2 tbsp (25 mL) other ingredients recommended (see left) for this condition to the following:

Juices
- Blue Water, page 165
- Celery, page 184
- Cranberry Juice, page 168
- Gooseberry Berry, page 169
- Nip of Goodness, page 192

Smoothies
- Cran-Orange, page 302
- Watermelon Smoothie, page 308

Teas
- Free Flow Tea, page 279

Tonics
- Barley Water, page 268

Uterine Fibroids

Uterine fibroids are benign growths that are stimulated by estrogen. They can cause pain, heavy menstrual bleeding, anemia and bladder problems. With the drop in estrogen that occurs at menopause, fibroids usually shrink. Plenty of exercise to improve pelvic circulation is helpful.

Healing Foods

Fruits and vegetables
apples, beets, carrots, celery, leafy greens, watercress

Herbs
burdock root, chasteberry, cinnamon, dandelion leaf and root, garlic, ginger, red clover, red raspberry leaf, stinging nettle, yarrow*, yellow dock

Other
kelp, tofu, whole grains

* Do not take yarrow if you are pregnant.

What to Do

Maximize
- Sea herbs to reduce fibroid growth
- Fiber from fresh fruits and vegetables and whole grains to improve the elimination of toxins
- Hormone-balancing herbs (chasteberry), liver-supporting herbs (dandelion root, burdock root, milk thistle seed) and vegetables (beets, carrots)
- Organic foods

Eliminate
- Caffeine (found in coffee, black and green tea, chocolate and soft drinks), which increases estrogen levels
- Fried foods, margarine and oils (except extra-virgin olive oil)
- Alcohol
- Artificial food additives, preservatives and colorings, which contribute to the accumulation of toxins and hormone imbalance

Other Recommendations
- Correct anemia if present (see Anemia, page 30).
- Correct constipation if present (see Constipation, page 41).

Healing Drinks

Add 1 tsp (5 mL) herbs and up to 2 tbsp (25 mL) other ingredients recommended (see left) for this condition to the following:

Juices
- Beet (add ½-inch/1 cm piece ginger), page 180
- Carrot Apple, page 183
- Kelp, page 190
- Leafy Greens, page 191

Teas
- Circulation Tea, page 249
- Cleansing Tea, page 274
- Hormone Balancing Tea, page 222
- Relax Tea, page 265

Coffee Substitutes
- Easy Root Coffee, page 335

Varicose Veins & Hemorrhoids

Healing Foods

Fruits and vegetables
berries (blueberries, strawberries, raspberries, blackberries), cherries, citrus fruits, pears, red grapes, broccoli, cabbage, leafy greens, onions, watercress

Herbs
alfalfa, burdock seed and root, cayenne, dandelion leaf and root, garlic, ginger, horse chestnut, parsley*, witch hazel, yarrow**

Other
buckwheat, dulse, kelp, legumes, nuts, oats, extra-virgin olive oil, soy products, seeds (flax, sunflower, pumpkin, sesame), wheat germ, whole grains

* If you are pregnant, limit your intake of parsley to ½ tsp (2 mL) dried or one sprig fresh per day. Do not take parsley if you are suffering from kidney inflammation.

** Do not take yarrow if you are pregnant.

Varicose veins develop in the legs when there is a restriction in blood flow to the heart, causing blood to pool and stretch the veins. Age and genetic predisposition are factors. Possible causes include heart-valve damage, which alters the flow of blood; high blood pressure, which causes blockage; blood-flow restriction (from tight clothing); excess weight; and lack of exercise. The risk increases during pregnancy and with age. Keep veins in good shape with a diet full of natural foods.

Hemorrhoids are varicose veins around the anus. They may be caused by constipation, pregnancy, obesity, lack of exercise or standing for long periods of time, all of which put extra pressure on the perineal area.

What to Do

Maximize
- Foods that are high in vitamin E (whole grains, wheat germ, legumes, nuts, seeds, leafy greens, sea herbs, soy products) to improve circulation
- Foods that are high in vitamin C (citrus fruits, red and green bell peppers, berries, leafy greens) to strengthen blood vessels

Other Recommendations
- Remedy constipation (see Constipation, page 41), which worsens hemorrhoids.
- Eat oily fish (salmon, sardines, mackerel, tuna) two or three times a week to provide essential fatty acids, which maintain elasticity of veins and help circulation.
- Exercise daily, according to your fitness level.
- Avoid hot baths, which relax the veins, or tone the veins immediately afterward by rinsing your legs with cold water and wiping gently with witch hazel.
- Do not massage varicose veins.
- Avoid standing for long periods of time.
- Raise feet whenever possible.

92 Health Conditions

Add 1 tsp (5 mL) herbs and up to 2 tbsp (25 mL) other ingredients recommended (see page 92) for this condition to the following:

Juices

- Berry Best, page 163
- Berry Fine Cocktail, page 310
- C-Blend, page 166
- C-Blitz, page 166
- C-Green, page 184
- Cherry Juice, page 166
- Gingered Broccoli, page 187
- Green Goddess, page 188
- Leafy Greens, page 191
- Orange Zinger, page 173
- Raspberry Juice, page 174

- Strawberry-Orange Lemonade, page 176
- Sunrise Supreme, page 177

Smoothies

- Blue Cherry (use 3 tbsp/ 45 mL buckwheat instead of banana), page 300
- Sea-Straw Smoothie, page 306
- Spa Special (use any recommended herb in place of milk thistle), page 307

Teas

- Circulation Tea, page 249
- Cleansing Tea, page 274
- Varicosi Tea, page 287

Water Retention
Edema

Healing Foods

Fruits and vegetables
blueberries, cantaloupe, grapes, strawberries, watermelon, asparagus, beets, broccoli, cabbage, carrots, celery, corn, cucumbers, leafy greens, squash, watercress

Water retention can be a symptom of a serious condition, such as high blood pressure, heart disease, kidney disease or liver disease. Or it may simply be the result of medications, poor circulation, allergies, anemia or protein deficiency. Consult with your health-care practitioner to determine the cause.

Cases of water retention in the late stages of pregnancy must always be referred to a doctor. Strong diuretics and water-loss diets can reduce water retention in the short term but may result in kidney damage over the long term. Water retention can result from too much (or too little) dietary protein, insufficient water intake or as a side effect of premenstrual syndrome (PMS) or menopause. Consult with your health-care practitioner in all cases of water retention.

Healing Foods

Herbs
burdock leaf, root and seeds; dandelion leaf and root; garlic; parsley*; stinging nettle

Other
adzuki beans and other legumes, fish oils, whole grains

* If you are pregnant, limit your intake of parsley to ½ tsp (2 mL) dried or one sprig fresh per day. Do not take parsley if you are suffering from kidney inflammation.

What to Do

Maximize
- Water intake (drink at least eight large glasses daily)
- Raw fruits and vegetables

Minimize
- Table salt, sea salt, soy sauce and salted snacks, which can cause water retention
- Tea and coffee, which are strong diuretics that can cause kidney strain if used excessively

Eliminate
- Food allergies and intolerances (see Appendix A: Food Allergies, page 359). Dairy products and wheat can cause water retention

- Sugar
- Refined flour

Other Recommendations
- Exercise daily, according to your fitness level, to improve circulation and reduce water retention.
- Use stronger diuretics (parsley*, celery) only occasionally.
- Include tonic diuretics (dandelion root, stinging nettle, asparagus, corn, grapes, cantaloupe, cucumbers, watermelon) regularly in your diet. The herbs can be made into teas, which can be used as liquid bases of smoothies.

Healing Drinks

Add 1 tsp (5 mL) herbs and up to 2 tbsp (25 mL) other ingredients recommended (see left) for this condition to the following:

Juices
- ABC Juice, page 179
- Berry Best, page 163
- Blue Water, page 165
- Brocco-Carrot, page 181
- Cabbage Cocktail, page 311

- C-Green, page 184
- Green Goddess, page 188
- Leafy Greens, page 191
- Liquid Lunch, page 191
- Popeye's Power, page 246

Teas
- Cleansing Tea, page 274
- Nettle Tea, page 284

Coffee Substitutes
- Easy Root Coffee, page 335
- Root Coffee Blend, page 338

Healthy Foods

Healthy Foods for Juicing

Buy Fresh

When choosing fruits and vegetables, make sure they are firm and ripe. Herbs should show no signs of wilting, yellowing or rust. Buy only what you plan to use in the next day or two because longer storage will destroy the live enzymes in the plants. Ideally you should shop daily for the fresh fruits, vegetables and herbs you need to make the recipes in this book. If this is impractical, store produce in the refrigerator for no more than 2 days.

As a rule of thumb, 1 lb (500 g) produce yields roughly 1 to 1½ cups (250 to 375 mL) fresh juice.

Buy Organic

The USDA National Organic Program defines sustainable agriculture as, "optimizing the health and productivity of interdependent communities of soil life, plants, animals, and people. Management practices are carefully selected with an intent to restore and then maintain ecological harmony on the farm, its surrounding environment and ultimately the whole planetary ecosystem."

Organic agriculture is a holistic method of farming based on ecological principles with the primary goal of creating a sustainable agricultural system. Organic farmers use the principles of recycling, interdependency and diversity in their farm design and farming practices. Organic agriculture is about much more than growing food without synthetic fertilizers and chemical biocides. Organic agriculture uses practices that benefit the planet as well as our bodies.

Because juicing uses fresh fruits, vegetables and herbs almost exclusively, organic produce is clearly the best choice.

For more information, visit www.organicfood.com.

Wash well

All fruits, vegetables and herbs — even if organic — should be washed, scrubbed or soaked in a sink of cool water to which 2 tbsp (25 mL) of food-grade peroxide or vinegar has been added. This will remove any soil, as well as bacteria that may have developed during transportation and handling. Spinach and leeks should be soaked to remove grit. In most cases, organic produce can be juiced with the skin on. Exceptions are noted below.

If you can't find organically grown produce, you can use the conventional variety, but only if you wash as directed above and remove the peel. However, because pesticide concentrations are particularly high in non-organic apples, Chilean grapes, cucumbers, peaches, strawberries and apricots, you might consider refraining from using them in juices.

Fruits

Fruit supplies the body with natural sugar that it uses for fuel. This sugar comes in the form of fructose. We use some fruits, such as apples, grapes and mangoes, in vegetable juices to make those juices more palatable. The fiber in fresh raw fruit is important in maintaining digestion and for this reason, it is important to eat both fruits and vegetables whole in addition to juicing them.

Caution
Diabetics and people prone to yeast infections and hypoglycemia need to watch how much fruit they use because they cause a rapid rise in blood sugar.

Açai

Euterpe oleraceae

A small, round, dark purple berry from an Amazon palm tree, available in frozen form from whole and natural foods stores. The flavor of the berries is an unusual blend of chocolate and blueberry.

Actions: Antioxidant, anticancer

Uses: Due to an exceptionally high concentration of phenolic pigments and anthocyanins with antioxidant properties, açai is being researched for its role in the prevention of numerous human disease conditions. The berry is high in omega-6 and omega-9 fatty acids, fiber, calcium, copper, iron, magnesium, phosphorus, potassium and zinc.

Buying and Storing: Açai is available in several forms: dried pulp purée; bottled liquid pulp purée; frozen whole or puréed berries; and freeze-dried capsules. Look for whole pulp pure organic açai berries for juicing or pulping.

For Juicing: Açai adds a creamy texture and deep purple color to juices. Thaw and use ½ to 1 cup (125 to 250 mL) in fruit juice blends.

For Pulping: Often used in fruit smoothies, açai helps thicken the mixture and add a fresh fruit flavor. Use ½ cup (125 mL) for every 2 cups (500 mL) of smoothie.

Açai Recipes:
- Açai Berry Combo, page 255
- Berry Yogurt Flip, page 240
- Brazilian Berry Smoothie, page 230

Apples

Malus pumila

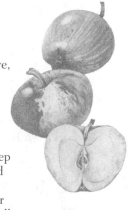

Actions: Tonic, digestive, diuretic, detoxifying, laxative, antiseptic, lower blood cholesterol, antirheumatic, liver stimulant.

Uses: Fresh apples help cleanse the system, lower blood cholesterol levels, keep blood sugar level up and aid digestion. The French use the peels in preparations for rheumatism and gout, as well as in urinary tract remedies. Apples are also very useful components in cleansing fasts because they help eliminate toxins. Apples are good sources of vitamin A. They also contain vitamins B and C and riboflavin and are high in two important phytochemicals: pectin and boron.

Buying and Storing: Look for blemish-free apples with firm, crisp flesh and smooth, tight skin. Because of the widespread use of pesticides on apples, choose organic whenever possible or peel before using. Apples will keep in a cool, dark, dry place (or the crisper drawer of your refrigerator) for one month or more.

For Juicing: Apples are the most versatile fruit for juicing and can be blended with any vegetable juice to give it a natural sweetness. The greener the apple, the sharper its juice. Use the peel (if organic) and core (but not the seeds) when juicing. One pound (500 g), about 4 medium apples, yields about 1 cup (250 mL) juice.

For Pulping: One apple, peeled and cored, yields approximately 1 cup (250 mL) roughly chopped. Homemade or commercially packaged applesauce may also be used in smoothies.

Apple Recipes:
- Apple Beet Pear, page 162
- Apple Fresh, page 162
- Apple Pear, page 162

Apricots

Prunus armeniaca

Actions: Antioxidant, anticancer.

Uses: Apricots are very high in beta carotene, a precursor of vitamin A, which may prevent the formation of cholesterol deposits in the arteries, thus preventing heart disease (three small fresh apricots deliver 2,770 IU of vitamin A; 1/2 cup/125 mL dried apricots contain 8,175 IU). Apricots are also high in vitamin B_2, potassium, boron, iron, magnesium and fiber. Apricots help normalize blood pressure and heart function and maintain normal body fluids. They contain virtually no sodium or fat, so fresh or dried apricots are especially recommended for women because they are good sources of calcium and excellent sources of vitamin A.

Buying and Storing: Choose firm, fresh apricots that range in color from dark yellow to orange. Keep in a cool, dry place for up to one week.

For Juicing: Choose firm, fresh, dark yellow to orange apricots. Leave peel on if organic but do not use the pit. Apricot juice blends well with berry juice. One pound (500 g), about 4 apricots, yields about 1 1/2 cups (375 mL) juice.

For Pulping: Dried apricots provide extra sweetness to smoothies. Look for sulfate-free dried apricots, especially if allergies exist.

Apricot Recipes:

Bananas

Musa cavendishii, syn. *M. chinensis*

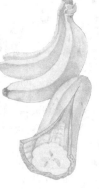

Actions: Antiulcer, antibacterial, boost immunity, lower blood cholesterol levels.

Uses: Due to their ability to strengthen the surface cells of the stomach lining and protect them against acids, bananas are recommended when ulcers or the risk of ulcers is present. High in potassium and vitamin B6, bananas help prevent heart attacks, strokes and other cardiovascular problems.

Buying and Storing: Look for ripe bananas: they are soft, yellow and slightly speckled with brown. Store in a cool, dark, dry place.

For Pulping: Often used in fruit smoothies, bananas thicken the mixture and add a fresh fruit flavor. Use one whole banana for every 2 cups (500 mL) of smoothie.

Banana Recipes:

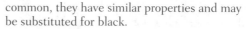
Blackberries

Rubus species

Actions: Antioxidant.

Uses: Blackberries are an excellent source of vitamin C and fiber and have high levels of potassium, iron, calcium and manganese.

Buying and Storing: Choose plump, richly colored berries with firm flesh. They're best used immediately (if necessary, store for one day only in the refrigerator). Wash just before using.

For Juicing: Use immediately upon picking or purchasing. If necessary, store for 1 day only in the refrigerator. Wash just before using. One pint (2 cups/500 mL) yields about ¾ cup (175 mL) juice.

For Pulping: Use fresh, frozen or canned blackberries in smoothies.

Blackberry Recipes:
- Berry Combo (punch), page 321
- Berry Fine, page 209
- Berry Young, page 229
- Black Pineapple, page 164
- Gooseberry Berry, page 169
- Mandarin Orange, page 223
- Purple Power, page 247
- Star Berry, page 176
- Tart and Tingly, page 205

Black Currants

Ribes nigrum

Actions: Antioxidant, antibacterial, antidiarrheal, anticancer, boost immunity, promote healing.

Uses: Black currant flesh is extremely high in vitamin C — 200 mg in 3 oz (90 g). Black-currant skins and the outer layers of flesh closest to the skin contain anthocyanins, which have been proven to prevent the growth of bacteria such as *E. coli*. Black currants (especially the seeds) are high in gamma linolenic acid (GLA), which is important for heart health and a number of bodily functions. For these reasons, whole currants are used in smoothies more often than their juice. Although red currants are not as common, they have similar properties and may be substituted for black.

Buying and Storing: Currants are not widely available but are sometimes found at farmer's markets. While not as fragile as blackberries or raspberries, fresh currants must be stored in the refrigerator, where they will keep for up to one week. Wash just before using.

For Juicing: Use fresh or frozen red or black currants, including the seeds. The flavor is tart, so blend with other, sweeter juices such as apples, apricots and bananas. Add the pulp to salsas, quick breads, spreads, dips, slaws and fruit pestos. One pint (2 cups/500 mL) yields about ½ cup (125 mL) juice.

For Pulping: Use fresh, frozen or dried black or red currants and include the seeds.

Black Currant Recipes:
- Pine-Berry, page 174

Blueberries

Vaccinium species

Actions: Antidiarrheal, antioxidant, antibacterial, antiviral.

Uses: High concentrations of tannins are found in blueberries. They kill bacteria and viruses and help prevent (or relieve) bladder infections. Anthocyanins protect blood vessels against cholesterol buildup. High in pectin, vitamin C, potassium and natural acetylsalicylic acid, blueberries also add extra fiber to smoothies.

Buying and Storing: A silvery "bloom" on blueberries indicates freshness. Choose plump, firm, dark blue berries with smooth skin. Pick over and discard split or soft berries. Blueberries are best used immediately but can be stored in the refrigerator for up to three days. Wash just before using.

For Juicing: Use immediately upon picking or purchasing. If necessary, store for 1 day only in the refrigerator. Wash just before using. Flavor can be tart, especially in wild varieties, treat as black currants. To prevent or treat bladder infections, juice at least ½ cup (125 mL), add to other ingredients and take daily for a minimum of 3 weeks. One pint (2 cups/500 mL) yields about ½ cup (125 mL) juice.

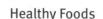

For Pulping: Add ¼ to ½ cup (50 to 125 mL) to smoothies for extra healing benefits.

Blueberry Recipes:

Cantaloupes

See Melons, page 104

Cherries

Prunus species

Actions: Antibacterial, antioxidant, anticancer.

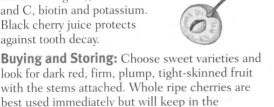

Uses: Cherries are high in ellagic acid (a potent anticancer agent), vitamins A and C, biotin and potassium. Black cherry juice protects against tooth decay.

Buying and Storing: Choose sweet varieties and look for dark red, firm, plump, tight-skinned fruit with the stems attached. Whole ripe cherries are best used immediately but will keep in the refrigerator for up to two days.

For Juicing: Do not use the seeds One pound (500 g), 2 cups (500 mL), yields about ⅔ cup (150 mL) juice.

For Pulping: When fresh cherries are not available, use pitted frozen, dried or canned cherries in smoothies.

Cherry Recipes:

Citrus Fruits

Citrus species
Oranges, lemons, limes, grapefruit, tangerines

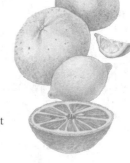

Actions: Antioxidant, anticancer.

Uses: All citrus fruits are high in vitamin C and limonene, which is thought to inhibit breast cancer. Red grapefruit is high in cancer-fighting lycopene. Oranges are a good source of choline, which improves mental function. The combination of carotenoids, flavonoids, terpenes, limonoids and coumarins makes citrus fruits an excellent all-around cancer-fighting package.

Buying and Storing: Purchase plump, juicy fruits that are heavy for their size and yield slightly to pressure. Although citrus fruits will keep for at least a couple of weeks if kept moist in the refrigerator, they are best if used within one week. Organic is preferable — you can be certain the fruits are not injected with gas for transportation.

For Juicing: Remove the peel because it contains bitter elements, but leave as much of the white pith surrounding the sections as possible. The pith contains pectin and bioflavonoids, which help the body to absorb vitamin C and are powerful antioxidants, and they strengthen the body's capillaries, assisting circulation and enhancing the skin. If you have a centrifugal extractor, use the seeds; they contain limonoids (protect against cancer), calcium, magnesium and potassium.

Citrus juice from a centrifugal extractor is more balanced, thicker, with more of the pith, sweeter tasting and less acidic than juice from a cone juicer. One pound (500 g), about 3 oranges, yields about 1¼ cups (300 mL) juice.

Note: If saving citrus pulp for sauces or breads, remove as much of the bitter white pith as possible before juicing.

For Pulping: Make fresh citrus juice with a citrus press or juicing machine, or use citrus fruit whole in smoothies. Canned oranges or grapefruit may be used if fresh are not available.

Citrus Recipes:
- Apple-Orange Punch, page 320
- Carrot Fennel Orange, page 165
- C-Blend, page 166
- C-Blitz, page 166
- Cherry Sunrise, page 167
- Citrus Cocktail, page 313
- Cran-Orange, page 302
- Diabetic Breakfast, page 221
- Endo-Cran, page 221
- Eye Opener, page 169
- Folic Plus, page 187
- Gardener's Lemonade, page 323
- Grapefruit, page 169
- Grape Heart, page 202
- Lemon Aid, page 171
- Lemon Ice, page 350
- Lemon Lime, page 171
- Lemon Sauce, page 295
- Mandarin Orange, page 223
- Orange Cream Cocktail, page 314
- Orange Crush, page 172
- Orange Pom, page 172
- Orange Star, page 172
- Orange Yogurt, page 224
- Orange Zinger, page 173
- Pineapple Citrus, page 174
- Razz-Man-Flax, page 236
- Strawberry Citrus, page 225
- Strawberry-Orange Lemonade, page 176
- Wake Up and Shine, page 205

Cranberries

Vaccinium macrocarpum

Actions: Antibacterial, antiviral, antioxidant, anticancer.

Uses: Cranberries are extremely useful in treating urinary tract and bladder infections. They work like elderberries, preventing the hooks on the bacteria from attaching to the cells of the bladder or urinary tract, rendering them ineffective. Best used as a preventive step against urinary tract and bladder infections, cranberry juice does not take the place of antibiotic drugs, which are more effective in eliminating bacteria once an infection has taken hold. High in vitamins A and C, iodine and calcium, cranberries also prevent kidney stones and deodorize the urine.

Buying and Storing: Choose bright red, plump cranberries that bounce. Keep in the crisper drawer of your refrigerator for two to three weeks.

For Juicing: Fresh cranberry juice is much more effective than the commercial variety, which has a high sugar content. In season during the fall, cranberries freeze very well and can be added frozen to smoothies or juiced without thawing. Wash just before using. Flavor is tart, so blend with sweeter juices such as apples, pineapple, apricots, grapes. To prevent or treat bladder infections, juice at least ½ cup (125 mL), blend with other juices as desired, and take every day for a minimum of 3 weeks. One pound (500 g) yields about ¾ cup (175 mL) juice.

For Pulping: Because their flavor is so tart, you may wish to cook cranberries with sugar, honey or stevia and a small amount of water or juice (see Cranberry Juice, page 168) before combining with other fruit (such as apples or oranges) and blending for smoothies.

Cranberry Recipes:
- Berry Combo (punch), page 321
- Berry Fine Cocktail, page 310
- Blue Water, page 165
- C-Blend, page 166
- Cran-Apple, page 167
- Cran Attack, page 231
- Cranberry, page 168
- Cranberry Juice, page 168
- Cran-Orange, page 302
- Deep Purple Heart, page 201
- Deep Red Heart, page 202
- Endo-Cran, page 221
- Mulled Cranberry, page 318
- Orange Crush, page 172
- Pineapple Cranberry Sizzler, page 318
- Plum Immune, page 236
- The Rio Thing, page 237
- Strawberry Sparkle, page 204
- Tart and Tingly, page 205

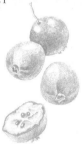

Crenshaw Melons

See Melons, page 104

Dates

Phoenix dactylifera

Actions: Boost estrogen levels, laxative

Uses: Dates are good sources of boron, which prevents calcium loss, so important in the fight against osteoporosis and weakening of bones. Dates contain vitamins A, B_1 (thiamin), B_2 (riboflavin), C and D and valuable mineral salts as well as fiber.

For Juicing: Dates have a low water content and do not juice well although date purée may be added to some vegetable juices to make them more palatable.

For Pulping: Use 3 or 4 dates to sweeten and thicken smoothies.

Date Recipes:
- Date and Nut Shake, page 331
- Date Milk, page 328
- Hot Carob, page 331
- Hot Spiced Apples, page 317
- Sea-Straw Smoothie, page 306

Elderberries

Sambucus nigra

Actions: Diuretic, laxative, diaphoretic.

Uses: Elderberries support detoxification by promoting bowel movements, urination, sweating and mucus secretion. They are effective in combating viruses, such as those that cause colds and flu.

Buying and Storing:
Elderberries are still mainly harvested in the wild (although some are now grown commercially in the United States and Canada). They are usually available at farmer's markets from mid- to late summer. Look for plump deep purple–black berries with tight, shiny skin and firm flesh. Use immediately or, if necessary, store for one day in the refrigerator. Wash just before using.

For Juicing: Use up to ¼ cup (50 mL) fresh elderberries with sweet fruits such as apples, pineapple, cherries and grapes.

For Smoothies: Elderberries add a dark blue color and a sweet-to-slightly-tart taste to smoothies. Use fresh or frozen elderberries, about ½ cup (125 mL) per smoothie recipe or 1 to 2 tbsp (15 to 25 mL) elderberry syrup or jam per smoothie.

Figs

Ficus carica

Actions: Antibacterial, anticancer, antiulcer, digestive, demulcent, laxative.

Uses: Figs contain benzaldehyde, a cancer-fighting agent. They are also high in potassium, B vitamins, calcium and magnesium.

Caution: Dried figs can trigger headaches in some people.

Buying and Storing: Dried figs are readily available in supermarkets throughout the year. In summer and early fall, some supermarkets and most Middle Eastern grocery stores carry fresh figs. When purchasing fresh figs, choose soft, plump, dark brown fruit with thin skins.

For Juicing: Figs have a low water content and do not juice well.

For Pulping: Fresh figs can be found in some supermarkets and most Middle Eastern food markets in summer and early fall. Choose soft, plump figs, remove skin and blend the flesh and seeds.

Use dried or fresh figs or Fig Milk (see page 328) to sweeten and thicken smoothies.

Fig Recipes:
- Figgy Duff, page 302
- Fig Milk, page 328
- Hot Carob, page 331

Gooseberries

Ribes grossularia

Actions: Protect skin and gums, laxative.

Uses: High in vitamin C, potassium and pectin, a natural fiber.

For Juicing: The tartness of gooseberries requires that they be sweetened by combining them with apples, grapes, or date purée.

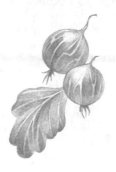

For Pulping: Add ½ cup (125 mL) to smoothies for extra healing benefits.

Gooseberry Recipes:
• Gooseberry Berry, page 169

Grapefruits

See Citrus Fruits, page 100

Grapes

Vitis vinifera

Actions: Antioxidant, antiviral, anticancer.

Uses: Grapes contain large amounts of ellagic and caffeic acids, which deactivate carcinogens, and are a good source of potassium. The flavonoids in grape juice protect the heart, and the resveratrol found in red wine and red grape juice has a protective effect on the cardiovascular system. Grapes also contain boron, which helps maintain estrogen levels (thus preventing calcium loss) and may be instrumental in preventing osteoporosis.

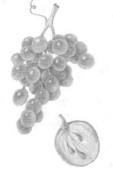

Buying and Storing: Organic grapes are preferable due to the large amounts of pesticides used on non-organic crops. When purchasing grapes, always look for bright color, firm flesh and unwrinkled skin. Wash in food-grade hydrogen peroxide (or other produce cleaner) and store in the crisper drawer of your refrigerator for three or four days.

For Juicing: Common varieties for juicing include Thompson seedless, concord, red and green seedless grapes. Wash thoroughly and juice whole with skin and seeds intact. Two cups (500 mL) yields about ¾ cup (175 mL) juice.

For Pulping: Use fresh, seedless grapes or raisins in smoothies and blended drinks.

Grape Recipes:
• Apple Fresh, page 162
• Apple Pear, page 162
• Apricot Peach, page 163
• Berry Best, page 163
• Berry Fine, page 209
• Blueberry, page 165
• Cherry Juice, page 166
• Cranberry, page 168
• Cucumber Cooler, page 185
• Deep Purple Heart, page 201
• Grape Heart, page 202
• Grape Power, page 170
• Great Grape, page 212
• Mint Julep, page 171
• Pear Pineapple, page 173
• Peppered Fruit, page 214
• Purple Power, page 247
• Razzy Orange (red grapes and raisins), page 236
• Summer Swizzle, page 177
• Sunrise Supreme, page 177

Honeydew Melons

See Melons, page 104

Kiwifruits

Actinidia chinesis

Actions: Antioxidant, anticancer, aid digestion.

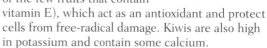

Uses: Kiwis are often used as part of cleansing regimens or to aid digestion. They are high in vitamins C and E (they are one of the few fruits that contain vitamin E), which act as an antioxidant and protect cells from free-radical damage. Kiwis are also high in potassium and contain some calcium.

Buying and Storing: Choose ripe fruits that yield to gentle pressure. Kiwis will ripen in a brown paper bag at room temperature after two or three days. They will keep for at least one week in the crisper drawer of the refrigerator.

For Juicing: Choose ripe fruit that yield to gentle pressure. Peel and feed flesh and seeds through juicer. One pound (500 g), about 4 kiwifruits, yields about ⅓ cup (75 mL) juice.

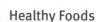

For Pulping: Use fresh, peel and cut in half or quarters before blending.

Kiwi Recipes:
- Before Dinner Mint, page 207
- C-Blitz, page 166
- Kiwi Kick, page 208
- Orange Sunrise, page 203
- Papaya Punch, page 208
- Pineapple-Kiwi Cocktail, page 315
- Seedy Kiwi, page 225
- Tart and Tingly, page 205
- Tropics, page 308

Lemons

See Citrus Fruits, page 100

Limes

See Citrus Fruits, page 100

Mangoes

Mangifera indica

Actions: Antioxidant, anticancer.

Uses: High in vitamin A (there are 8,000 IU of beta carotene in one mango), vitamin C, potassium, niacin and fiber, mangoes help protect against cancer and arteriosclerosis. They also help the body fight infection and maintain bowel regularity.

Buying and Storing: Choose large, firm, unblemished yellow to yellow-red fruit with flesh that gives slightly when gently squeezed. Store in the crisper drawer of your refrigerator for three or four days.

For Juicing: Choose large, firm unblemished fruit, yellow to yellow-red in color. Remove peel and stone before using. Handle carefully since its sap can irritate the skin. Mangoes add a creamy texture to juices.

For Pulping: Add one whole mango to smoothie recipes for added vitamin A.

Mango Recipes:
- Brazilian Berry Smoothie, page 230
- Creamy Pineapple, page 207
- Deep Orange Heart, page 201
- Gold Star, page 243
- Liquid Gold, page 304
- Mango Madness, page 304
- Oaty Orange, page 257
- Tropical Shake, page 332
- Tropi-Cocktail, page 307

Melons

Cucumis melo
Cantaloupe, honeydew, crenshaw, Spanish, musk

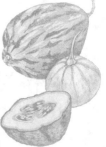

Actions: Antioxidant, anticancer, anticoagulant (cantaloupe and honeydew).

Uses: Adenosine is an anticoagulant chemical found in melons that lessens the risks of heart attack and stroke. Melons are a good source of vitamin A and contain vitamin C and calcium.

Buying and Storing: Ripe melons are heavy for their size and give off a full, sweet perfume. Avoid soft, blemished fruit.

For Juicing: Choose ripe melons. Peel, cut into wedges, and juice with the seeds. Two cups (500 mL) melon chunks yields about ⅔ cup (150 mL) juice.

For Pulping: Use 1 or 2 peeled wedges per smoothie recipe and coarsely chop the flesh before adding to the blender.

Melon Recipes:
- Berry Best, page 163
- Beta Blast, page 164
- Beta Boost, page 299
- Beta Whiz, page 330
- Burdock and Melon, page 230
- Calming Chamomile Smoothie, page 301
- Citrus Cocktail, page 313
- Deep Orange Heart, page 201
- De-Vine Fruits, page 202
- Melon Cocktail, page 313
- Melon Mania, page 203
- Melon Morning Cocktail, page 313
- Melon Nightcap, page 264
- Orange Star, page 172
- Sass in a Glass, page 176
- Stinging Bs, page 253
- Tropi-Cocktail, page 307

Musk Melons

See Melons, page 104

Nectarines

Prunus persica var. *nectarina*

Actions: Antioxidant, anticancer.

Uses: A good source of vitamins A and C and potassium, nectarines are an ancient fruit and not, as many people think, a cross between a peach and a plum.

Buying and Storing: Choose fruit with some bright red areas that are smooth and tight, with no soft patches. Nectarines should be heavy for their size (which means they are full of juice) and firm when pressed. They should not be hard.

For Juicing: Choose fruit that are smooth and tight without soft patches. Cut in half, remove pit, and juice with skin on. Nectarines are sweeter than peaches and can replace them in juicing recipes. One pound (500 g), about 3 nectarines, yields about 1 cup (250 mL) juice.

For Pulping: Cut in quarters, remove pit, and add to the blender with other ingredients.

Nectarine Recipes:
• Melon Nightcap, page 264
• Summer Flower Nectar (punch), page 326
• Summer Nectar, page 177

Oranges

See Citrus Fruits, page 100

Papayas

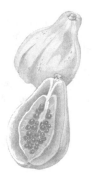

Carica papaya

Actions: Antioxidant, anticancer, aid digestion.

Uses: High in vitamins A and C and potassium.

Buying and Storing: Choose large, firm, unblemished yellow fruit with flesh that gives slightly when gently squeezed. Store in the crisper drawer of your refrigerator for three or four days.

For Juicing: Choose yellow fruit that yields to gentle pressure. Peel, avoiding too much contact with the skin. It is not necessary to remove the seeds before juicing.

For Pulping: Papayas blend well with other fruits in drinks and serve as a sweet addition that gives a creamy texture to smoothies. Use the seeds, since they contain protein.

Papaya Recipes:
• After Dinner Cocktail Smoothie, page 209
• Orange Sunrise, page 203
• Papaya Marinade, page 295
• Papaya Punch, page 208
• Spiced Papaya Tea, page 216
• Taste of the Tropics, page 307
• Tropical Twister, page 208
• Tropi-Cocktail, page 307
• Tropics, page 308

Peaches

Prunus persica

Actions: Antioxidant, anticancer.

Uses: Rich in vitamin A and potassium, peaches contain boron, niacin, some iron and vitamin C. They help protect against cancer, osteoporosis and heart disease, and their sugar content is low (about 9%).

Buying and Storing: Fruit that is full and heavy for its size, with fuzzy down and lightly firm flesh, is preferable. Store in the crisper drawer of your refrigerator for up to four days. Freestone varieties (such as Loring and Redhaven) are easier to pit than clingstone varieties.

For Juicing: Choose firm, full-colored fruit that yields to gentle pressure. Cut in half, remove and discard pit and juice with the skin intact. One pound (500 g), about 4 peaches, yields about ⅔ cup (150 mL) juice.

For Pulping: Canned peaches add extra nutrients to winter smoothies. Drain and add sliced peaches to winter smoothies.

Peach Recipes:
• Apricot Peach, page 163
• Autumn Refresher, page 163

- Beta-Carro, page 164
- Cucumber Fuzz, page 186
- Liquid Gold, page 304
- Summer Flower Nectar (punch), page 326
- Summer Nectar, page 177
- Summer Swizzle, page 177

Pears

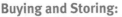

Pyrus communis

Actions: Protect the colon.

Uses: Perhaps one of the oldest cultivated fruits, pears are a good source of vitamin C, boron and potassium. Pears are also a sweet source of fiber.

Buying and Storing: Pears should be lightly firm, unblemished and sweetly pear-scented. They are often available before they are fully ripe, in which case they can be ripened in a brown paper bag at room temperature for one to three days. Ripe pears can be stored in the crisper drawer of your refrigerator for three or four days.

For Juicing: Use varieties such as Bartlett, Comice, Seckel and Bosc. Choose firm unblemished pears and juice the whole fruit. One pound (500 g), about 3 pears, yields about ½ cup (125 mL) juice.

For Pulping: Drain and use sliced canned pears in smoothie recipes.

Pear Recipes:
- Apple Beet Pear, page 162
- Apple Pear, page 162
- Autumn Refresher, page 163
- Breath of Autumn, page 256
- Carrot Head, page 183
- Hot Spiced Pear Nectar, page 317
- Pear Fennel, page 173
- Pear Pineapple, page 173
- Pear-Pom, page 224
- Thorny Pear, page 196

Pineapples

Ananas comosus

Actions: Aid digestion.

Uses: Pineapples are a good source of potassium and contain some vitamin C and iron.

Buying and Storing: Choose large, firm fruits (heaviness indicates juiciness) that are yellow all over. Heaviness in ripe pineapples indicates juiciness. Cut off leaves and outer rind of the fruit.

For Juicing: Cut in half and then in wedges without trimming away the woody core. One pound (500 g), about ⅓ medium pineapple, yields about ½ cup (125 mL) juice.

For Pulping: One fresh wedge of pineapple equals approximately 1 cup (250 mL) chopped. Frozen, canned or dried pineapple may be substituted for fresh in smoothies.

Pineapple Recipes:
- After Dinner Cocktail Smoothie, page 209
- Avocado Pineapple, page 299
- Black Pineapple, page 164
- Cherries Jubilee, page 301
- Cranberry, page 168
- Creamy Pineapple, page 207
- Great Grape, page 212
- Kiwi Kick, page 208
- Melon Morning Cocktail, page 313
- Orange Cream Cocktail, page 314
- Pear Pineapple, page 173
- Pinea-Colada, page 251
- Pineapple Citrus, page 174
- Pineapple Cranberry Sizzler, page 318
- Pineapple-Kiwi Cocktail, page 315
- Pineapple Sage Frappé, page 346
- Pine-Berry, page 174
- Sass in a Glass, page 176
- Taste of the Tropics, page 307
- Tropical Shake, page 332
- Tropical Twister, page 208

Plums

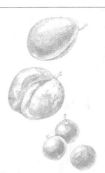

Prunus species

Actions: Antibacterial, antioxidant.

Uses: A good source of vitamin A, plums contain calcium and a small amount of vitamin C.

Buying and Storing: Ripe plums are firm, with no soft spots or splits. Look for brightly colored (yellow, black or red) plums with tight skins that are heavy for their size and smell sweet. Keep in the crisper drawer of your refrigerator for up to four days.

For Juicing: Use yellow, black or red sweet plums. Pit and juice plums with skin intact. One pound (500 g), about 4 large, yields about ¾ cup (175 mL) juice.

For Pulping: Use whole, fresh plums or prunes in smoothies and blended drinks. If using for constipation, use 4 to 6 prunes for every 1 cup (250 mL) smoothie.

Prunes are dried plums and are high in pectin and other insoluble fiber, and low in sugar. They act as a natural laxative, and the pectin in them fights colon cancer. Use plump, pitted stewed prunes in juicing or two or three pitted dried prunes per smoothie recipe.

Plum Recipes:
- Blue Star, page 229
- Deep Purple Heart, page 201
- Green Tea and Blueberries, page 233
- Hot Spiced Apples, page 317
- Plum Immune (black plums and prunes), page 236
- Plum Lico, page 305
- Pomegranate Plus, page 204
- Pom Pom, page 174
- Prune Smoothie (prunes), page 305
- Purple Power, page 247
- Razz-Man-Flax (prunes), page 236
- Razzy Strawberry, page 237
- Red Horizon, page 175
- Summer Nectar, page 177
- 3PO, page 178

Pomegranates

Punica granatum

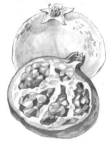

Actions: Antidiarrheal, antifever, astringent

Uses: High levels of antioxidant-rich tannins and flavonoids in the juice and peel make pomegranates beneficial in helping to prevent some forms of cancer. Traditionally used to reduce fevers.

Buying and Storing: Select firm, bright red fruits that are free of bruising and feel heavy. Whole, un-peeled pomegranates keep for up to 2 months in the crisper of the refrigerator. Whole seeds may be frozen and stored for up to 3 months (thaw slightly before juicing).

For Juicing: Peel and remove as much of the white membrane as possible before juicing the seeds. Use the seeds from 1 or 2 whole pomegranates in combination with other fruits.

For Pulping: Use the juice for pulping.

Pomegranate Recipes:
- Fruit of Life, page 232
- Granate Berry, page 212
- Orange Pom, page 172
- Pear-Pom, page 224
- Pomegranate Plus, page 204
- Pom Pom, page 174
- Red Horizon, page 175
- Strawberry Sparkle, page 204
- Wake Up and Shine, page 205

Raspberries

Rubus idaeus

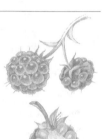

Actions: Enhance immunity.

Uses: Raspberries are rich in potassium and niacin and also contain iron and some vitamin C (see also Red Raspberry, page 144).

Buying and Storing: Buy or pick in peak season and choose whole, plump, brightly colored berries. Sort and discard soft or broken berries. Store in the crisper drawer of your refrigerator for one day. Wash just before using.

For Juicing: Do not store long. Wash just before juicing. Raspberries blend with other berries in juices and the taste is enhanced with a small amount of citrus juice. One pint (2 cups/500 mL) yields about ½ cup (125 mL) juice.

For Pulping: Substitute frozen, dried or canned raspberries for fresh in blended drinks. You can also add up to ¼ cup (50 mL) raspberry jam to smoothies.

Raspberry Recipes:
- Berry Fine Cocktail, page 310
- Berry Young, page 229
- Black Pineapple, page 164
- Blueberry, page 165
- Cran Attack, page 231
- Deep Red Heart, page 202
- Fruit Punch, page 322
- Gooseberry Berry, page 169
- Granate Berry, page 212
- Raspberry Juice, page 174
- Raspberry Relaxer, page 264

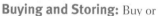

Rhubarb

Rheum species

Actions: Laxative.

Uses: Rhubarb is actually a vegetable that is almost always used as a fruit. It is high in potassium and contains a fair amount of iron. The calcium in 1 cup (250 mL) of cooked rhubarb is twice that of the same amount of milk.

Caution: Never use rhubarb leaves, which are toxic and inedible due to their high concentration of oxalic acid.

Buying and Storing: If you do not have a rhubarb patch in your garden, look for rhubarb in farmer's markets in the spring.

Choose thin, firm stalks that are at least 90% red. Rhubarb should snap when bent. Store in a cool, dry place or the crisper drawer of your refrigerator for no longer than two days.

For Juicing: Use stalks and root, but not the leaves, which contain toxic concentrations of oxalic acid. Rhubarb can be juiced fresh or frozen. To soften its tartness, combine rhubarb with sweeter fruits or juices.

For Pulping: Blend chunks with sweeter fruits, or stew it with maple sugar, honey, stevia or sugar, and then use with other fresh fruit in smoothies.

Rhubarb Recipes:
- Berry Combo (punch), page 321
- Rhubarb, page 175
- Roo-Berry Pie, page 175

Spanish Melons

See Melons, page 104

Star Fruits

Averrhoa carambola

A tropical fruit that grows in the shape of a star.

Actions: Antioxidant

Uses: High in vitamin C, potassium, proanthocyanidins, epicatechins and carotene, star fruit is traditionally used to treat arthritis, coughs, diarrhea, hangovers, hemorrhoids, bladder stones, kidney stones and toothache.

Caution: People who suffer from gout or with kidney or other renal problems and/or diabetes should avoid star fruit due to its oxalic acid.

Buying and Storing: Star fruit is delicate, with 5 pointed ribs and should be handled with care. The skin is thin, smooth and waxy. Ripe fruit is golden in color with little or no green. Keep in the crisper section of the refrigerator for up to 4 days.

For Juicing or Pulping: Star fruit juice is refreshingly thirst quenching with a tart and slightly citrus flavor. Use 1 or 2 whole, even-colored and yellow fruits in combination with other fruits in juices and smoothies.

Star Fruit Recipes:
- Blue Star, page 229
- Gold Star, page 243
- Orange Star, page 172
- Sass in a Glass, page 176
- Star Berry, page 176
- Tropical Shake, page 332

Strawberries

Fragaria species

Actions: Antioxidant, antiviral, anticancer.

Uses: Effective against kidney stones, gout, rheumatism and arthritis, strawberries are also used in cleansing juices and as a mild tonic for the liver. Strawberries are high in cancer-fighting ellagic acid and vitamin C. They are also a good source of vitamin A and potassium, and contain some iron. Both the leaves and the fruit are used medicinally. Strawberry leaf tea can be used to treat diarrhea and dysentery.

Buying and Storing: Pick your own or choose brightly colored firm berries with the hulls attached. They are best used immediately but may be stored for no more than two days in the refrigerator. Wash just before using.

For Juicing: Wash just before juicing. Strawberries add a sweet and powerful flavor to juices. They are best blended with only one or two other fruits, although they blend well with other berries in juices. The taste is enhanced with a small amount of citrus juice. One pint (2 cups/500 mL) yields about $1/2$ cup (125 mL) juice.

For Pulping: Strawberries blend well with banana and other fruit in blended drinks. The traditional smoothie combination includes strawberry, banana and orange juice.

Strawberry Recipes:
- Berry Young, page 229
- Cabbage Patch, page 200
- Citrus Cocktail, page 313
- Cran Attack, page 231
- Deep Red Heart, page 202
- De-Vine Fruits, page 202
- Eye Opener, page 169
- Frozen Strawberry Yogurt, page 355
- Fruit Punch, page 322
- Orange Slushie, page 258
- Razzy Strawberry, page 237
- Rhubarb, page 175
- Roo-Berry Pie, page 175
- Strawberry Citrus, page 225
- Strawberry-Orange Lemonade, page 176
- Strawberry Shake, page 332
- Strawberry Sparkle, page 204
- Sunrise Supreme, page 177
- Wake Up and Shine, page 205
- Watermelon Cooler, page 178
- Watermelon Strawberry, page 178

Tangerines

See Citrus Fruits, page 100

Watermelons

Citrullus vulgaris

Actions: Antibacterial, anticancer.

Uses: Watermelons contain vitamins A and C, iron and potassium. Their high water content makes them good summer refreshments.

Buying and Storing: A watermelon should have a bright green rind and firm flesh (no blemishes or soft spots) and feel heavy for its size. Store in a cool dark place or in the refrigerator for two or three days.

For Juicing: Peel the rind. Use flesh and seeds, which contain protein, zinc, vitamin E and essential fatty acids. Watermelon is a refreshing summer juice on its own or blended with other fruits as a thirst quencher. Two cups (500 mL) chunked watermelon yields about 1 cup (250 mL) juice.

For Pulping: One $1/2$-inch slice watermelon yields approximately 1 cup (250 mL) chopped fruit. Use 1 cup (250 mL) chopped watermelon for every blended drink.

Watermelon Recipes:
- Blue Water, page 165
- Lemon Aid, page 171
- Summer Swizzle, page 177
- Watermelon Cooler, page 178
- Watermelon Smoothie, page 308
- Watermelon Strawberry, page 178

Top Common Antioxidant Fruits

ORAC (Oxygen Radical Absorbance Capacity) is a testing system that measures antioxidant capability of fruits and vegetables. A total of 1,670 ORAC units would be the average equivalent of eating five mixed servings of fruits and vegetables a day; however, juicing or pulping with fruits and vegetables known to be high in antioxidants, or with a high ORAC value, will add much more protection from damaging free radicals.

Fruits	Amount	ORAC Value*
Açai	½ cup (125 mL)	16,140
Pomegranates	2 whole	10,500
Blueberries	1 cup (250 mL), whole cultivated	9,019
Cranberries	1 cup (250 mL) whole	8,983
Blackberries	1 cup (250 mL), cultivated	7,701
Prunes	½ cup (125 mL)	7,291
Raspberries	1 cup (250 mL)	6,058
Strawberries	1 cup (250 mL)	5,938
Red Delicious Apple	1	5,900
Sweet Cherries	1 cup (250 mL)	4,873
Black Plum	1	4,844

*Source: USDA data on foods with high levels of antioxidants.

Vegetables

Asparagus

Asparagus officinalis

Actions: Antioxidant, anticancer, anti-cataracts, diuretic, promotes healing.

Uses: Asparagus is one of only four vegetables that are high in vitamin E. It is also a source of vitamins A and C, as well as potassium, niacin and some iron.

Buying and Storing: Look for tight buds at the tips and smooth green stalks with some white at the very bottoms. Fresh asparagus will snap at the point where the tender stalk meets the tougher end. Store stalks upright in ½ inch (1 cm) of water in the refrigerator for up to two days.

For Juicing: Wash spears (no need to trim them) and feed through tube stalk end first. One pound (500 g) of asparagus yields about ¾ cup (175 mL) juice.

For Pulping: Trim off tough stem bottoms and cook in boiling water for 3 minutes. Drain, cool to room temperature and coarsely chop before adding to smoothies. Frozen or canned asparagus with juices may be substituted when fresh is not available.

Asparagus Recipes:
- ABC Juice, page 179
- Folic Plus, page 187
- Spring Celebration, page 195

Avocados

Persea americana

Actions: Antioxidant.

Uses: Avocados (which are technically fruits) contain more potassium than many other fruits and vegetables (bananas are just slightly higher). High in essential fatty acids, avocados also contain 17 vitamins and minerals, including vitamins A, C and E; all the B vitamins, except B12, and including riboflavin; iron; calcium; copper; phosphorus; zinc; niacin; and magnesium.

They also have the largest amount of protein of any fruit. One avocado blended into a smoothie adds creamy texture and exceptional nutritional value.

Buying and Storing: Look for ripe, heavy avocados that have dull dark green skin with no dents. Ripe avocados give slightly when gently squeezed. Avocados are often sold unripe, but you can ripen them in a paper bag at room temperature and store them in the refrigerator for just over one week once ripe.

For Juicing: Avocados contain little water and do not juice well.

For Pulping: Peel and cut in half. Remove pit and cut flesh into pieces. Blend with other fruits or vegetables. Brush with lemon juice to keep flesh from turning brown.

Avocado Recipes:
- Avocado Gazpacho, page 292
- Avocado Pineapple, page 299
- Avocado Shake, page 329
- Ginger Smoothie, page 256

Beans

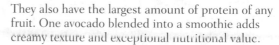

Phaseolus vulgaris
Green, yellow wax, Italian, snap and string beans; also green peas, snow peas

Actions: Improve memory, antioxidant.

Uses: Green beans and peas are the same botanically as dry beans because they are all leguminous plants, meaning that they produce their seeds in pods. However, fresh beans have lower nutrient levels than dried legumes. A good source of choline, which improves mental function, beans also contain vitamin A and potassium, as well as some protein, iron, calcium and vitamins B and C. The amino acids in beans and peas make them a valuable food for vegetarians.

Buying and Storing: Buy fresh peas and beans with firm pods that show no signs of wilting. The bigger the pea or bean inside the pod the older the vegetable. Fresh yellow or green beans should be pliant but still snap when bent. Store unwashed fresh peas (in their pods) and beans in a plastic bag in the refrigerator for two or three days. Parboiled fresh beans and peas freeze well.

For Juicing: Fresh green or yellow beans may be juiced but because of their low water content, peas work best in smoothies.

For Pulping: Raw or blanched green peas thicken blended drinks. Wash, shell and add to other fruits or vegetables in the blender in ¼-cup (50 mL) amounts. Reconstituted beans such as red beans, chickpeas and lentils are an excellent addition to smoothies because they add protein and thicken the drink.

Bean Recipes:
- Green Bean, page 243
- Peas and Carrots, page 192
- Peas Please, page 193
- Soft Salad (sprouts), page 195

Beets

Beta vulgaris

Actions: Antibacterial, antioxidant, tonic, cleansing, laxative.

Uses: Beets (the root of the beet plant) are high in vitamin A and the enzyme betaine, which nourishes and strengthens the liver and gallbladder. Beets are also an excellent source of potassium and are cleansing for the liver, kidneys and gallbladder.

Buying and Storing: Bright, glossy, crisp beet greens indicate fresh beets (see Leafy Greens, page 117, for how to use beet greens in smoothies). Buy firm unblemished small beets with greens intact, if possible. To store, cut off tops and treat as leafy greens. Store unwashed beets in a plastic bag in the refrigerator. Beets will keep for up to 1½ weeks. Wash just before cooking.

For Juicing: Scrub roots and leave skin on. Feed tops through juicer first and follow with roots, tapping them through the tube. One pound (500 g), 2 medium beets with greens, yields about 1 cup (250 mL) juice.

For Pulping: Use cooked fresh, frozen or canned beets with juices.

Beet Recipes:
- Apple Beet Pear, page 162
- Apple-Orange Punch, page 320
- Beet, page 180
- Beet Retreat, page 260
- Blazing Beets, page 180

- Green Beet, page 188
- Heart Beet, page 203
- Hypo-Health, page 223
- Leafy Greens, page 191
- Lights Out, page 263
- Mulled Cranberry (beet juice), page 318
- Popeye's Power, page 246
- Red Devil, page 193
- Root Combo, page 194
- Slippery Beet, page 194
- Spring Celebration, page 195
- Tomato Tang, page 197

Broccoli

Brassica oleracea var. *italica*

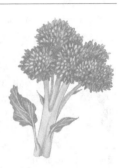

Actions: Antioxidant, anticancer, promotes healing, anti-cataracts.

Uses: Broccoli is one of only four vegetables that are high in vitamin E. It is also high in cancer-fighting indoles and glucosinolates and has fair amounts of vitamins A, B and C.

Buying and Storing: Broccoli yellows as it ages, so deep green color and firm tight buds are signs of freshness. Thin stalks are more tender than thick or hollow ones. Store in a vented plastic bag in the crisper drawer of the refrigerator for up to three days.

For Juicing: Use thick stalks and leaves as well as tops. Wash and cut into spears.

For Pulping: Use cooked fresh, frozen or canned broccoli with juices.

Broccoli Recipes:
- ABC Juice, page 179
- Allium Antioxidant, page 227
- Bone Builder, page 241
- Brocco-Artichoke, page 181
- Brocco-Carrot, page 181
- Cauliflower Cocktail, page 312
- Cream of Broccoli Smoothie, page 242
- Cream of the Crop, page 256
- Cruciferous, page 185
- Cruciferous Chiller, page 221
- Gingered Broccoli, page 187
- Green Gift, page 232
- Green Goddess, page 188
- Hypo-Health, page 223
- Live Young, page 235

- Red Pepper, page 237
- Rust Proofer #1, page 238
- Spiced Carrot, page 195

Brussels Sprouts

See Cabbage, below

Cabbage

Brassica oleracea var. *capitata*
Green, red, Savoy, bok choy and Chinese cabbage; kohlrabi; and Brussels sprouts

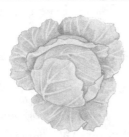

Actions: Antibacterial, anticancer, helps memory, antioxidant, detoxifying, diuretic, anti-inflammatory, tonic, antiseptic, restorative, antiulcer, boosts immunity, anti-cataracts, promotes healing.

Uses: High in cancer-fighting indoles and a good source of choline, which improves mental function, cabbage is one of only four vegetables that are high in vitamin E. An excellent remedy for anemia, cabbage has also been used as a nutritive tonic to restore strength in cases of debility and during convalescence. Beneficial to the liver, cabbage is also effective in preventing colon cancer and may be of help to diabetics by reducing blood sugar levels. Cabbage juice is especially effective in preventing and healing ulcers.

Buying and Storing: Fresh cabbage has loose outer leaves around a firm center head. Stored cabbage does not have the outer wrapper leaves and tends to be paler in color. Cabbage will keep for up to two weeks in a plastic bag in the refrigerator. Wash and cut or slice just before using.

For Juicing: Wash and cut into wedges, leaving dark green outer leaves and core intact. Juice Brussels sprouts whole. One pound (500 g) of cabbage (about ⅓ head) yields about 1 cup (250 mL) juice.

For Pulping: Shred or cut fresh or frozen cabbage into chunks for blending into smoothies.

Cabbage Recipes:
- Artichoke Eight, page 180
- Cabbage Cocktail, page 311
- Cabbage Head, page 209
- Cabbage Patch, page 200
- Cabbage Rose, page 181
- Cabbage Salad, page 293
- Carrot Head, page 183
- Cauli-Slaw, page 184
- Cruciferous, page 185
- Dandelion Slam Dunk, page 210
- Green Bean, page 243
- Green Magic, page 190
- Peppery Cabbage, page 215
- Spiced Cabbage, page 215
- Vidalia Vigor, page 216

Carrots

Daucus carota ssp. *sativus*

Actions: Antioxidant, anticancer, protect arteries, expectorant, antiseptic, diuretic, boost immunity, antibacterial, lower blood cholesterol levels, prevent constipation.

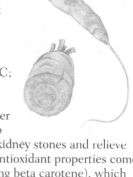
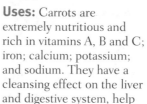

Uses: Carrots are extremely nutritious and rich in vitamins A, B and C; iron; calcium; potassium; and sodium. They have a cleansing effect on the liver and digestive system, help prevent the formation of kidney stones and relieve arthritis and gout. Their antioxidant properties come from carotenoids (including beta carotene), which have been shown to cut cancer risk, protect against arterial and cardiac disease, and lower blood cholesterol. Carrots enhance mental function and decrease the risk of cataracts and macular degeneration.

Buying and Storing: The green tops continue to draw nutrients out of the carrot, so choose fresh carrots that are sold loose without the tops, or remove the tops immediately after purchase. Choose firm well-shaped carrots with no cracks. If stored unwashed in a cold, moist place, carrots should not shrivel. Keep for up to two weeks in a vented plastic bag in the crisper drawer of your refrigerator.

For Juicing: Carrots are the sweetest most versatile vegetable, and can be used in almost any juicing recipe. The deeper the color, the higher the concentration of carotene. Do not use carrot greens for juicing. One pound (500 g), about 6 medium, yields approximately 1 cup (250 mL) or more juice.

For Pulping: Cooking frees up carotenes (precursors to vitamin A), the anti-cancer agents in carrots. Steam or simmer carrots just until tender, then add to the blender with other fruits or vegetables.

Carrot Recipes:
- Artichoke Carrot, page 179
- Beet, page 180
- Beet Retreat, page 260
- Beta Blast, page 164
- Beta-Carro, page 164
- Brocco-Carrot, page 181
- Cabbage Rose, page 181
- Carrot Allium, page 183
- Carrot Apple, page 183
- Carrot Fennel Orange, page 165
- Carrot Head, page 183
- Cauli-Slaw, page 184
- Gallstone Solvent, page 187
- Gout Buster, page 188
- Hot Spiced Carrots, page 263
- Immunity, page 190
- Liquid Lunch, page 191
- Moist & Juicy, page 192
- Orange Crush, page 172
- Orange Zinger, page 173
- Peas and Carrots, page 192
- Root Combo, page 194

Cauliflower

Brassica oleracea var. *botrytis*

Actions: Antioxidant, anticancer.

Uses: Like all cruciferous vegetables (cabbage, Brussels sprouts, broccoli, collard greens, kohlrabi), cauliflower is rich in cancer-fighting indoles. Cauliflower contains vitamin C and potassium, as well as some protein and iron.

Buying and Storing: Fresh cauliflower has dense, tightly packed florets, and the head is surrounded by crisp green leaves. Keep loosely covered in a perforated plastic bag in the refrigerator for no longer than one week.

For Juicing: Wash and cut into pieces, leaving core and leaves intact. One pound (500 g) flowerets yields approximately 1 cup (250 mL) juice.

For Pulping: Cut into pieces and cook before blending. Use some of the core if it is not too woody.

Cauliflower Recipes:
- Carrot Head, page 183
- Cauliflower Cocktail, page 312
- Cauli-Slaw, page 184
- Cream of Broccoli Smoothie, page 242
- Cream of the Crop, page 256
- Cruciferous, page 185
- Cruciferous Chiller, page 221

Celery

Apium graveolens var. *dulce* and *Celeriac Apium graveolens* var. *rapaceum*

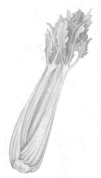

Actions: Mild diuretic, anticancer.

Uses: Sometimes used as a treatment for high blood pressure (two to four stalks per day), celery also helps detoxify carcinogens (see also Celery Seeds, page 128, for their healing properties).

Buying and Storing: Fresh celery has crisp green leaves and firm, crisp ribs. (The leaves are removed from older stalks.) Store for up to two weeks in a vented plastic bag in the refrigerator.

For Juicing: Use stalks and leaves. One stalk yields about ¼ cup (50 mL) juice. Cut celeriac to fit the diameter of the feed tube.

For Pulping: Use celery stalks and leaves in vegetable cocktails to add natural saltiness. Cut into chunks before adding to the blender. Celeriac, the root of a different variety of celery than common table celery, adds a stronger celery flavor to smoothies. Peel off the tough outer skin, then slice and chop before adding to the blender.

Celery Recipes:
- Artichoke Eight, page 180
- Blazing Beets, page 180
- Carrot Apple, page 183
- Cauli-Slaw, page 184
- Celery, page 184
- The Chiller, page 185
- Cucumber Fuzz, page 186
- The Curl, page 243
- Gallstone Solvent, page 187

Celeriac

See Celery, page 114

Chile Peppers

Capsicum annuum

See also Cayenne, page 127; Chiles: The Culinary Firebrands, page 182

Actions: Stimulant, tonic, diaphoretic, rubefacient, carminative, antiseptic, antibacterial, expectorant, anti-bronchitis, anti-emphysema, decongestant, blood thinner.

Uses: Chiles are hot peppers that contain the active element capsaicin. They are high in vitamin A and contain some vitamin C, calcium, iron, magnesium, phosphorus and potassium. Chile peppers help people with bronchitis and related problems by irritating the bronchial tubes and sinuses, causing the secretion of fluid that thins the constricting mucus and helps move it out of the body. Capsaicin also blocks pain messages from the brain, making it an effective pain reliever. In addition, it also helps prevent heart attacks (if taken on a consistent basis), as it has clot-dissolving properties. Cayenne (see page 127) is a variety of chile. It appears in the Herb Profiles section because it is used medicinally, as well as in cooking.

Buying and Storing: Look for firm, crisp chile peppers with smooth skin and no blemishes. Store in a paper bag in the crisper drawer of your refrigerator for up to four days. Peppers freeze well and may be added frozen to smoothies. When purchasing dried chile peppers, make sure they are clean and fully dried. Store them in a cool, dry place.

For Juicing: Wash peppers and remove stems. Wash hands thoroughly after handling, since capsaicin will irritate skin and is very painful if it contacts the eyes, lips or nasal passages. When first using chile peppers for juicing, juice after all other ingredients have been put through the machine and keep the juice separate. Add it to vegetable juice blends 1 tsp (5 mL) at a time until you reach the level of heat with which you are comfortable. Alternatively, whisk in a drop of hot or jerk sauce (or ¼ tsp/1 mL powdered cayenne) to juices and blended drinks.

For Pulping: Use fresh, reconstituted or dried or canned chiles in smoothies. Adding yogurt to chile drinks helps extinguish the fire.

Chile Pepper Recipes:
- Blazing Beets, page 180
- Blazing Bullshot, page 316
- Flaming Antibiotic, page 186
- Hot Spiced Pear Nectar, page 317
- Liquid Salsa, page 191

Collard Greens

See Leafy Greens, page 117

Cucumbers

Cucumis sativus

Actions: Diuretic.

Uses: Moderate sources of vitamin A, iron and potassium, cucumbers are high in water, making them good vegetables for smoothies. Cucumbers contain sterols, which may help the heart by reducing cholesterol.

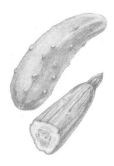

Buying and Storing: Choose shiny, bright green, firm cucumbers. Avoid those with yellow spots (although this is a sign of ripeness, the seeds will be bitter and the flesh too soft) and wax on the skin (which is not good to eat and usually a sign of age). Store in the crisper drawer of the refrigerator for four or five days.

For Juicing: Peel if skin has been waxed. Use whole or cut in half lengthwise and leave seeds intact. One pound (500 g), about 1 large, yields approximately 1¼ cups (300 mL) juice.

For Pulping: Cut into cubes but leave the seeds intact for blending into smoothies.

Cucumber Recipes:
- Beet Retreat, page 260
- The Chiller, page 185
- Cucumber Cooler, page 185
- Cucumber Fuzz, page 186
- Flaming Antibiotic, page 186
- Green Goddess, page 188
- Lemon Aid, page 171
- Liquid Lunch, page 191
- Peppers Please, page 193
- Thorny Pear, page 196

Fennel

Foeniculum vulgare

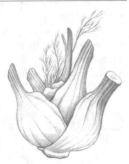

Actions: Antioxidant, seeds are digestive.

Uses: A bulb-like vegetable similar to celery but with a distinctly sweet anise taste, fennel is a good source of vitamin A.

Buying and Storing: Avoid wilted or browning stalks on fennel. The bulb should be firm and white with a light green tinge. Remove leaves and keep for up to one week in the refrigerator.

For Juicing: Use the leaves if attached to the stalks. Use only one-quarter of the bulb (or less) per serving of juice. Larger amounts will make the flavor overpowering.

For Pulping: Use one quarter chopped raw, cooked or frozen fennel bulb in smoothies.

Fennel Recipes:
- Brocco-Artichoke, page 181
- Carrot, Fennel & Orange Frappé, page 345
- Celery, page 184
- Cherry Juice, page 166
- Digestive Cocktail Juice, page 210
- Fennel Fantasy, page 207
- Ginger Smoothie, page 256
- Kelp, page 190
- Nip of Goodness, page 192
- Pear Fennel, page 173
- Peas and Carrots, page 192

- Spiced Cabbage, page 215
- Vidalia Vigor, page 216
- Watermelon Cooler, page 178

Garlic

See page 133

Garlic Recipes:
- Allium Antioxidant, page 227
- Avocado Gazpacho, page 292
- Cabbage Cocktail, page 311
- Cajun Cocktail, page 312
- Cajun Salsa, page 294
- Digestive Cocktail Juice, page 210
- Flaming Antibiotic, page 186
- Gout Buster, page 188
- Immunity, page 190
- Peppery Cabbage, page 215
- Peppery Tomato Cocktail, page 314
- Pumpkin Heart, page 204
- Slippery Beet, page 194
- Tomato Juice Cocktail, page 315
- Tomato Sauce, page 297

Jerusalem Artichoke

Helianthus tuberosus

Actions: Antibacterial

Uses: Jerusalem artichokes are the tuberous roots of a plant related to the sunflower (which is why they are often sold as "sunchokes.") Their sweet, nutty flavor blends well in juices. Diabetics easily digest the inulin, a type of carbohydrate found in Jerusalem artichokes. They are also a source of calcium, iron and magnesium.

For Juicing: Scrub well and cut larger tubers in half. One cup (250 mL) tubers yields about ½ cup (125 mL) juice.

For Pulping: Blanch in boiling water for 3 minutes, cool and chop coarsely before adding to blended drinks.

Artichoke Recipes:
- Artichoke Carrot, page 179
- Artichoke Eight, page 180
- Brocco-Artichoke, page 181

Kale

See Leafy Greens, below

Kohlrabi

See Cabbage, page 113

Leafy Greens

Kale, Swiss chard, collard greens, mustard greens, turnip greens, lettuce

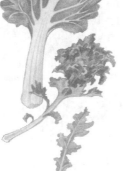

Actions: Antioxidant, anticancer.

Uses: Excellent sources of vitamin A and chlorophyll, leafy greens are also good sources of vitamin C, with some calcium, iron, folic acid and potassium, as well.

Buying and Storing: Buy bright green, crisp (not wilted) greens and store unwashed in a vented plastic bag in the crisper drawer of your refrigerator. Leafy greens are very tender and will sag and yellow (or brown) when not stored or handled properly. Store away from fruits.

For Juicing: Wash, roll along stem into a long cylinder and feed through tube by tapping.

For Pulping: Remove tough ribs and stems, shred or chop coarsely before adding to the blender.

Greens Recipes:
- Bitter Bite, page 218
- Bone Builder, page 241
- Cruciferous, page 185
- Cruciferous Chiller, page 221
- The Curl, page 243
- Deep Green Heart, page 201
- Folic Plus, page 187
- Gout Buster, page 188
- Green Gift, page 232
- Green Peace, page 262
- Kelp, page 190
- Leafy Greens, page 191
- Lights Out, page 263
- Live Young, page 235
- Lofty Leaves, page 245
- Mighty Mineral Smoothie, page 245
- Moist & Juicy, page 192
- Popeye's Power, page 246
- Soft Salad, page 195
- Spring Green Bitters, page 219
- Swiss Knife, page 254

Leeks

Allium ampeloprasum

Actions: Expectorant, diuretic, relaxant, laxative, antiseptic, digestive, hypotensive.

Uses: Easily digested, leeks are used in tonics, especially during convalescence from illness. They can be blended into toddies for relief from sore throats, thanks to their warming, expectorant and stimulating qualities.

Buying and Storing: Bright green ends showing no signs of slime or wilt, with crisp white roots intact, means that leeks are fresh. Unwashed and kept in a vented plastic bag in the refrigerator, leeks should last for one to two weeks.

For Juicing: Leave roots and dark green leaves intact, split and wash inner layers well. Use one-half to one leek per serving.

For Pulping: Trim and wash well and cut into chunks before adding to the blender.

Leek Recipes:
- Artichoke Eight, page 180
- Moist & Juicy, page 192

Lettuce

See Leafy Greens, left

Mustard Greens

See Leafy Greens, left

Onions

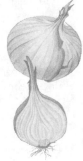

Allium species

Actions: Antibacterial, anticancer, antioxidant, circulatory and digestive stimulant, antiseptic, detoxifying, lower blood cholesterol levels, hypotensive, lower blood sugar level, diuretic, cardioprotective.

Uses: Onions help prevent thrombosis, reduce high blood pressure, lower blood sugar, prevent inflammatory responses and prohibit the growth of cancer cells. Shallots and yellow or red onions are the richest dietary sources of quercetin, a potent antioxidant and cancer-inhibiting phytochemical.

Buying and Storing: Examine each onion to make sure it has dry, tight skin and is firm. Avoid onions with woody centers in the neck and black powdery patches. If stored in a cool, dry place with good air circulation, onions will keep for up to two weeks (one month or more in the refrigerator).

For Juicing: Leave skin on and cut in half if necessary to fit feed tube. Blend with other juices. One medium onion yields approximately 3 tbsp (45 mL) juice.

For Pulping: Vidalia or red onions are preferable for smoothies because they are milder in flavor. Peel and chop before adding to the blender.

Onion Recipes:
- Allium Antioxidant, page 227
- Cauli-Slaw, page 184
- Cream of the Crop, page 256
- Cruciferous Chiller, page 221
- Curry Sauce, page 294
- Heart Beet, page 203
- Peas and Carrots, page 192
- Tomato Tango, page 205
- Vidalia Vigor, page 216

Parsnips

Pastinaca sativa

Actions: Anti-inflammatory, anticancer.

Uses: Parsnips are best fresh after frost has concentrated their carbohydrates into sugar, making them sweeter. Good sources of vitamins C and E and potassium, they also contain some protein, iron and calcium. Parsnips, like other root vegetables, keep well and are excellent in winter smoothies.

Buying and Storing: Look for firm flesh with no evidence of shriveling, soft spots or cuts. Parsnips should snap when bent. Small thin parsnips with tops still intact are preferable. Keep them in a plastic bag in the refrigerator for up to 1½ weeks.

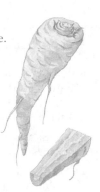

For Juicing: Choose firm, small parsnips. Juice with both ends intact. One pound (500 g) yields approximately 1 cup (250 mL) juice.

For Pulping: Pair with apples and/or carrots in smoothies. Steam or blanch before adding to ingredients in smoothies.

Parsnip Recipes:
- Artichoke Eight, page 180
- Cabbage Cocktail, page 311
- Nip of Goodness, page 192
- Peas and Carrots, page 192
- Root Combo, page 194
- Watercress, page 197

Peas

See Beans, page 111

Peppers

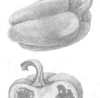

Capsicum annuum
Bell or sweet pepper: green, red, yellow and orange

Actions: Antioxidant, anticancer, cardioprotective.

Uses: Use green, yellow, orange, purple and red peppers in vegetable cocktails and blended drinks — they are all high in vitamins A and C and contain some potassium.

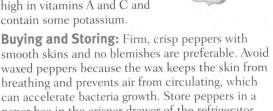

Buying and Storing: Firm, crisp peppers with smooth skins and no blemishes are preferable. Avoid waxed peppers because the wax keeps the skin from breathing and prevents air from circulating, which can accelerate bacteria growth. Store peppers in a paper bag in the crisper drawer of the refrigerator for up to four days. Peppers freeze well and may be added to smoothies without thawing.

For Juicing: Choose thick, fleshy, smooth-skinned peppers. Wash before using. Discard stem, but use seeds. One pound (500 g) yields about 1½ cups (375 mL) juice.

For Pulping: Frozen, canned, or reconstituted dried peppers may be used in place of fresh in smoothies.

Pepper Recipes:
- Bone Builder, page 241
- The Chiller, page 185
- Grape Power, page 170
- Green Goddess, page 188
- Hormone Healthy, page 223
- Peppered Fruit, page 214
- Peppers Please, page 193
- Peppery Cabbage, page 215
- Peppery Tomato Cocktail, page 314
- Red Devil, page 193
- Red Pepper, page 237
- Suite Vegetables, page 266
- Thorny Pear, page 196
- 3PO, page 178
- Vidalia Vigor, page 216
- Watercress, page 197

Pumpkin

See Squash, page 120

Radishes

Raphanus sativum
Red, white and Japanese daikon

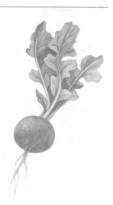

Uses: A good source of potassium and iron, radishes lend a pleasantly hot taste to juices.

For Juicing: Scrub, leaving root and stem on, but discard leaves.

Radish Recipes:
- Dandelion Tonic, page 186
- Gallstone Solvent, page 187
- Red Devil, page 193

Spinach

Spinacea oleracea

Actions: Anticancer, improves memory, antioxidant, promotes healing, anti-cataracts, anti-anemia.

Uses: A good source of choline, which improves mental function, and folic acid, a heart protector, spinach is one of only four vegetables that are high in vitamin E. It is also high in cancer-fighting lutein, chlorophyll and vitamins A and C, and is a good source of calcium, iron, protein and potassium.

Buying and Storing: Choose loose spinach, which is fresher than prepackaged, when available. However, be sure to wash it thoroughly, as it tends to be gritty. Look for broad, crisp, deep green leaves with no signs of yellowing, wilting or softness. Spinach keeps for up to three days in a perforated plastic bag in the crisper drawer of the refrigerator. Pick over and remove yellow or wilted leaves of prepackaged spinach before using.

For Juicing: Wash well. Roll into a long cylinder along stem and feed through tube by tapping.

For Pulping: Use fresh, frozen or canned spinach in blended drinks. Remove tough ribs and stems, and coarsely chop the leaves before adding to the blender.

Spinach Recipes:
- Artichoke Eight, page 180
- Bitter Bite, page 218
- Cabbage Rose, page 181
- Carrot Allium, page 183
- C-Green, page 184
- Cream of Broccoli Smoothie, page 242
- Folic Plus, page 187
- Green Bean, page 243
- Green Beet, page 188
- Green Energy, page 303
- Green Magic, page 190
- Green Peace, page 262
- Hormone Healthy, page 223
- Hot Spiced Carrots, page 263
- Leafy Greens, page 191
- Popeye's Power, page 246
- Smart Smoothie, page 306
- Spiced Carrot, page 195
- Spin Doctor, page 247
- Spring Celebration, page 195

Squash

Cucurbita species
Acorn, butternut,
Hubbard, pumpkin,
turban

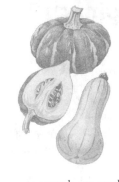

Actions: Antioxidant,
anticancer.

Uses: Squash is a good
winter vegetable that is
high in vitamin A.

Buying and Storing: Summer squash are small
and tender, with pliable skins and seeds. Winter
squash have been allowed to mature on the vine, and
their rinds and seeds are tough and woody. Keep
whole squash in a cold, moist place or in a perforated
plastic bag in the refrigerator. Winter squash may
keep for up to one month if stored properly. Cooked
squash freezes well for use in smoothies.

For Juicing: Scrub and remove stem. Use skin (if
not too thick or waxed) and juice with seeds (high
in cancer-fighting chemicals). One pound (500 g),
about half a medium squash, yields about ½ cup
(125 mL) juice.

For Pulping: Frozen, canned or leftover cooked
squash is the easiest to use in smoothies.

Squash Recipes:
- Breakfast Cocktail, page 311
- Green Magic, page 190
- Pumpkin Heart, page 204
- Sea Herb Surprise, page 194
- Squash Special, page 196
- Thyme Pumpkin Bread, page 296

Swiss Chard

See Leafy Greens, page 117

Tomatoes

Lycopersicon esculentum

Actions: Antioxidant, anticancer.

Uses: High in lycopene and glutathione, two
powerful antioxidants, tomatoes are thought to
reduce the risk of many cancers. Lycopene is also
thought to help maintain mental and physical
functions and is absorbed by the body more
efficiently when tomatoes are juiced (or cooked).

Tomatoes also contain glutamic acid, which is
converted in the body to gamma-aminobutyric acid
(GABA), a calming agent known to be effective in
reducing kidney hypertension. Drink tomato juice or
smoothies made with tomatoes to relax after a
stressful day.

Buying and Storing: Vine-ripened heritage
varieties are the most flavorful. Tomatoes are best
bought fresh only when in season (use canned or
reconstituted dried at other times). Local tomatoes
are not treated with ethylene gas to force reddening.
Plump, heavy, firm-skinned, bright red tomatoes
keep for two or three days at room temperature.
When almost overripe, store tomatoes in the
refrigerator for only one or two more days.

For Juicing: Wash. Discard stem and leaves. Use
skin and seeds. Twelve ounces (375 g), about 3 small
tomatoes, yields 1 cup (250 mL) or more juice.

For Pulping: Skin and seeds are blended fine in
smoothies and do not need to be removed.

Tomato Recipes:
- Blazing Bullshot, page 316
- Cajun Cocktail, page 312
- Cajun Salsa, page 294
- Cauliflower Cocktail, page 312
- De-Vine Fruits, page 202
- Digestive Cocktail Juice, page 210
- Gallstone Solvent, page 187
- Liquid Salsa, page 191
- Peppery Tomato Cocktail, page 314
- Red Devil, page 192
- Rust Proofer #2, page 238
- Spin Doctor, page 247
- Suite Vegetables, page 266
- Tomato Juice Cocktail, page 315
- Tomato Sauce, page 297
- Tomato Tang, page 197
- Tomato Tango, page 205
- Tree Trimming Tomato Warmer, page 319
- Zippy Tomato, page 197

Turnips

Brassica rapa

Actions: Tonic, decongestant, antibacterial,
anticancer, diuretic.

Uses: Turnips have a beneficial effect on the
urinary system, purify the blood and aid in the

elimination of toxins. For this reason, they make a good addition to cleansing smoothies. Both the root and the green tops (see Leafy Greens, page 117) are high in glucosinolates, which are thought to block the development of cancer. Good sources of calcium, iron and protein, small tender turnips are available in the spring and sometimes in the fall.

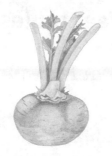

Buying and Storing: Small firm white turnips with dark green leaves that show no signs of wilting or yellowing are best. Turnips will keep for up to one week in a plastic bag in the refrigerator.

For Juicing: Choose fresh turnips with tops intact. Remove tops and wash. Scrub bulbs and juice alternately with tops.

For Pulping: Cooked fresh spring turnip is a pleasant addition to smoothies. Treat young turnips the same way as parsnips.

Turnip Recipes:
• Nip of Goodness, page 192

Watercress

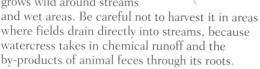

Rorippa nasturtium-aquaticum

Actions: Antioxidant, diuretic, anticancer, tonic, antibiotic, cleansing.

Uses: High in fiber and vitamin C and a good source of vitamin A, watercress grows wild around streams and wet areas. Be careful not to harvest it in areas where fields drain directly into streams, because watercress takes in chemical runoff and the by-products of animal feces through its roots.

Buying and Storing: Pick watercress just before using. If purchasing, choose crisp bright green sprigs with intact leaves. Sort through and remove any yellow or wilted stems. Watercress is fragile and should be used immediately. Wrapped in a towel in the crisper drawer of the refrigerator, it will keep for one or two days.

For Juicing: Wash well and feed through tube alternately with other vegetables. Watercress adds a slightly hot bite to juice drinks.

For Pulping: Use sparingly. Add up to 3 sprigs watercress (leaves and stems) to blended drinks.

Watercress Recipes:
• C-Green, page 184
• Dandelion Tonic, page 186
• Gallstone Solvent, page 187
• Peppery Tomato Cocktail, page 314
• Spring Celebration, page 195
• Watercress, page 197

Wild Greens

Dandelion, mustard, sorrel, turnip, wild garlic and wild leek (ramp)

See Leafy Greens, page 117

Zucchinis

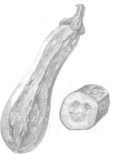

Cucurbita pepo
Italian, yellow straightneck, yellow crookneck

Actions: Antioxidant.

Uses: A good source of vitamins A and C, potassium and niacin, zucchinis are mild tasting and blend well with stronger vegetables.

Buying and Storing: Although zucchinis grow quite large, the smaller they are, the more tender. Look for soft thin skin with no cuts or bruises, and intact stem ends.

For Juicing: Choose small, firm zucchini. Scrub well, leaving skin and blossom end on. Ten ounces (300 g), about 1 medium zucchini, yields about 1 cup (250 mL) of juice.

For Pulping: Coarsely chop before adding to the blender.

Zucchini Recipes:
• The Chiller, page 185
• Tomato Juice Cocktail, page 315

Top Common Antioxidant Vegetables

ORAC (Oxygen Radical Absorbance Capacity) is a testing system that measures the antioxidant capability of fruits and vegetables. A total of 1,670 ORAC units would be the average equivalent of eating five mixed servings of fruits and vegetables a day; however, juicing or pulping with fruits and vegetables known to be high in antioxidants, or with a high ORAC value, will add much more protection from damaging free radicals.

Vegetables	Amount	ORAC Value*
Red Beans	½ cup (125 mL)	13,727
Red Kidney Beans	½ cup (125 mL)	13,259
Pinto Beans	½ cup (125 mL)	11,864
Artichoke Hearts	1 cup (250 mL) cooked	7,904
Russet Potato	1, cooked	4,649
Black Beans	½ cup (125 mL)	4,181
Kale	1 cup (250 mL)	2,540

*Source: USDA data on foods with high levels of antioxidants.

Herbs

Some herbal practitioners recommend using whole fresh herbs for juicing. This is because only the whole fresh juice, taken immediately, captures the entire synergistic complex of healing ingredients locked within the cellular structure of the living plant. (Sigfried Gursche, *Healing with Herbal Juices,* Alive Books, 1993.)

Most herbalists work with the dried form of herbs for medicinal teas because dried herbs are the most widely available and are the easiest to store, transport and work with. For the same reasons, with some exceptions, dried herbs are recommended for use in the tea recipes and some of the juice recipes in this book. However, if fresh herbs are available, be sure to use them.

For each measure of dried herbs called for in a recipe, use 3 times the quantity of fresh.

Most of the herbs profiled in the following section are available dried from whole or natural foods stores. Many can be grown in pots or in your garden and some can be wildcrafted (gathered from the wild). See the Sources section (page 368) for information on how to obtain herbs, tinctures and flower essences by mail.

For the greatest medicinal value, dried herbs should be as fresh as possible. Purchase organic dried herbs from a farm or health/alternative store in small quantities and store for up to 8 or 10 months. If you store your herbs and spices for longer periods, you may not experience the desired effect from them.

Tinctures

A popular and widely available method of herbal medication is the herbal tincture. Tinctures are highly concentrated liquid extracts of the healing herbal properties of medicinal herbs. Tinctures are easy to make and high-quality organic preparations are available from whole or natural foods stores.

Water or vinegar may be used but alcohol is the most popular method of extracting the active components in herbs. Alcohol tinctures will last for many years. For each herb listed below, we have given the medicinal dose for using the tincture of that herb.

Alfalfa

Medicago sativa

A hardy perennial easily grown in most parts of North America.

Parts Used
Leaves, flowers and sprouted seeds.

Healing Properties
Actions: Tonic, nutritive, lowers blood cholesterol, antianemia.
Uses: Alfalfa is a cell nutritive and overall tonic for the body. It promotes strong teeth, bones and connective tissues. Alfalfa is one of the best sources of chlorophyll, which stimulates new skin growth; heals wounds and burns; diminishes the symptoms of arthritis, gout and rheumatism; lowers blood cholesterol level; reduces inflammation; and improves the body's resistance to cancer.

Caution
Alfalfa seeds and sprouts are rich in the amino acid canavanine, which can contribute to inflammation in rheumatoid arthritis, systemic lupus erythematosus and other rheumatoid and inflammatory conditions. Alfalfa leaves are not a source of canavanine and can be used for inflammatory and rheumatic conditions.

Availability
Whole or cut dried leaves are available in alternative/health stores. Sprouted seeds are readily available in supermarkets.

How to Use in Juicing
Whole fresh sprigs: Roll in a ball and feed through tube along with other ingredients. Use about 6 sprigs for each 1 cup (250 mL) of juice.
Dried leaf and flowers: Crush to a fine powder and whisk into fresh juice or add to ingredients in blended drinks. Use 1 tbsp (15 mL) for each 1 cup (250 mL) of juice.
Infusion: Pour ¼ cup (50 mL) boiling water over 2 tbsp (25 mL) fresh or 2 tsp (10 mL) dried cut or powdered leaf. Steep for 10 minutes. Strain, discard herb, and add liquid to 1 cup (250 mL) of juice.
Tincture: Add 1 tsp (5 mL) tincture to 1 cup (250 mL) of juice.

Astragalus

Astragalus membranaceus

A hardy shrub-like perennial native to eastern Asia but grown in temperate regions.

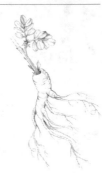

Parts Used
Root.

Healing Properties
Actions: Immunostimulant, antimicrobial, cardiotonic, diuretic, promotes tissue regeneration.
Uses: Used throughout Asia as a tonic, astragalus is a powerful immune-system stimulator for virtually every kind of immune-system activity. It has also been shown to alleviate the adverse effects of steroids and chemotherapy on the immune system, and can be used during traditional cancer treatment.

Availability
While more and more North American herb farms are growing this exceptional medicinal herb, the most-reliable sources for the dried root are Asian herb stores in large urban areas. However, alternative/health stores carry cut or ground dried astragalus, as well as the tincture form.

How to Use in Juicing
Powder: Add 1 tsp (5 mL) dried powder to 1 cup (250 mL) of juice or add to ingredients in blended drinks.
Decoction: In a small saucepan, combine ¼ cup (50 mL) boiling water and 1 dried root stick or 1 tsp (5 mL) dried chopped root. Simmer with lid on 10 minutes and steep 10 minutes. Strain, discard herb, and add liquid to 1 cup (250 mL) of juice.
Tincture: Add 10 to 20 drops to 1 cup (250 mL) of juice.

Basil

Oscimum basilicum

A bushy annual with large, waxy, deep green leaves and small tubular flowers on long spikes.

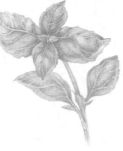

Parts Used
Leaves and flowering tops.

Healing Properties
Actions: Antispasmodic, soothing digestive, antibacterial, antidepressant, adrenal gland stimulant.
Uses: Indigestion, nervous tension, stress, tension headaches.

Availability
Fresh sprigs are sold in season at farmer's markets and supermarkets. Sifted chopped dried leaves are available at alternative/health stores.

How to Use in Juicing
Whole fresh sprigs: Roll in a ball and feed through tube along with other ingredients. Use about 6 sprigs for each 1 cup (250 mL) of juice.

Black Cohosh

Cimicifuga racemosa

A tall, wild woodland perennial native to North America with broad leaves and spikes of fragrant white flowers.

Parts Used
Root and rhizome.

Healing Properties
Actions: Antirheumatic, antispasmodic, mild pain reliever, estrogenic, sedative, anti-inflammatory, uterine stimulant.
Uses: A bitter, tonic herb that soothes aches and pains, black cohosh is used to treat rheumatoid arthritis, sciatica, bronchial spasms, menstrual cramps, menopausal problems, and labor and postpartum pains.

Caution
Do not take black cohosh if you are pregnant or breastfeeding unless otherwise advised by your health-care practitioner. Excessive doses can cause headaches.

Availability
Seeds, rootlets and plants are available for growing. Dried roots and tinctures are available at alternative/health stores.

How to Use in Juicing
Do not take more often than once daily.
Decoction: In a small saucepan, combine ¼ cup (50 mL) boiling water and ½ tsp (2 mL) dried cut or powdered root. Simmer with lid on 10 minutes. Steep 10 minutes. Strain, discard herb, and add liquid to 1 cup (250 mL) of juice.
Tincture: Add 8 drops to 1 cup (250 mL) of juice.

Borage

Borago officinalis

A self-seeding annual with a branching, hollow stem that supports alternating long oval leaves. Small blue star-shaped flowers hang in wide, drooping clusters. The whole plant is covered with prickly silver hairs.

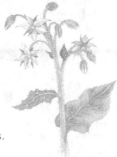

Parts Used
Leaves and flowering tops.

Healing Properties
Actions: Adrenal gland restorative, expectorant, increases milk in breastfeeding.
Uses: Coughs, depression, stress, to strengthen adrenal glands after treatment with corticosteroid drugs.

Caution
Borage leaves contain very small amounts of pyrrolizidine alkaloids, which can be toxic to the liver but are considered safe for occasional use under the supervision of a qualified health-care practitioner.

Availability
Easy to grow in containers or gardens, fresh borage is not readily available to purchase. Dried leaves are sometimes available in alternative/health stores. Use fresh whenever possible, as dried leaves have lost most of their medicinal effectiveness.

How to Use in Juicing
Whole fresh sprigs: Roll in a ball and feed through tube along with other ingredients. Use about 4 sprigs for each 1 cup (250 mL) of juice.
Dried leaf and flowers: Crush to a fine powder and whisk into fresh juice or add to ingredients in blended drinks. Use 1 tbsp (15 mL) for each 1 cup (250 mL) of juice.
Infusion: In a teapot, pour ¼ cup (50 mL) boiling water over 1 tbsp (15 mL) fresh or 1 tsp (5 mL) dried borage. Steep for 10 minutes. Strain, discard herb and add liquid to 1 cup (250 mL) of juice.

Buchu

Barosma betulina

A small green shrub native to South Africa. Plants in this genus have attractive flowers and aromatic bright green ovate leaves that make them popular as ornamentals.

Parts Used
Leaves.

Healing Properties
Actions: Diuretic, urinary antiseptic.
Uses: Used to treat urinary disorders, such as painful urination, cystisis, prostatitis and urethritis. Research indicates that buchu contains properties that block ultraviolet light, which could be helpful in skin preparations.

Availability
Dried leaves and tinctures are available in alternative/health stores.

How to Use in Juicing
Dried leaves: Whisk 1 tsp (5 mL) powdered dried leaves into juices or add to ingredients before blending smoothies or shakes.
Infusion: Pour ¼ cup (50 mL) boiling water over 1 tsp (5 mL) dried cut or powdered leaf. Steep 10 minutes. Strain, discard herb, and add liquid to 1 cup (250 mL) of juice.
Tincture: Add 20 to 40 drops tincture to 1 cup (250 mL) of juice.

Burdock

Arctium lappa

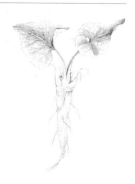

A hardy biennial that produces fruiting heads covered with hooked burrs that catch on clothing and animal fur. Grows wild extensively in North America. Due to its wide availability in rural and urban waste areas, burdock can be easily foraged. Avoid collecting it from roadsides, ditches, streams close to field runoff, or other areas likely to be polluted by car exhaust or chemical runoff.

Parts Used
Root, stalk, leaves and seeds.

Burdock Leaf

Healing Properties
Actions: Mild laxative, diuretic.
Uses: Leaves may be used in the same way that the root is (see Burdock Root, page 126), though they are less effective.

Availability

Dried leaves and tinctures are available in alternative/health stores.

How to Use in Juicing

Whole fresh leaves: Roll in a ball and feed through tube along with other ingredients. Use one leaf for each 1 cup (250 mL) of juice.

Dried leaf: Crush to a fine powder and whisk into fresh juice or add to ingredients in blended drinks. Use 1 to 2 tsp (5 to 10 mL) for each 1 cup (250 mL) of juice.

Infusion: Pour ¼ cup (50 mL) boiling water over 1 tbsp (15 mL) fresh or 1 tsp (5 mL) dried cut or powdered leaf. Steep 10 minutes. Strain, discard herb, and add liquid to 1 cup (250 mL) of juice.

Tincture: Add 10 to 40 drops tincture to 1 cup (250 mL) of juice.

Burdock Root

Healing Properties

Actions: Mild laxative, antirheumatic, antibiotic, diaphoretic, diuretic, skin and blood cleanser, soothing demulcent, tonic, soothes kidneys, lymphatic cleanser.

Uses: Burdock root is used as a cleansing, eliminative remedy. It helps remove toxins that cause skin problems (including eczema, acne, rashes and boils), digestive sluggishness and arthritis pain. It supports the liver, lymphatic glands and digestive system.

Availability

Dig roots in the wild in the fall. Scrub and chop, then dry for storage. Chopped dried root and tinctures are available in alternative/health stores.

How to Use in Juicing

Whole fresh root: Scrub and feed through tube along with other ingredients. Use 2 to 3 inches (5 to 7.5 cm) fresh root per 1 cup (250 mL) of juice.

Dried root: Crush to a fine powder and whisk into fresh juice or add to smoothie ingredients. Use 1 tsp (5 mL) for each 1 cup (250 mL) of juice.

Decoction: Gently simmer 1 tsp (5 mL) dried root in ¼ cup (50 mL) of water for 15 minutes. Strain, discard herb, and add liquid to 1 cup (250 mL) of juice.

Tincture: Add 10 to 20 drops tincture to 1 cup (250 mL) of juice.

Burdock Seeds

Healing Properties

Actions: Antipyretic, anti-inflammatory, antibacterial, reduce blood sugar level.

Uses: Lymphatic cleanser, soothing demulcent, tonic, soothe kidneys.

Availability

Seeds can be gathered easily in the wild in late summer and early fall (see Burdock, page 125). They are not always available in alternative/health stores, but burdock tinctures are.

How to Use in Juicing

Infusion: In a teapot, pour ¼ cup (50 mL) boiling water over 1 tsp (5 mL) bruised fresh or dried seeds. Steep with lid on for 10 minutes. Strain, discard herb and add liquid to 1 cup (250 mL) of juice.

Tincture: Add 10 to 40 drops to 1 cup (250 mL) of juice.

Calendula

Calendula officinalis

A prolific annual easily grown from seed, with bright yellow to orange marigold-like flowers.

Parts Used

Petals.

Healing Properties

Actions: Astringent, antiseptic, antifungal, anti-inflammatory, heals wounds, menstrual regulator, stimulates bile production.

Uses: Calendula acts as a digestive aid and general tonic. It improves menopausal problems, menstrual pain, gastritis, peptic ulcers, gallbladder problems, indigestion and fungal infections.

Availability

Whole dried flower heads are available in alternative/health stores.

How to Use in Juicing

Infusion: Pour ¼ cup (50 mL) boiling water over 1 tbsp (15 mL) fresh or 1 tsp (5 mL) dried petals. Steep 10 minutes if using dried, 15 minutes if using fresh petals. Strain, discard herb, and add liquid to 1 cup (250 mL) of juice.

Tincture: Add 5 to 20 drops tincture to 1 cup (250 mL) of juice.

Cardamom

Elettaria cardamomum

A rhizomatous perennial with
large lanceolate leaves originally
from the Indian rain forests. For
centuries it has been exported to
Europe, mainly for its fragrance.
When coaxed into bloom, the
flowers are white with dark pink–striped lips.

Parts Used
Seeds.

Healing Properties
Actions: Antispasmodic, carminative, digestive
stimulant, expectorant.
Uses: A pungent herb with stimulating, tonic effects
that work best on the digestive system, cardamom
relaxes spasms, stimulates appetite and relieves
flatulence.

Availability
Whole or ground dried seeds are widely available in
supermarkets and alternative/health stores.

How to Use in Juicing
Dried seeds: Whisk 1 tsp (5 mL) ground
cardamom seeds into 1 cup (250 mL) of juice or
add to smoothie ingredients.
Infusion: In a teapot, pour ¼ cup (50 mL) boiling
water over 1 tsp (5 mL) lightly crushed seeds. Steep
with lid on 10 minutes. Strain, discard herb, and
add liquid to 1 cup (250 mL) of juice.

Catnip

Nepeta cataria

A hardy perennial — and a
favorite of cats — with erect
branched stems that bear gray-
green toothed ovate leaves and
whorls of white tubular flowers.

Parts Used
Leaves, stems and flowers.

Healing Properties
Actions: Antispasmodic, astringent, carminative,
diaphoretic, cooling, sedative.
Uses: Catnip lowers fever, relaxes spasms, increases
perspiration and is often taken at night to ensure
sleep. It is also used for diarrhea, stomach upsets,
colic, colds, flu, inflammation, pain and
convulsions. It is especially useful for lowering
children's fevers.

Availability
Catnip is easily grown in North America, but
dried leaves, stems and flowers are available in
alternative/health stores.

How to Use in Juicing
Whole fresh sprigs: Roll in a ball and feed through
tube along with other ingredients. Use about
4 sprigs for each 1 cup (250 mL) of juice.
Dried leaf and flowers: Crush to a fine powder
and whisk into fresh juice or ingredients in blended
drinks. Use 1 tsp (5 mL) for each 1 cup (250 mL)
of juice.
Infusion: Pour ¼ cup (50 mL) boiling water over
1 tbsp (15 mL) fresh or 1 tsp (5 mL) dried cut or
powdered catnip. Steep 10 minutes. Strain, discard
herb, and add liquid to 1 cup (250 mL) of juice.

Cayenne

Capsicum annum and
Capsicum frutescens

A tropical perennial grown
as an annual in temperate
zones (see also Chile Peppers,
page 115). Although many
varieties of chile peppers are
used in cooking to add flavor
and heat, the cayenne pepper
is also used frequently
as an herb because of its healing powers.

Parts Used
Red pepper fruit.

Healing Properties
Actions: Stimulant, tonic, carminative, diaphoretic,
rubefacient, antiseptic, antibacterial.
Uses: Cayenne stimulates blood circulation, purifies
the blood, promotes fluid elimination and sweating,
and is most often used as a stimulating nerve tonic.
Applied externally, over-the-counter creams and
ointments that contain active capsaicin extract are
often effective in relieving the pain of osteoarthritis,
rheumatoid arthritis and shingles, as well as the
burning pain in the toes, feet and legs caused by
diabetic neuropathy and fibromyalgia.

Caution
Cayenne contains an irritating compound that,
when applied externally, heals inflammations on
unbroken skin by bringing blood to the surface.
If used on broken skin, cayenne will irritate the
wound and not be as effective. Natural-medicine
practitioners often advise that capsicum not be
taken internally in cases of chronic inflammation of

the intestinal tract, such as in irritable bowel syndrome, ulcerative colitis and Crohn's disease. It should be used sparingly during pregnancy.

Availability

Fresh whole cayenne peppers are available in Latin American markets, supermarkets and alternative/ health stores. Dried whole cayenne peppers and ground cayenne pepper are widely available.

How to Use in Juicing

Fresh: See Chile Peppers, page 115.
Dried: Whisk 1/8 to 1/4 tsp (1 mL) dried ground cayenne pepper into 1 1/2 cups (375 mL) juice or add to ingredients in blended drinks.

Celery Seeds

Apium graveolens

A biennial with a bulbous, fleshy root and thick, grooved stems. Although the stalk, leaves and, sometimes, the seeds are used in cooking (see Celery, page 114), it is the seeds collected from wild celery that are used for medicinal purposes.

Parts Used
Seeds.

Healing Properties

Actions: Anti-inflammatory, antioxidant, carminative, sedative, urinary antiseptic.
Uses: Celery seeds are an aromatic, tonic herb that relieves muscle spasms and are used to treat gout, inflammation of the urinary tract, cystitis, osteoarthritis and rheumatoid arthritis.

Caution

Do not use celery seeds if you are pregnant.

Availability

Purchase celery seeds from herbalists or alternative/ health stores only.

How to Use in Juicing

Whole fresh stalks and leaves: See Celery, page 114.
Dried seeds: Crush to a fine powder and whisk into fresh juice or add to ingredients in blended drinks. Use 1/4 tsp (1 mL) for each 1 cup (250 mL) of juice.
Infusion: In a teapot, pour 1/4 cup (50 mL) boiling water over 1/4 tsp (1 mL) dried lightly crushed seeds. Steep 10 minutes. Strain, discard herb, and add liquid to 1 cup (250 mL) of juice.

Chamomile

See German Chamomile

Chickweed

Stellaria media

A low, spreading annual with diffusely branched stems, ovate leaves and white star-shaped flowers found in most parts of North America.

Parts Used

Roots, leaves, flowers and stems.

Healing Properties

Actions: Anticancer, anti-inflammatory, antirheumatic, astringent, heals wounds, demulcent.
Uses: Chickweed is used internally to treat rheumatism, constipation, mucus in the lungs, coughs, colds, tumors and blood disorders. It is used externally to treat eczema, psoriasis and other skin conditions.

Availability

A common weed, chickweed may be wildcrafted from summer through fall. Dried aerial parts (stem, leaves and flowers) and roots are available in alternative/health stores.

How to Use in Juicing

Whole fresh sprigs: Roll in a ball and feed through tube along with other ingredients. Use about 6 sprigs for each 1 cup (250 mL) of juice.
Dried leaf and flowers: Crush to a fine powder and whisk into fresh juice or add to ingredients in blended drinks. Use 2 tsp (10 mL) for each 1 cup (250 mL) of juice.
Infusion: In a teapot, pour 1/4 cup (50 mL) boiling water over 2 tbsp (25 mL) fresh or 2 tsp (10 mL) dried cut or powdered chickweed. Steep 10 minutes. Strain, discard herb, and add liquid to 1 cup (250 mL) of juice.

Cinnamon

Cinnamomum zeylanicum and *C. cassia*

The dried smooth inner bark of a cultivated laurel-like tree that grows in the hot, wet tropical regions of India, Brazil, the East and West Indies, and islands in the Indian Ocean.

Parts Used

Bark.

Healing Properties

Actions: Carminative, diaphoretic, astringent, stimulant, antimicrobial.
Uses: Cinnamon is a warming carminative used to promote digestion and relieve nausea, vomiting and diarrhea. It is used for upset stomach and to treat irritable bowel syndrome (see page 69). Recent research has shown that cinnamon helps the body use insulin more efficiently, which may be helpful in the management of diabetes.

Availability

Dried rolled sticks are sold in 2- to 18-inch (5 to 45 cm) lengths. Powdered cinnamon and ground cinnamon, which is coarser, are widely available.

How to Use in Juicing

Powder: Whisk ¼ tsp (1 mL) powdered cinnamon into 1 cup (250 mL) of juice or add to ingredients for blended drinks.
Infusion: In a teapot, pour ¼ cup (50 mL) boiling water over a 1-inch (2.5 cm) stick of cinnamon, broken in pieces. Steep with lid on 5 minutes. Strain, discard herb, and add liquid to 1 cup (250 mL) of juice.

Clove

Syzygium aromaticus

The pink unopened flower buds of an evergreen tree native to Indonesia that's now grown in Zanzibar, Madagascar, the West Indies, Brazil, India and Sri Lanka.

Parts Used

Dried buds.

Healing Properties

Actions: Antioxidant, anesthetic, antiseptic, anti-inflammatory, anodyne, antispasmodic, carminative, stimulant, antiemetic, antihistamine, warming.
Uses: Cloves are used to treat asthma, bronchitis, nausea, vomiting, flatulence, diarrhea and hypothermia. Some studies indicate that cloves may have anticoagulant properties and may stimulate the production of enzymes that fight cancer. Clove oil is the active ingredient in some mouthwashes, toothpastes, soaps, insect repellents, perfumes,

foods and veterinary medications, as well as many over-the-counter toothache remedies.

Availability

Whole and ground dried cloves are widely available.

How to Use in Juicing

Powder: Whisk ¼ tsp (1 mL) powdered cloves into 1 cup (250 mL) of juice or add to ingredients in blended drinks.
Infusion: In a teapot, pour ¼ cup (50 mL) boiling water over ¼ tsp (1 mL) lightly crushed cloves. Steep with lid on 10 minutes. Strain, discard herb and add liquid to 1 cup (250 mL) of juice.

Coriander Seeds

Coriandrum sativum

A hardy annual with slender, erect branched stems that bear aromatic pinnate parsley-like leaves. Small flat umbels of tiny white to pale mauve flowers yield round green berries (seeds) that ripen to a brownish yellow.

Parts Used

Seeds.

Healing Properties

Actions: Soothing digestive, appetite stimulant, improve digestion and nutrient absorption.
Uses: Digestive problems, flatulence.

Availability

Dried seeds are readily available in alternative/health stores and Indian markets.

How to Use in Juicing

Dried seeds: Crush to a powder and whisk ½ tsp (2 mL) into 1 cup (250 mL) of juice or add to ingredients in blended drinks.
Infusion: In a teapot, pour ¼ cup (50 mL) boiling water over 1 tsp (5 mL) lightly crushed seeds. Steep with lid on 10 minutes. Strain, discard herb, and add liquid to 1 cup (250 mL) of juice.

Cumin

Cuminum cyminum

A slender annual with dark green leaves found wild from the Mediterranean to Sudan in Africa and in central Asia. Umbels of tiny white or pink flowers are followed by bristly oval seeds.

Parts Used
Seeds.

Healing Properties
Actions: Stimulant, soothing digestive, antispasmodic, diuretic, increases milk in breastfeeding.
Uses: Indigestion, flatulence.

Availability
Dried seeds are readily available in alternative/health stores and Indian markets.

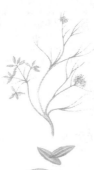

How to Use in Juicing
Dried Seeds: Crush to a powder and whisk ½ tsp (2 mL) powder into 1 cup (250 mL) of juice or add to ingredients in blended drinks.
Infusion: In a teapot, pour ¼ cup (50 mL) boiling water over ½ tsp (2 mL) lightly crushed seeds. Steep with lid on 10 minutes. Strain, discard herb and add liquid to 1 cup (250 mL) of juice.

Dandelion

Taraxacum officinale

A hardy herbaceous perennial commonly found in most parts of North America.

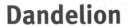

Parts Used
Roots, stems, leaves and flowers.

Dandelion Leaf

Healing Properties
Actions: Diuretic, liver and digestive tonic.
Uses: Dandelion is used for liver, gallbladder, kidney and bladder ailments, including hepatitis and jaundice. It is also used as a diuretic. The leaves are used specifically to support the kidneys.

Availability
Whole plants are easily foraged from spring through fall. Look for fresh leaves in some supermarkets, farmer's markets and alternative/health stores; chopped dried leaves are available in alternative/health stores.

How to Use in Juicing
Whole fresh leaves: Roll in a ball and feed through tube along with other ingredients. Use 4 to 6 leaves for each 1 cup (250 mL) of juice.
Dried leaf: Whisk 1 tsp (5 mL) chopped, dried leaf into 1 cup (250 mL) of juice or add to ingredients in blended drinks.

Infusion: In a teapot, pour ¼ cup (50 mL) boiling water over 1 tbsp (15 mL) fresh or 1 tsp (5 mL) dried dandelion leaf. Steep for 10 minutes. Strain, discard herb, and add liquid to 1 cup (250 mL) of juice.

Dandelion Root

Healing Properties
Actions: Liver tonic, promotes bile flow, diuretic, mild laxative, antirheumatic.
Uses: Dandelion is used for liver, gallbladder, kidney and bladder ailments, including hepatitis and jaundice. It is also used as a diuretic. The root is used specifically to support the liver.

Availability
Dig fresh roots in the fall. Chopped dried roots and tinctures are available in alternative/health stores.

How to Use in Juicing
Whole fresh root: Scrub and feed through tube along with other ingredients. Use 2 to 3 inches (5 to 7.5 cm) fresh root per 1 cup (250 mL) of juice.
Dried root: Crush to a fine powder and whisk into fresh juice or add to smoothie ingredients. Use 1 tsp (5 mL) for each 1 cup (250 mL) of juice.
Decoction: Gently simmer 1 tsp (5 mL) chopped dried root in ¼ cup (50 mL) of water for 10 minutes. Strain, discard herb, and add liquid to 1 cup (250 mL) of juice.
Tincture: Add 1 tsp (5 mL) to 1 cup (250 mL) of juice.

Dill

Anethum graveolens

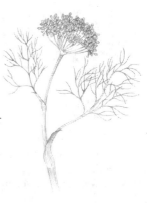

A tall top-heavy annual with a long hollow stem growing out of a spindly taproot. Terminal flower heads, which grow out of the top of the stem, appear in a wide, flat umbel of numerous yellow flowers. Branches along the stem support feathery blue-green leaflets.

Parts Used
Seeds.

Healing Properties
Actions: Soothing digestive, antispasmodic, increases milk in breastfeeding.
Uses: Flatulence, infant colic, bad breath.

Availability

Easy to grow, dill seeds can be harvested from late summer through early fall. Dried seeds are readily available in alternative/health stores and supermarkets.

How to Use in Juicing

Dried seeds: Crush to a powder and ½ tsp (2 mL) into 1 cup (250 mL) of juice or add to ingredients in blended drinks.

Infusion: In a teapot, pour ¼ cup (50 mL) boiling water over 1 tsp (5 mL) lightly crushed seeds. Steep with lid on 10 minutes. Strain, discard herb, and add liquid to 1 cup (250 mL) of juice.

Echinacea

Echinacea angustifolia or *E. purpurea*

A hardy perennial also known as coneflower that is native to North America, with bright purple petals surrounding a brown cone.

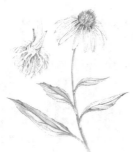

Parts Used

Leaves, seeds, flowers, roots, stems.

Healing Properties

Actions: Immune modulating, anti-inflammatory, antibiotic, antimicrobial, antiseptic, analgesic, antiallergenic, lymphatic tonic.

Uses: Echinacea is used clinically to prevent and treat infections in the respiratory, urinary and digestive systems. It is useful in chronic candida and sinus infections and to support the health of patients undergoing chemotherapy. Externally, echinacea speeds healing of skin infections and wounds. Evidence shows that echinacea is effective because it increases the activity of phagocytes, which play an important role in preventing and overcoming bacterial, viral and fungal infections. Test-tube studies of its antiviral properties indicate that the above ground parts of *E. purpurea* may be effective in inhibiting the viruses that cause herpes, influenza and polio. The roots of *E. angustifolia*, *E. pallida* and *E. purpurea* may be effective in defending the body against the herpes simplex and influenza viruses.

Availability

Whole or chopped dried root, stems and leaves are available in alternative/health stores. Echinacea is also available in tincture and tablet form.

How to Use in Juicing

Decoction: Gently simmer 1 tsp (5 mL) chopped dried root in ¼ cup (50 mL) of water for 10 minutes. Strain and add to 1 cup (250 mL) of juice.
Tincture: Add ½ tsp (2 mL) of tincture to 1 cup (250 mL) of juice.

Elder

Sambucus nigra

A fast-growing hardy perennial shrub common in many parts of North America.

Parts Used

Bark, flowers and berries.

Healing Properties

Actions: (Flowers) Expectorant, reduce phlegm, circulatory stimulant, diaphoretic, diuretic, topically anti-inflammatory. (Berries) Diaphoretic, diuretic, laxative. (Bark) Purgative, large doses are emetic, diuretic.

Uses: (Flowers) Elderflowers can be taken early in allergy season to strengthen the upper respiratory tract and help prevent hay fever. (Berries) Elderberries support detoxification by promoting bowel movements, urination, sweating and mucus secretion. Elderberries are effective in combating viruses, including those that cause colds and flu.

Availability

Fresh elderberries are found in season at farmer's markets. Dried flowers, fresh or dried berries and elder tinctures are available in alternative/health stores.

How to Use in Juicing

Infusion, flowers: In a teapot, pour ¼ cup (50 mL) boiling water over 1 tbsp (15 mL) fresh or dried flowers. Steep 10 minutes if using dried flowers, 15 minutes if using fresh flowers. Strain and add to 1 cup (250 mL) of juice.
Fresh berries: Add up to ¼ cup (50 mL) fresh berries to other fruits in juicer.
Infusion, berries: Pour ¼ cup (50 mL) boiling water over 1 tbsp (15 mL) fresh or 1 tsp (5 mL) lightly crushed dried berries. Steep 10 minutes. Strain, discard herb, and add liquid to 1 cup (250 mL) of juice.
Tincture: Add 1 tsp (5 mL) of tincture to 1 cup (250 mL) of juice.

Evening Primrose

Oenothera biennis

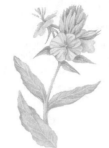

An erect biennial with a rosette of basal leaves. In summer, yellow flowers open at night. Downy pods that contain tiny black seeds follow blooms.

Parts Used
Seed oil.

Healing Properties
Actions: Anticoagulant, anti-inflammatory, improves blood circulation, nutritive, the essential fatty acids in the seed oil help repair tissues.
Uses: Acne, anxiety, arthritis, asthma, breast tenderness, diabetes, dry skin, eczema, hangover, inflammation, high blood pressure, hyperactivity in children, migraines, multiple sclerosis, premenstrual syndrome.

Availability
Evening primrose oil is widely available in gel capsule form and sometimes in bulk in alternative/health stores.

How to Use in Juicing
Oil: Whisk 1 tsp (5 mL) oil into 1 cup (250 mL) of juice or add to ingredients in blended drinks.

Fennel Seeds

Foeniculum vulgare

The fennel plant looks like a larger version of dill. Stout, solid stems support bright yellow, large umbel clusters of flowers. Thread-like, feathery green leaves alternately branch out from joints on the stem. Flowers appear in summer, followed by gray-brown seeds, which are used for medicinal purposes.

Parts Used
Seeds.

Healing Properties
Actions: Soothing diuretic, anti-inflammatory, antispasmodic, soothing digestive, increases milk in breastfeeding, mild expectorant.
Uses: Indigestion, flatulence, increases milk in breastfeeding, relieves colic in babies when taken by nursing mother. Fennel seed infusion is safe to treat colic and coughs in babies and children.

Caution
Avoid large doses if you are pregnant, as fennel seeds are a uterine stimulant.

Availability
Fennel grows wild in Mediterranean Europe and Asia and has become naturalized in many other parts of the world, where the fleshy bulb is harvested and used as a vegetable (see page 116). Harvest seeds in late summer and early fall. Dried seeds are readily available in alternative/health stores and supermarkets.

How to Use in Juicing
Fresh bulb: See Fennel, page 116.
Dried seeds: Crush to a powder and whisk ¼ tsp (1 mL) into 1 cup (250 mL) of juice or add to ingredients in blended drinks.
Infusion: In a teapot, pour ¼ cup (50 mL) boiling water over ¼ to ½ tsp (1 to 2 mL) lightly crushed seeds. Steep with lid on 15 minutes. Strain, discard herb, and add liquid to 1 cup (250 mL) of juice.

Fenugreek

Trigonella foenum-graecum

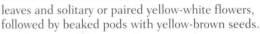

Grown as a fodder crop in southern and central Europe, fenugreek is widely naturalized from the Mediterranean to southern Africa to Australia. This annual has aromatic trifoliate leaves and solitary or paired yellow-white flowers, followed by beaked pods with yellow-brown seeds.

Parts Used
Aerial parts (stem, leaves and flowers) and seeds.

Healing Properties
Actions: Expectorant, soothing digestive, protects intestinal surfaces, reduces blood sugar level, increases milk in breastfeeding.
Uses: Bronchitis, coughs, diabetes, diverticular disease, ulcerative colitis, Crohn's disease, menstrual pain, peptic ulcers, stomach upsets.

Availability
Dried seeds are available in alternative/health stores.

How to Use in Juicing
Decoction: Simmer gently 1 to 2 tsp (5 to 10 mL) crushed seeds in 1 cup (250 mL) of water for 10 minutes. Strain, discard herb, and add liquid to 1 cup (250 mL) of juice.

Feverfew

Tanacetum parthenium

A perennial that appears throughout northern temperate regions. Bright green oblong leaves contain pungent volatile oils that may cause unpleasant reactions if handled or consumed in excess. Flowers are small and daisy-like.

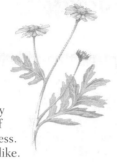

Parts Used
Leaves.

Healing Properties
Actions: Anti-inflammatory, vasodilator, digestive.
Uses: Prevention of migraine headaches, inflammatory arthritis, menstrual pain.

Caution
Do not take feverfew if you are pregnant, since it stimulates the uterus. Fresh leaves may cause mouth ulcers in sensitive people.

Availability
Easily grown, fresh leaves may be harvested from June through late fall. Chopped dried leaves are available in alternative/health stores.

How to Use in Juicing
Whole fresh leaves: Roll in a ball and feed through tube along with other ingredients. Use 1 or 2 large leaves for each 1 cup (250 mL) of juice.
Dried leaf: Crush to a fine powder and whisk into fresh juice. Use 1 tsp (5 mL) for each 1 cup (250 mL) of juice.
Tincture: Add 5 to 20 drops of tincture to 1 cup (250 mL) of juice.

Garlic

Allium sativum

A hardy perennial with an onion-like bulb that's easily grown in North America.

Parts Used
Bulb or "bud" at the root of the plant.

Healing Properties
Actions: Antimicrobial, antibiotic, cardioprotective, hypotensive, anticancer, diaphoretic, anticoagulant, lowers blood cholesterol level, lowers blood sugar level, expectorant, digestive stimulant, diuretic, antihistamine, antiparasitic.

Uses: Research has shown that garlic inhibits cancer-cell formation and proliferation. It lowers total and low-density lipoprotein (LDL) cholesterol in humans and reduces blood clotting, thereby reducing the risks of blocked arteries and heart disease. Garlic is also an antioxidant and stimulates the immune system. It has strong antibiotic and anti-inflammatory properties, making it a good topical medicine. Garlic protects organs from damage inflicted by synthetic drugs, chemical pollutants and radiation.

Availability
Buy fresh whole organic bulbs at farmer's markets and supermarkets.

How to Use in Juicing
Only the fresh cloves have medicinal value. Add one or two fresh cloves to other vegetables when juicing.

German Chamomile

Matricaria recutita

A low-growing hardy annual easily grown in North America. Flowers have daisy-like petals that surround rounded yellow centers.

Parts Used
Flower heads and petals.

Healing Properties
Actions: Gentle sedative, anti-inflammatory, mild antiseptic, antiemetic, antispasmodic, carminative, nervine, emmenagogue, mild pain reliever.
Uses: Anxiety, insomnia, indigestion, peptic ulcer, motion sickness, inflammation (such as gastritis) and menstrual cramps. Chamomile also reduces flatulence and gas pains.

Availability
Whole dried flower heads and tinctures are available in alternative/health stores.

How to Use in Juicing
Infusion: In a teapot, pour ¼ cup (50 mL) boiling water over 1 tbsp (15 mL) fresh or 1 tsp (5 mL) dried flower heads. Steep for 10 minutes. Strain, discard herb, and add liquid to 1 cup (250 mL) of juice.
Tincture: Add 1 tsp (5 mL) of tincture to 1 cup (250 mL) of juice.

Ginger

Zingeber officinalis

A tender perennial edible rhizome native to Southeast Asia.

Parts Used
Root.

Healing Properties
Actions: Antinausea, relieves headaches and arthritis, anti-inflammatory, circulatory stimulant, expectorant, antispasmodic, antiseptic, diaphoretic, anticoagulant, peripheral vasodilator, anti-emetic, carminative, antioxidant.

Uses: Gingerroot calms nausea and morning sickness and prevents vomiting. It is a cleansing, warming herb. Ginger stimulates blood flow to the digestive system and increases nutrient absorption. It increases the action of the gallbladder while protecting the liver against toxins and preventing the formation of ulcers. Studies show that ginger gives some relief from the pain and swelling of arthritis without side effects. Ginger is also used to control flatulence, circulation problems and impotence, and to prevent nausea after chemotherapy.

Caution
Ginger can be irritating to the intestinal mucosa and should be taken with or after meals. Ginger is contraindicated for people who are suffering from kidney disease.

Availability
Fresh gingerroot and ground dried ginger are widely available in supermarkets, Asian and Indian markets, and alternative/health stores.

How to Use in Juicing
Fresh root: Add ½- to 1-inch (1 to 3 cm) piece to fruits or vegetables when juicing. Leave peel on if organic.

Infusion: In a teapot, pour ¼ cup (50 mL) boiling water over 1 tsp (5 mL) grated fresh ginger. Steep for 10 minutes. Strain, discard herb, and add liquid to 1 cup (250 mL) of juice.

Dried powder: Whisk 1 tsp (5 mL) powdered ginger into 1 cup (250 mL) of juice or add to ingredients in blended drinks.

Ginkgo

Ginkgo biloba

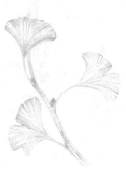

A deciduous tree and one of the oldest trees to survive to the present day, ginkgo originated in central China but is grown as an ornamental in central North America. Light green fan-shaped leaves with two lobes turn yellow in autumn.

Parts Used
Leaves.

Healing Properties
Actions: Antioxidant, circulatory stimulant, increases blood flow to the brain, relieves bronchial spasms.

Uses: Asthma, tinnitus, cold hands and feet, varicose veins, hemorrhoids, headache, hangover, age-related memory loss, hearing loss, eyesight changes, Alzheimer's disease, Raynaud's disease, retinopathy, impotence.

Availability
Leaves can be gathered when yellow in the fall. Dried ginkgo leaves are available in alternative/health stores.

How to Use in Juicing
Dried leaf: Crush to a fine powder and whisk into fresh juice or add to ingredients in blended drinks. Use 1 tsp (5 mL) for each 1 cup (250 mL) of juice.

Infusion: In a teapot, pour ¼ cup (50 mL) boiling water over 1 tbsp (15 mL) fresh or 1 tsp (5 mL) dried leaves. Steep for 10 minutes. Strain, discard herb, and add liquid to 1 cup (250 mL) of juice.

Liquid extract: Add 40 drops to 1 cup (250 mL) of juice.

Ginseng

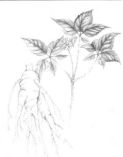

Siberian: *Eleutherococcus senticosis,* North American: *Panax quinquefolius,* Asian: *Panax ginseng*

A hardy perennial native to cool wooded areas of eastern and central North America.

Parts Used
Root (from plants more than four years old) and leaves (if organic).

Healing Properties
Actions: Antioxidant, adaptogen, tonic, stimulant, regulates blood sugar and cholesterol levels, stimulates the immune system.

Uses: Ginseng helps the body resist and adapt to stress. It is a mild stimulant and, as a tonic, promotes long-term overall health. Along with increasing resistance to diabetes, cancer, heart disease and various infections, ginseng is also credited with improving memory, increasing fertility, protecting the liver against toxins and protecting the body against radiation. It is also used to treat impotence and depression.

Caution
Avoid ginseng if you have a fever, asthma, bronchitis, emphysema, high blood pressure or cardiac arrhythmia. Do not take ginseng if you are pregnant or if you drink coffee, and never give ginseng to a hyperactive child. Do not take continuously for a period of more than four weeks.

Availability
Whole or chopped dried root, tea, powdered and tinctures are all available in alternative/health stores and Asian grocery stores. In its native North American woodlands, ginseng has been harvested to near extinction. Please do not collect it in the wild or purchase wildcrafted North American ginseng.

How to Use in Juicing
Fresh root: Add 2- to 3-inch (5 to 7.5 cm) piece to juicing ingredients. Only use organic ginseng and leave peel on.

Dried root: Grate finely and whisk ¼ tsp (1 mL) powder into 1 cup (250 mL) of juice or add to ingredients in blended drinks.

Decoction: Gently simmer 1 tsp (5 mL) chopped dried root in ¼ cup (50 mL) of water for 10 minutes. Strain and add to 1 cup (250 mL) of juice.

Tincture: Add 10 to 20 drops of tincture to 1 cup (250 mL) of juice.

Goldenrod

Solidago virgaurea

A perennial with upright stems, oval leaves and yellow flowers that appear in late summer. Goldenrod is indigenous to North America, with a long history of use by native peoples.

Parts Used
Aerial parts (stem, leaves and flowers).

Healing Properties
Actions: Anticatarrhal, anti-inflammatory, antiseptic to mucous membranes, urinary antiseptic, diuretic, diaphoretic.

Uses: Bronchitis, coughs, respiratory congestion, urethritis, tonsillitis, prostatitis, kidney and bladder problems.

Availability
Goldenrod is widely available in the wild and in waste lands. Harvest from July through fall. Chopped dried leaves, stems and flowers are available in alternative/health stores.

How to Use in Juicing
Whole fresh sprigs: Roll in a ball and feed through tube along with other ingredients. Use 2 to 4 sprigs for each 1 cup (250 mL) of juice.

Dried leaf and flowers: Crush to a fine powder and whisk into fresh juice or add to ingredients in blended drinks. Use ¼ to ½ tsp (1 to 2 mL) for each 1 cup (250 mL) of juice.

Infusion: In a teapot, pour ¼ cup (50 mL) boiling water over 1 tbsp (15 mL) fresh or 1 tsp (5 mL) dried goldenrod. Steep for 10 minutes. Strain, discard herb, and add liquid to 1 cup (250 mL) of juice.

Gotu Kola

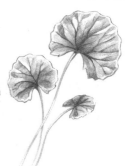

Hydrocotyle asiatica

A small, creeping tropical perennial, this plant has been used for centuries in India for its rejuvenating properties.

Parts Used
Aerial parts.

Healing Properties
Actions: Blood tonic, digestive, central nervous system relaxant, laxative, strengthens adrenal glands

Uses: Exhaustion, age-related memory loss, nervous disorders, Parkinson's disease, stress

Caution
Gotu Kola is not to be used in pregnancy or epilepsy. Do not use for longer than 6 weeks without a break. May aggravate itching. In large doses, may cause headache.

Availability
Dried aerial parts may be available at health/alternative stores. Tincture is available where tablets are sold.

How to Use in Juicing
Dried leaf and flowers: Crush to a fine powder and whisk into fresh juice or add to ingredients in blended drinks, use ½ tsp (2 mL) for each 1 cup (250 mL) of juice.
Infusion: In a teapot, pour ¼ cup (50 mL) of boiling water over ½ tsp (2 mL) gotu kola. Steep for 10 minutes. Strain, discard herb, and add liquid to 1 cup (250 mL) of juice.
Tincture: Add ½ to 1 tsp (2 to 5 mL) to 1 cup (250 mL) of juice.

Green Tea

Camellia sinensis

Green and black tea leaves come from a shrub or small tree indigenous to the wet forests of Asia. It is now cultivated commercially in Asia, Africa, South America and North America.

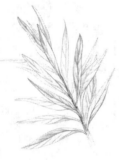

Parts Used
Leaves.

Healing Properties
Actions: Antioxidant, diuretic, recently found to have anticancer properties.
Uses: Cancer prevention, protection against radiation if taken daily at least a week before exposure.

Caution
Green tea contains caffeine, so minimize your intake of it if you have a health condition that is aggravated by caffeine.

Availability
Available dried in bulk in Asian grocery stores and alternative/health stores, or individually wrapped in supermarkets.

How to Use in Juicing
Dried leaf: Crush to a fine powder and whisk into fresh juice or add to ingredients in blended drinks, use 1 tsp (5 mL) for each 1 cup (250 mL) of juice.
Infusion: In a teapot, pour ¼ cup (50 mL) of boiling water over 1 tsp (5 mL) dried green tea. Steep for 3 to 5 minutes. Strain, discard herb, and add liquid to 1 cup (250 mL) of juice.

Hawthorn

Crataegus monogyna and *C. oxyacanthoides*

A thorny shrub found throughout northern temperate regions, hawthorn grows wild in hedgerows in Europe and the northeastern United States and Canada. Scented white flowers bear dark red oval fruit with stony pits.

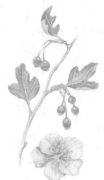

Parts Used
Flowering tops and fruit.

Healing Properties
Actions: Heart tonic, improves coronary circulation.
Uses: Angina, hypertension, poor circulation.

Caution
Consult your health-care practitioner before taking hawthorn if you are taking other heart medications.

Availability
Harvest flowering tops in the spring and fresh fruit in late summer and dry for medicinal use. Dried hawthorn "berries" are available in alternative/health stores.

How to Use in Juicing
Fresh berries: For a wonderful heart tonic, add ¼ to ½ cup (50 to 125 mL) fresh berries to any fresh berry or other fruit juice recipe.
Infusion: In a teapot, pour ¼ cup (50 mL) of boiling water over 1 to 2 tsp (5 to 10 mL) bruised fresh or dried hawthorn blossoms or lightly crushed fresh or dried berries. Steep with lid on 10 minutes. Strain, discard herb and add liquid to 1 cup (250 mL) of juice.
Tincture: Add 10 to 20 drops to 1 cup (250 mL) of juice.

Horse Chestnut

Aesculus hippocastanum

A large tree common in North America and southeastern Europe with palmate leaves and long spikes of white flowers that appear in the spring. Globular green-brown spiny fruits replace flowers in summer.

Parts Used
Bark and seeds.

Healing Properties

Actions: Astringent, anti-inflammatory, circulatory tonic, strengthens and tones veins.
Uses: Varicose veins, hemorrhoids, phlebitis. Horse chestnut tea can be used externally to treat bruises and leg ulcers.

Availability

Dried bark and seeds are available in alternative/health stores.

How to Use in Juicing

Infusion: In a teapot, pour ¼ cup (50 mL) boiling water over ½ tsp (2 mL) lightly crushed bark and seeds. Steep with lid on 15 minutes. Strain, discard herb, and add liquid to 1 cup (250 mL) of juice.
Tincture: Add 30 drops to 1 cup (250 mL) of juice.

Hyssop

Hyssopus officinalis

A bushy evergreen woody perennial native to central and southern Europe, western Asia and northern Africa. The square, upright stems have linear opposite leaves and dense spikes at the tops that bear whorls of purple flowers.

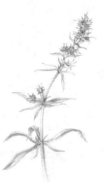

Parts Used

Leaves and flowering tops.

Healing Properties

Actions: Antispasmodic, expectorant, diaphoretic, mild pain reliever, diuretic, antiviral against herpes simplex, reduces phlegm, soothing digestive.
Uses: Asthma, bronchitis, colds, coughs, influenza, fevers, flatulence.

Availability

Hyssop is easy to grow and can be harvested from May through fall in central and northern North America. Dried leaves are available in alternative/health stores.

How to Use in Juicing

Whole fresh sprigs: Roll in a ball and feed through tube along with other ingredients. Use 4 to 6 sprigs for each 1 cup (250 mL) of juice.
Dried leaf and flowers: Crush to a fine powder and whisk into fresh juice or add to ingredients in blended drinks. Use 1 tsp (5 mL) for each 1 cup (250 mL) of juice.

Kava Kava

Piper methysticum

An evergreen shrub grown and used in Polynesia that belongs to the pepper (*Piper*) genus of plants.

Parts Used

Root and rhizome.

Healing Properties

Actions: Antimicrobial, especially to the genitourinary system; antispasmodic; nerve and muscle relaxant; diuretic; stimulant.
Uses: Stress; anxiety; chronic fatigue syndrome; fibromyalgia; insomnia; infections of the kidneys, bladder, vagina, prostate or urethra.

Caution

Do not use kava kava if you are pregnant or breastfeeding. Consult with your health-care practitioner before taking kava kava with other drugs that act on the nervous system. Do not take for a period of more than three months unless advised to do so by your health-care practitioner. Do not drive or operate heavy machinery while taking kava kava and do not use if you drink alcohol or take drugs that affect the liver.

Availability

Dried root and liquid extracts are available in alternative/health stores.

How to Use in Juicing

Decoction: In a small saucepan, combine ½ cup (125 mL) boiling water with 1 tsp (5 mL) dried root. Simmer with lid on for 10 minutes or until decoction is colored light brown. Strain, discard herb, and add liquid to 1 cup (250 mL) of juice.
Liquid extract: Add ½ to 1 tsp (2 to 5 mL) to 1 cup (250 mL) of juice.

Lavender

Lavandula spp

A shrub-like plant with dense, woody stems from which linear pine-like gray-green leaves grow. Whorls of tiny flowers grow on spikes that branch off the long stems.

Parts Used

Leaves, stems and flowering tops.

Healing Properties

Actions: Relaxant, antispasmodic, antidepressant, nervous system tonic, circulatory stimulant, antibacterial, antiseptic, carminative, promotes bile flow.
Uses: Colic, depression, exhaustion, indigestion, insomnia, stress, tension headaches.

Caution

Avoid large doses if you are pregnant because it is a uterine stimulant.

Availability

Easily grown in temperate climates, lavender can be harvested from June through fall. Dried flower buds are available at alternative/health stores.

How to Use in Juicing

Whole fresh flowers: Feed through tube along with other ingredients. Use 2 to 4 sprigs for each 1 cup (250 mL) of juice.
Dried flowers: Crush to a fine powder and whisk into fresh juice or add to ingredients in blended drinks. Use 1 tsp (5 mL) for each 1 cup (250 mL) of juice.
Infusion: In a teapot, pour ¼ cup (50 mL) boiling water over 1 tbsp (15 mL) fresh or 1 tsp (5 mL) dried flower buds. Steep for 15 minutes. Strain, discard herb, and add liquid to 1 cup (250 mL) of juice.

Lemon Balm

Melissa officinalis

A bushy perennial with strongly lemon-scented opposite oval leaves that grow on thin, square stems. White or yellow tubular flowers grow in clusters at the base of the leaves.

Parts Used

Leaves and flowering tops.

Healing Properties

Actions: Antioxidant, antihistamine, carminative, antispasmodic, antiviral, antibacterial, nerve relaxant, antidepressant, stimulates bile flow, hypotensive.
Uses: Anxiety, depression, stress, flatulence, indigestion, insomnia.

Availability

An easily grown perennial, lemon balm leaves and flowers can be harvested from June through autumn. Dried leaves are available in alternative/health stores.

How to Use in Juicing

Whole fresh sprigs: Roll in a ball and feed through tube along with other ingredients. Use 4 to 6 sprigs for each 1 cup (250 mL) of juice.
Dried leaf and flowers: Crush to a fine powder and whisk into fresh juice or add to blended drinks, use 1 tsp (5 mL) for each 1 cup (250 mL) of juice.
Infusion: In a teapot, pour ¼ cup (50 mL) boiling water over 1 tbsp (15 mL) fresh or 1 tsp (5 mL) dried lemon balm. Steep for 10 minutes. Strain, discard herb, and add liquid to 1 cup (250 mL) of juice.

Lemon Verbena

Aloysia triphylla

A fast-growing deciduous shrub native to South America that grows to a height of over six feet (180 cm) in zones 8 to 10. Long, pointed green leaves grow on erect stems that grow out of green-to-brown bark and turn woody when mature. Tiny lavender-colored flowers grow in spikes.

Parts Used

Leaves.

Healing Properties

Actions: Antispasmodic, digestive.
Uses: Indigestion, flatulence.

Availability

Dried leaves may be available in alternative/health stores.

How to Use in Juicing

Whole fresh sprigs: Roll in a ball and feed through tube along with other ingredients. Use 4 to 6 sprigs for each 1 cup (250 mL) of juice.
Dried leaf: Crush to a fine powder and whisk into fresh juice or add to ingredients in blended drinks. Use 1 tsp (5 mL) for each 1 cup (250 mL) of juice.
Infusion: In a teapot, pour ¼ cup (50 mL) boiling water over 1 tsp (5 mL) dried or 1 tbsp (15 mL) fresh, bruised leaves. Steep for 10 minutes. Strain, discard herb, and add liquid to 1 cup (250 mL) of juice.

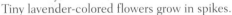

Licorice

Glycyrrhiza glabra

A tender perennial, native to the Mediterranean region and southwest Asia.

Parts Used
Root.

Healing Properties
Actions: Gentle laxative, tonic, anti-inflammatory, antibacterial, anti-arthritic, soothes gastric and intestinal mucous membranes, expectorant.

Uses: Licorice root is considered one of the best tonic herbs because it provides nutrients to almost all body systems. It detoxifies, regulates blood sugar level and recharges depleted adrenal glands. It has also been shown to heal peptic ulcers, soothe irritated membranes and loosen and expel phlegm in the upper respiratory tract. It is also used to treat sore throats, urinary tract infections, coughs, bronchitis, gastritis and constipation.

Caution
Large amounts taken over long periods of time may cause fluid retention and lower blood potassium levels. Avoid if you have high blood pressure.

Availability
Whole or ground dried root is available in alternative/health stores.
Note: Extracts lack the tonic action.

How to Use in Juicing
Decoction: Gently simmer 1 tsp (5 mL) chopped dried root in ¼ cup (50 mL) of water for 10 minutes. Strain and add to 1 cup (250 mL) of juice.

Linden Flower

(Lime Flowers) *Tilia cordata* or *T. eurpoea*

A deciduous tree with shiny dark green heart-shaped leaves and yellow-white flowers that appear in midsummer. Found throughout northern temperate regions, linden is often grown as an ornamental in North American cities.

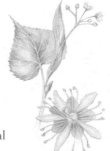

Parts Used
Leaves and flowering tops.

Healing Properties
Actions: Antispasmodic, diaphoretic (hot tea), diuretic (warm tea), hypotensive, relaxant, mild astringent.

Uses: Linden flower tea is a pleasant-tasting, relaxing remedy for stress, anxiety, tension headache and insomnia. It relaxes and nourishes blood vessels, making it a useful treatment for high blood pressure and heart disease. Because it promotes sweating, it is helpful in treating colds, flu and fevers. The tea can be given to children as a calming remedy or to reduce fever.

Availability
Harvest flowers in mid-June and leaves from early summer through fall. Dried leaves and flowers are available in alternative/health stores. Linden tea bags are often available in supermarkets.

How to Use in Juicing
Dried leaf and flowers: Part of linden's actions are due to its essential oils, which are only released with heat. For this reason, dried or fresh linden is not added to juices except as a cooled tea.

Infusion: In a teapot, pour ¼ cup (50 mL) boiling water over 1 tbsp (15 mL) fresh or dried flowering tops; steep for 10 minutes. Strain, discard herb, and add liquid to 1 cup (250 mL) of juice.

Marshmallow

Althaea officinalis

A robust perennial with a fleshy taproot and upright stems that bear toothed oval leaves and pale pink flowers. Marshmallow is partial to wet ground and is often found in the wild in the United States, southern Canada, western Europe, central Asia and northern Africa. Hollyhock (*A. rosea*) is in the same genus.

Parts Used
Flowers, leaves and root.

Healing Properties
Actions: (Root and leaves) Soothes mucous membranes; diuretic; expectorant; soothes, cleanses and heals external wounds. (Flower) Expectorant.

Uses: The high mucilage content of marshmallow root makes it useful for soothing inflammation in the digestive tract, kidneys and bladder; peptic ulcers; ulcerative colitis; Crohn's disease; urethritis; hiatal hernia; cystitis; diarrhea; and gastritis. Marshmallow leaves are used to treat bronchial inflammations, such as bronchitis, and in teas for internal ulcerative conditions. Marshmallow flower is used in expectorant cough syrups.

Availability
Gather leaves and flowers from mid-June through fall and harvest roots in the fall. Dried root is available in alternative/health stores.

How to Use in Juicing
Whole fresh sprigs: Roll in a ball and feed through tube along with other ingredients. Use 4 to 6 sprigs for each 1 cup (250 mL) of juice.

Dried leaf and flowers: Crush to a fine powder and whisk into fresh juice or add to ingredients in blended drinks. Use 1 tsp (5 mL) for each 1 cup (250 mL) of juice.

Infusion: In a teapot, pour ¼ cup (50 mL) boiling water over 1 tbsp (15 mL) fresh or 1 tsp (5 mL) dried aerial parts. Steep for 10 minutes. Strain, discard herb, and add liquid to 1 cup (250 mL) of juice.

Whole fresh root: Feed through tube along with other ingredients. Use a 2- to 3-inch (5 to 7.5 cm) piece for each 1 cup (250 mL) of juice.

Decoction: In a small saucepan, pour ¼ cup (50 mL) of water over 1 tsp (5 mL) chopped dried root. Stand overnight. Strain, discard herb, and add liquid to 1 cup (250 mL) of juice.

Tincture: Add 10 to 20 drops to 1 cup (250 mL) of juice.

Meadowsweet

Filipendula ulmaria

A hardy herbaceous perennial found in moist or boggy soils throughout Europe, North America and temperate Asia. Toothed pinnate leaves grow on upright stems. Creamy white almond-scented flowers appear from midsummer to early autumn.

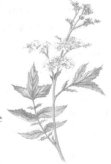

Parts Used
Aerial parts (stem, leaves and flowers).

Healing Properties
Actions: Antacid, anti-inflammatory, anticoagulant, astringent, antirheumatic, diuretic, liver supportive, diaphoretic.

Uses: The anti-inflammatory and antacid actions of meadowsweet are useful in treating rheumatoid arthritis, cystitis, peptic ulcer, hyperacidity and gastric reflux. As an astringent, it is used to treat some types of diarrhea. Meadowsweet contains salicylic acid and can be used instead of Aspirin as an anti-inflammatory. Because it protects the mucous membranes of the digestive tract, unlike Aspirin, long-term use does not cause stomach bleeding.

Availability
Harvest leaves and flowers from mid-July through fall. Dried leaves and flowers are available in alternative/health stores.

How to Use in Juicing
Dried leaf and flowers: Crush to a fine powder and whisk into fresh juice or add to ingredients in blended drinks. Use 1 tsp (5 mL) for each 1 cup (250 mL) of juice.

Infusion: In a teapot, pour ¼ cup (50 mL) boiling water over 1 tbsp (15 mL) fresh or 1 tsp (5 mL) dried aerial parts. Steep for 15 minutes. Strain, discard herb, and add liquid to 1 cup (250 mL) of juice.

Tincture: Add 40 drops to 1 cup (250 mL) of juice.

Milk Thistle

Silybum marianus

One of two species in this genus (Blessed Thistle is the other), milk thistle is a stout annual or biennial with large oblong leaves and purple flowers. Black seeds, each bearing a tuft of white hairs, appear in mid- to late summer.

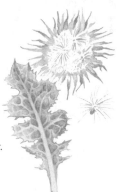

Parts Used
Seeds.

Healing Properties
Actions: Antioxidant, promotes bile production and flow, protects the liver by promoting development of new liver cells and repairing existing liver cells, detoxifies, increases milk in breastfeeding.

Uses: Milk thistle's strong liver-protective action is important in treating diseases such as alcoholism, cirrhosis and hepatitis, as well as in chronic conditions that cause liver congestion, such as constipation, bloating and premenstrual syndrome.

Availability

Seeds may be collected in the wild in midsummer but are widely available in alternative/health stores.

How to Use in Juicing

Dried seeds: Crush to a fine powder and whisk into fresh juice or add to ingredients in blended drinks. Use 1 tsp (5 mL) for each 1 cup (250 mL) of juice.
Infusion: In a teapot, pour ¼ cup (50 mL) boiling water over 1 tsp (5 mL) dried ground seeds. Steep for 15 minutes. Strain, discard herb, and add liquid to 1 cup (250 mL) of juice.
Tincture: Add 10 to 20 drops to 1 cup (250 mL) of juice.

Motherwort

Leonurus cardiaca

A strong-smelling perennial found throughout temperate Europe, Asia and North America. Deeply lobed palmate leaves grow out of purple stems. Mauve-pink to white flowers grow in whorls from single stems from midsummer to mid-autumn.

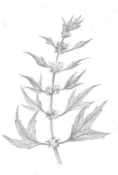

Parts Used

Aerial parts (stem, leaves and flowers).

Healing Properties

Actions: Antispasmodic, nerve and heart sedative, hypotensive, uterine stimulant.
Uses: Motherwort has long been used to ease menstrual pain. It eases hot flashes and other menopausal symptoms, as well as the anxiety associated with premenstrual syndrome. As a heart tonic, motherwort is especially useful for palpitations and other heart conditions in which anxiety and tension play a part. Its relaxing action makes it helpful in reducing withdrawal symptoms from antidepressant drugs.

Caution

Do not take if you are pregnant or during heavy menstrual bleeding.

Availability

Gather aerial parts (stem, leaves and flowers) from midsummer to mid-fall. Dried leaves and flowers are available in alternative/health stores.

How to Use in Juicing

Whole fresh sprigs: Roll in a ball and feed through tube along with other ingredients. Use 4 to 6 sprigs for each 1 cup (250 mL) of juice.

Dried leaf and flowers: Crush to a fine powder and whisk into fresh juice or add to ingredients in blended drinks. Use 1 tsp (5 mL) for each 1 cup (250 mL) of juice.
Infusion: In a teapot, pour ¼ cup (50 mL) boiling water over 1 tbsp (15 mL) fresh or 1 tsp (5 mL) dried motherwort. Steep for 15 minutes. Strain, discard herb, and add liquid to 1 cup (250 mL) of juice.
Tincture: Add 1 tsp (5 mL) to 1 cup (250 mL) of juice.

Nutmeg

Myristica fragrans

A bushy evergreen tree native to the tropical rain forests in the Moluccas and the Banda Islands that is now grown commercially in Asia, Australia, Indonesia and Sri Lanka. Pale yellow flowers produced in axillary clusters are followed by fleshy yellow globe- to pear-shaped fruits (generally called seeds).

Parts Used

Dried kernel of the nutmeg fruit.

Healing Properties

Actions: Anti-inflammatory, antispasmodic, carminative, digestive stimulant, sedative.
Uses: Colic, diarrhea, flatulence, nausea, vomiting, muscle tension.

Caution

Do not use in medicinal doses if you are pregnant, as nutmeg has strong volatile oil components.

Availability

Whole, dried nutmeg seeds are available in alternative/health stores, specialty stores and many supermarkets. Ground nutmeg is widely available.

How to Use in Juicing

Dried seeds: Grate to a fine powder and whisk into juice or add to ingredients in blended drinks. Use ¼ tsp (1 mL) per serving.

Oats

Avena sativa

A grain commonly grown throughout North America.

Parts Used
All, including seeds.

Healing Properties
Actions: Antioxidant, nerve restorative, antidepressant, nourishes brain and nerves, improves stamina, can increase libido if taken regularly.
Uses: Anxiety, depression, stress, withdrawal from alcohol and antidepressant drugs.

Availability
Oat seeds, oat straw and oatmeal are available at alternative/health stores. Oatmeal is available in supermarkets.

How to Use in Juicing
Dried seeds, leaf and straw: Crush to a fine powder and add to ingredients in blended drinks. Use 1 tsp (5 mL) per serving.
Infusion: In a teapot, pour ¼ cup (50 mL) boiling water over 1 tsp (5 mL) dried oat straw or seed. Steep for 15 minutes. Strain, discard herb, and add liquid to 1 cup (250 mL) of juice.

Oregon Grape

Berberis aquifolium

Also called mountain grape, Oregon grape is the state flower of Oregon. It bears holly-like leaves and bright yellow flowers that mature into grape-like berry clusters. It grows in the mountainous regions of the West Coast of the United States and southern British Columbia.

Parts Used
Root and rhizome.

Healing Properties
Actions: Laxative; blood tonic; increases bile flow; liver stimulant; digestive; antimicrobial in the digestive tract; stimulates salivary and stomach secretions, including hydrochloric acid.
Uses: Eczema, psoriasis, constipation, indigestion, liver and gallbladder problems, gum and tooth problems.

Availability
Dried root and powdered dried root are available in alternative/health stores or by mail order.

How to Use in Juicing
Powder: Whisk ¼ to ½ tsp (1 to 2 mL) powdered, dried root into 1 cup (250 mL) of juice or add to ingredients in blended drinks.
Decoction: In a small saucepan, combine ¼ cup (50 mL) boiling water and 1 dried root stick or ¼ to ½ tsp (1 to 2 mL) dried chopped root. Simmer with lid on for 20 minutes. Steep for 10 minutes. Strain, discard herb, and add liquid to 1 cup (250 mL) of juice.

Parsley

Petroselinum crispum

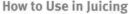

A hardy biennial native to the Mediterranean and grown as an annual in colder climates.

Parts Used
Leaves, stems and root.

Healing Properties
Actions: Antioxidant, tonic, digestive, diuretic.
Uses: As a diuretic, parsley helps the body expel excess water and flush the kidneys. Always look for and treat underlying causes of water retention. Parsley is one of the richest food sources of vitamin C.

Caution
Do not take large doses of parsley if you are pregnant because it is a uterine stimulant. Parsley is also contraindicated if you are suffering from kidney inflammation.

Availability
Fresh sprigs are available in most supermarkets year-round.

How to Use in Juicing
Whole fresh leaves: Roll in a ball and feed through tube along with other ingredients. Use 6 sprigs for each 1 cup (250 mL) of juice.
Dried leaf: Whisk 1 tsp (5 mL) powdered, dried leaf into 1 cup (250 mL) of juice or add to ingredients in blended drinks.
Infusion: In a teapot, pour ¼ cup (50 mL) boiling water over 1 tbsp (15 mL) fresh or 1 tsp (5 mL) dried parsley. Steep for 10 minutes. Strain, discard herb, and add liquid to 1 cup (250 mL) of juice.

Passionflower

Passiflora incarnata

A perennial climbing vine with deeply lobed leaves and showy, fragrant, white-to-purple flowers. Some 350 species of passionflower are native to the southeastern United States and Mexico. Other species grow in tropical Asia and Australia.

Parts Used

Leaves and flowers.

Healing Properties

Actions: Antispasmodic, mild sedative, mild pain reliever, central nervous system relaxant.
Uses: Anxiety, asthma, insomnia, restlessness, headache, Parkinson's disease, withdrawal from antidepressant drugs and alcohol.

Availability

Passionflower can be harvested from May through July in the wild or in cultivated gardens. Dried passionflower is available in alternative/health stores.

How to Use in Juicing

Dried leaf and flowers: Crush to a fine powder and whisk into fresh juice. Use ¼ tsp (1 mL) for each 1 cup (250 mL) of juice.
Infusion: In a teapot, pour ¼ cup (50 mL) boiling water over 1 tbsp (15 mL) fresh or ½ tsp (2 mL) dried passionflower. Steep for 15 minutes. Strain, discard herb, and add liquid to 1 cup (250 mL) of juice.
Tincture: Add 40 drops to 1 cup (250 mL) of juice.

Peppermint

Mentha piperita

An invasive hardy perennial native to Europe and Asia but easily grown in North America. It has aromatic bright green oval leaves on purple stems and small pink, white or purple flowers in elongated conical spikes at the tops of the stems.

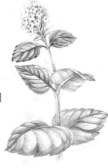

Parts Used

Leaves and flowers.

Healing Properties

Actions: Antispasmodic, digestive tonic, anti-emetic, carminative, peripheral vasodilator, diaphoretic, promotes bile flow, analgesic.
Uses: Taking peppermint before eating helps stimulate the liver and gallbladder by increasing bile flow to the liver and intestines. It is well known for its ability to quell nausea and vomiting. Peppermint is used to treat ulcerative colitis, Crohn's disease, diverticular disease, motion sickness, fevers, colds and flu, and to improve appetite.

Caution

Do not use if you are pregnant or give to a child.

Availability

Fresh sprigs appear in some farmer's markets and supermarkets year-round. Dried leaves are available in alternative/health stores. Peppermint tea in bulk and bags is widely available.

How to Use in Juicing

Whole fresh leaves: Roll in a ball and feed through tube along with other ingredients. Use 6 sprigs for each 1 cup (250 mL) of juice.
Dried leaf: Whisk 1 tsp (5 mL) powdered dried leaf into 1 cup (250 mL) of juice.
Infusion: In a teapot, pour ¼ cup (50 mL) boiling water over 1 tbsp (15 mL) fresh or 1 tsp (5 mL) dried peppermint. Steep for 10 minutes. Strain, discard herb, and add liquid to 1 cup (250 mL) of juice.

Plantain

Plantago major and *P. lanceolata*

Broad-leaved plantain and narrow-leaved plantain are common weeds found in waste areas throughout North America. Leaves grow in a basal rosette, and flowers top long cylindrical spikes that grow up to six inches (15 cm) above leaves.

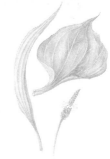

Parts Used

Leaves.

Healing Properties

Actions: Antibacterial, soothing expectorant, provides mucilage-rich protection to digestive tract, nutrient, antihistamine, astringent.
Uses: Coughs, bronchitis, allergies, irritable bowel syndrome, gastric ulcers.

Availability

The leaves can be collected throughout the summer. Dried leaves are available in alternative/health stores.

How to Use in Juicing

Whole fresh leaves: Roll in a ball and feed through tube along with other ingredients. Use 2 to 4 leaves for each 1 cup (250 mL) of juice.

Infusion: In a teapot, pour ¼ cup (50 mL) boiling water over 1 tbsp fresh (15 mL) or 1 tsp (5 mL) dried leaves. Steep for 15 minutes. Strain, discard herb, and add liquid to 1 cup (250 mL) of juice.

Psyllium

Plantago psyllium

The mucilage-rich seeds of *Plantago psyllium* (native to the Mediterranean) are similar to those of broad-leaved plantain (plantago major), common in Europe and naturalized in North America.

Parts Used

Seeds.

Healing Properties

Actions: Soothing, digestive, safe and gentle laxative, cholesterol-lowering

Uses: Constipation, irritable bowel syndrome, diverticular disease, detoxification, and obesity. The seeds act as a laxative by bulking-up the stool and lubricating the bowel. It is necessary to drink at least one large glass of water when taking 1 to 2 tsp (5 to 10 mL) of the seeds. Drink another 8 glasses of water throughout the day.

Availability

Psyllium seeds are widely available in pharmacies and health/alternative stores.

How to Use in Juicing

Whole seeds: Whisk 1 to 2 tsp (5 to 10 mL) seeds into 1 cup (250 mL) fresh juice or blended drink and drink immediately before they can absorb the moisture. Drink one large glass of water and eight more glasses over the course of the day.

Caution

Psyllium can cause an allergic reaction in sensitive individuals; discontinue immediately if a reaction develops. It should be avoided by asthmatics. Psyllium must not be taken in cases of bowel obstruction.

Red Clover

Trifolium pratense

A perennial with tubular pink-to-red flowers throughout the summer, red clover grows in fields throughout North America. Its three long oval leaflets distinguish it as a clover.

Parts Used

Flowering tops.

Healing Properties

Actions: Antispasmodic, expectorant, balances hormones, nutritive, anticoagulant, lymphatic cleanser.

Uses: Coughs, bronchitis, whooping cough, menstrual problems.

Caution

Because it helps thin the blood, don't use red clover during heavy menstrual flow.

Availability

The flowering tops can be harvested from May through September in the wild or in cultivated gardens. Dried flowers are available in alternative/health stores. Dried clover that has turned brown is of little use; be sure that the flowers are still pink.

How to Use in Juicing

Whole fresh sprigs: Roll flowering tops in a ball and feed through tube along with other ingredients. Use about 6 sprigs for each 1 cup (250 mL) of juice.

Dried leaf and flowers: Crush to a fine powder and whisk into fresh juice. Use 1 tsp (5 mL) for each 1 cup (250 mL) of juice.

Infusion: In a teapot, pour ¼ cup (50 mL) boiling water over 1 tbsp (15 mL) fresh or 1 tsp (5 mL) dried red clover. Steep for 15 minutes. Strain, discard herb, and add liquid to 1 cup (250 mL) of juice.

Red Raspberry

Rubus idaeus

A deciduous shrub with prickly stems and pinnately divided leaves that is widespread in Europe, Asia and North America. Small white flowers appear in clusters, and aromatic, juicy red fruit follow in early summer.

Parts Used

Leaves.

Healing Properties

Actions: Antispasmodic, astringent, increases milk in breastfeeding.

Uses: Red raspberry leaves have long been used to tone the uterus during pregnancy and labor, resulting in less risk of miscarriage, relief of morning sickness and safer, easier birth. As an astringent, raspberry leaves ease sore throat and diarrhea.

Availability

Harvest leaves from early summer through fall. Dried leaves are available in alternative/health stores.

How to Use in Juicing

Whole fresh leaves: Roll in a ball and feed through tube along with other ingredients. Use about 6 leaves for each 1 cup (250 mL) of juice.

Dried leaf: Crush to a fine powder and whisk into fresh juice or add to ingredients in blended drinks, use 1 tsp (5 mL) for each 1 cup (250 mL) of juice.

Infusion: In a teapot, pour ¼ cup (50 mL) boiling water over 1 tbsp (15 mL) fresh or 2 tsp (10 mL) dried bruised leaf. Steep for 15 minutes. Strain, discard herb and add liquid to 1 cup (250 mL) of juice.

Rose

Rosa

Cultivation of roses dates back thousands of years, with *R. rugosa*, *R. gallica*, *R. rubra* and *R. damascena* being among the oldest varieties. *R. rugosa* is a deciduous shrub with thorny stems and dark green oval leaves; dark pink or white flowers appear in summer and are followed by large globular bright red rose hips (fruit). Wild roses (including *R. canina* of North America) grow in northern temperate regions throughout the world.

Parts Used

Petals and hips.

Healing Properties

Actions: (Rose hips from *R. canina*) Contain vitamin C, diuretic, astringent, mild laxative. (Rose petals from *R. gallica*, *R. damascena*, *R. centifolia*, *R. rugosa*) Antidepressant, anti-inflammatory, astringent, blood tonic.

Uses: (Rose hips) The nutrient value of rose hips makes them useful in preventing the common cold. A tasty addition to herbal teas, rose hips improve immune function. As an astringent, they are used to treat diarrhea. (Rose petals) Add them to teas for their relaxing and uplifting fragrance. Used in baths, they ease the pain of rheumatoid arthritis.

Availability

Harvest petals from midsummer through fall and hips in the fall from pesticide-free bushes.

How to Use in Juicing

Dried flowers or hips: Crush to a fine powder and whisk into fresh juice or add to ingredients in blended drinks. Use ½ tsp (2 mL) for each 1 cup (250 mL) of juice.

Infusion: In a teapot, pour ¼ cup (50 mL) boiling water over 1 tbsp (15 mL) fresh petals or chopped fresh hips or 1 tsp (5 mL) dried petals or crushed dried hips. Steep for 10 minutes. Strain, discard herb, and add liquid to 1 cup (250 mL) of juice.

Rosemary

Rosmarinus officinalis

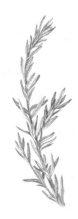

An evergreen shrub native to the Mediterranean that grows to a height of six feet (180 cm) in warm climates.

Parts Used

Leaves and flowers.

Healing Properties

Actions: Antioxidant, anti-inflammatory, astringent, nervine, carminative, antiseptic, diuretic, diaphoretic, promotes bile flow, antidepressant, circulatory stimulant, antispasmodic, nervous system and cardiac tonic.

Uses: An effective food preservative, rosemary may help prevent breast cancer and fight the deterioration of brain function. It is also useful in treating migraine and tension headaches, nervous tension, flatulence, depression, chronic fatigue syndrome and joint pain.

Caution

Do not take large amounts if you are pregnant, as rosemary contains strong volatile oil components.

Availability

Look for fresh sprigs in markets and supermarkets year-round. Dried whole and ground leaves are widely found in supermarkets and alternative/health stores.

How to Use in Juicing

Whole fresh leaves: Feed through tube along with other ingredients. Use 2 to 3 sprigs for each 1 cup (250 mL) of juice.

Infusion: In a teapot, pour $\frac{1}{4}$ cup (50 mL) boiling water over 1 tbsp (15 mL) fresh or 1 tsp (5 mL) dried rosemary. Steep for 10 minutes. Strain, discard herb, and add liquid to 1 cup (250 mL) of juice.

Sage

Salvia officinalis

A hardy evergreen woody perennial shrub native to the western United States and Mexico, with wrinkled gray-green oval leaves and purple, pink or white flowers.

Parts Used

Leaves and flowers.

Healing Properties

Actions: Antioxidant, antimicrobial, antibiotic, antiseptic, carminative, antispasmodic, anti-inflammatory, circulatory stimulant, estrogenic, peripheral vasodilator, reduces perspiration, uterine stimulant.

Uses: Sage's volatile oil kills bacteria and fungi — even those that are resistant to penicillin. It makes a very good gargle for sore throats, laryngitis and mouth ulcers. It is also used to reduce breast milk production and to relieve night sweats and hot flashes during menopause.

Caution

Sage can cause convulsions in very large doses. Do not use if you have high blood pressure or epilepsy or if you are pregnant.

Availability

Fresh sprigs can be found at some supermarkets and farmer's markets. Whole, rubbed or ground dried sage is available at most supermarkets.

How to Use in Juicing

Whole fresh leaves: Roll in a ball and feed through tube along with other ingredients. Use 3 to 4 sprigs for each 1 cup (250 mL) of juice.

Dried leaf and flowers: Crush to a fine powder and whisk into fresh juice or add to ingredients in blended drinks. Use $\frac{1}{2}$ tsp (2 mL) for each 1 cup (250 mL) of juice.

Infusion: In a teapot, pour $\frac{1}{4}$ cup (50 mL) boiling water over 1 tbsp (15 mL) fresh or 1 tsp (5 mL) dried sage. Steep for 10 minutes. Strain, discard herb, and add liquid to 1 cup (250 mL) of juice.

Saw Palmetto

Seranoa serrulata

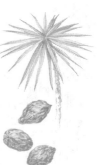

A clump-forming evergreen palm with long blue-green leaves and blue-black berries. It grows mainly along coastal areas of southeastern North America and forms dense thickets along the Atlantic coasts of Georgia and Florida.

Parts Used

Berries.

Healing Properties

Actions: Diuretic, urinary antiseptic, stimulates the hormone-secreting glands.

Uses: Benign prostate enlargement, low libido.

Availability

The berries can be harvested from September though January. Dried berries are available ground and in tablet form in alternative/health stores.

How to Use in Juicing

Powder: Whisk $\frac{1}{4}$ tsp (1 mL) powdered berries into 1 cup (250 mL) of juice or add to ingredients in blended drinks.

Infusion: In a teapot, pour $\frac{1}{4}$ cup (50 mL) boiling water over 1 tsp (5 mL) fresh or $\frac{1}{2}$ tsp (2 mL) dried lightly crushed berries. Steep for 10 minutes. Strain, discard herb, and add liquid to 1 cup (250 mL) of juice.

Liquid extract: Add 10 to 25 drops to 1 cup (250 mL) of juice.

Skullcap

Scutellaria laterifolia

A perennial member of the mint family that features hooded violet-blue flowers. It grows in wooded areas in most of the United States and southern Canada, except along the West Coast.

Parts Used
Aerial parts (stem, leaves and flowers).

Healing Properties
Actions: Antispasmodic, nourishes central nervous system, relaxant, sedative.
Uses: Drug addiction withdrawal, premenstrual tension, headaches, migraines, mental exhaustion, insomnia, stress.

Availability
Aerial parts (stem, leaves and flowers) can be collected while the plant is in flower. Dried skullcap is available in alternative/health stores.

How to Use in Juicing
Whole fresh sprigs: Roll in a ball and feed through tube along with other ingredients. Use 3 to 4 sprigs for each 1 cup (250 mL) of juice.
Dried leaf and flowers: Crush to a fine powder and whisk into fresh juice or add to ingredients in blended drinks. Use 1 tsp (5 mL) for each 1 cup (250 mL) of juice.
Infusion: In a teapot, pour ¼ cup (50 mL) boiling water over 1 tbsp (15 mL) fresh or 1 tsp (5 mL) dried skullcap. Steep for 10 minutes. Strain, discard herb, and add liquid to 1 cup (250 mL) of juice.
Tincture: Add 40 drops to 1 cup (250 mL) of juice.

Slippery Elm

Ulmus fulva

A deciduous tree found in moist woods in the eastern and midwestern United States and southeastern Canada.

Parts Used
Dried inner bark.

Healing Properties
Actions: Soothing digestive, antacid, nutritive, provides mucilage-rich protection to the digestive tract.
Uses: Peptic ulcers, indigestion, heartburn, hiatal hernia, Crohn's disease, ulcerative colitis, irritable bowel syndrome, diarrhea. A paste of slippery elm bark powder can be used to soothe and heal wounds and burns. It is one of the most useful herbs in herbal medicine.

Availability
Ground dried inner bark and lozenges are available in alternative/health stores.

How to Use in Juicing
Powder: Slippery elm powder does not blend easily into juices. It is best added to ingredients in blended drinks.
Infusion: In a teapot, pour ¼ cup (50 mL) boiling water over 1 tsp (5 mL) powdered slippery elm. Steep for 10 minutes. Add liquid to 1 cup (250 mL) of juice.

Spearmint

Mentha spicata

A hardy invasive perennial found in wet soil in most of North America. Like all mints, it has a square stem with bright green lanceolate leaves and lilac, pink, or white flowers that form in a terminal, cylindrical spike.

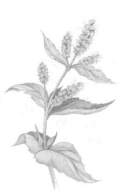

Parts Used
Leaves and flowering tops.

Healing Properties
Actions: Antispasmodic, digestive, diaphoretic.
Uses: Common cold, influenza, indigestion, flatulence, lack of appetite. Spearmint is milder than peppermint, so it is often used to treat children's colds and flus.

Availability
The leaves are best harvested just before the flowers open. Dried leaves are available in alternative/health stores.

How to Use in Juicing
Whole fresh sprigs: Roll in a ball and feed through tube along with other ingredients. Use 4 to 6 sprigs for each 1 cup (250 mL) of juice.
Dried leaf and flowers: Crush to a fine powder and whisk into fresh juice or add to ingredients in blended drinks. Use ½ tsp (2 mL) for each 1 cup (250 mL) of juice.
Infusion: In a teapot, pour ¼ cup (50 mL) boiling water over 1 tbsp (15 mL) fresh or 1 tsp (5 mL) dried spearmint. Steep for 10 minutes. Strain, discard herb, and add liquid to 1 cup (250 mL) of juice.

St. John's Wort

Hypericum perforatum

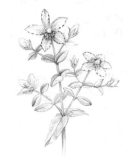

A perennial native of woodlands in Europe and temperate Asia that has also naturalized in temperate areas of the United States and Canada. It is an upright plant with straight stems that are woody at the base and has five-petaled yellow flowers growing from the tips of the branched stems. When rubbed, the yellow petals stain the fingers red.

Parts Used
Flowering tops.

Healing Properties
Actions: Astringent, antiviral, anti-inflammatory, antidepressant, nervous system tonic, sedative.
Uses: St. John's wort is widely used as an antidepressant. It has become popular because of its effectiveness and lack of side effects. As a sedative and nervous-system tonic, it is useful in treating neuralgia, shingles, sciatica, tension, anxiety, and emotional instability in premenstrual syndrome and menopause.

Caution
Recent studies suggest that St. John's wort increases the metabolism of certain drugs, reducing their effectiveness. If you are taking prescription drugs, consult with your herbalist, doctor or pharmacist about possible drug interactions before taking St. John's wort. Of particular concern are oral contraceptives, anticonvulsants, antidepressants (especially selective serotonin reuptake inhibitors), HIV drugs, anticoagulants (warfarin), cyclosporine (an immunosuppressant drug given after transplants) and digoxin.

Availability
Harvest flowering tops for two to three weeks in midsummer. Dried aerial parts (stem, leaves and flowers) and tinctures are available in alternative/health stores.

How to Use in Juicing
Dried leaf and flowers: Crush to a fine powder and whisk into fresh juice or add to ingredients in blended drinks. Use 1 tsp (5 mL) for each 1 cup (250 mL) of juice.
Infusion: In a teapot, pour ¼ cup (50 mL) boiling water over 1 tbsp (15 mL) fresh or 1 tsp (5 mL) dried St. John's wort. Steep for 15 minutes. Strain, discard herb, and add liquid to 1 cup (250 mL) of juice.
Tincture: Add 20 to 40 drops to 1 cup (250 mL) of juice.

Stevia

Stevia rebaudiana

A small tender shrub native to northeastern Paraguay and adjacent areas of Brazil.

Parts Used
Leaves.

Healing Properties
Actions: Energy booster, natural sweetener (without calories), tonic, digestive, diuretic.
Uses: Stevia's main benefit is that it is a safe sweetener and sugar alternative. With its powerful sweet licorice flavor (stevia is 200 to 300 times sweeter than sugar), it prevents cavities and does not trigger a rise in blood sugar. It increases energy and improves digestion by stimulating the pancreas without feeding yeast or fungi.

Availability
Cut and dried ground leaves and liquid extracts are available in alternative/health stores.

How to Use in Juicing
Whole fresh leaves: Roll in a ball and feed through tube along with other ingredients. Use 2 to 3 leaves for each 1 cup (250 mL) of juice.
Dried leaf: Whisk ⅛ tsp (0.5 mL) powdered, dried leaf into 1 cup (250 mL) of juice where required.
Infusion: In a teapot, pour ¼ cup (50 mL) boiling water over 1 tsp (5 mL) fresh or ¼ tsp (1 mL) dried stevia. steep for 10 minutes. Strain, discard herb, and add liquid to 1 cup (250 mL) of juice.
Liquid extract: Add 1 to 2 drops to 1 cup (250 mL) of juice.

Stinging Nettle

Urtica dioica

A perennial widespread in temperate regions of Europe, North America and Eurasia with bristly stinging hairs on the stems and toothed ovate leaves that cause minor skin irritation when touched.

Minute green flowers appear in clusters during the summer.

Parts Used
Leaves, root and seeds.

Healing Properties
Actions: (Leaves and flowers) Astringent, blood tonic, circulatory stimulant, diuretic, eliminates uric acid from the body, nutritive (high in iron, chlorophyll and vitamin C), increases milk in breastfeeding. (Fresh root) Astringent, diuretic.
Uses: (Leaves and flowers) A valuable herb, stinging nettle is useful as a general, everyday nourishing tonic, as well as for treatment of iron-deficiency anemia, gout, arthritis and kidney stones. It is also a good blood tonic to take during pregnancy or if you have diabetes, poor circulation or a chronic skin disease, such as eczema. (Fresh root) Fresh stinging nettle root has a strong effect on the urinary system. It is useful in treating water retention, kidney stones, urinary tract infections, cystitis, prostatitis and prostate enlargement.

Availability
Gather leaves and flowers while flowering in summer and root in fall. Use gloves to protect your hands from its uric acid, which dissipates with drying or cooking. Dried leaves and flowers are available in alternative/health stores.

How to Use in Juicing
Infusion: In a teapot, pour ¼ cup (50 mL) boiling water over 1 tbsp (15 mL) fresh or 1 tsp (5 mL) dried nettles. Steep for 15 minutes. Strain, discard herb, and add liquid to 1 cup (250 mL) of juice. Note: The sting dissipates when nettles are cooked or infused with boiling water.
Tincture: Add 1 tsp (5 mL) to 1 cup (250 mL) of juice.

Thyme

Thymus

A bushy low-growing shrub easily grown in North America.

Parts Used
Leaves and flowers.

Healing Properties
Actions: Antioxidant, expectorant, antiseptic, antispasmodic, astringent, tonic, antimicrobial, antibiotic, heals wounds, carminative, calms coughs, nervine.
Uses: Thyme is ideal for deep-seated chest infections, such as chronic coughs and bronchitis. It is also used to treat sinusitis, laryngitis, asthma and irritable bowel syndrome.

Caution
Do not take if you are pregnant. Children under two years of age and people with thyroid problems should not take thyme.

Availability
Fresh sprigs are available in season at farmer's markets and most supermarkets year-round. Dried whole leaves can be found in alternative/health stores.

How to Use in Juicing
Whole fresh leaves: Feed through tube along with other ingredients. Use 6 tender sprigs for each 1 cup (250 mL) of juice.
Dried leaf: Whisk ½ tsp (2 mL) powdered, dried leaf into 1 cup (250 mL) of juice or add to ingredients in blended drinks.
Infusion: In a teapot, pour ¼ cup (50 mL) boiling water over 1 tbsp (15 mL) fresh or 1 tsp (5 mL) dried thyme. Steep for 15 minutes. Strain, discard herb and add liquid to 1 cup (250 mL) of juice.

Turmeric

Curcuma longa

A deciduous tender perennial in the ginger family native to southeast Asia that is hardy to zone 10. The long rhizome resembles ginger but is thinner and rounder, with brilliant orange flesh.

Parts Used
Root.

Healing Properties
Actions: Antioxidant, anti-inflammatory, antimicrobial, antibacterial, antifungal, antiviral, anticoagulant, analgesic, lowers blood cholesterol, reduces postexercise pain, heals wounds, antispasmodic, protects liver cells, increases bile production and flow.

Uses: Turmeric appears to inhibit colon and breast cancer and is used to treat hepatitis, nausea and digestive disturbances. It also helps people whose gallbladders have been removed. It boosts insulin activity and reduces the risk of stroke. Turmeric is also used to treat rheumatoid arthritis, cancer, candida, AIDS, Crohn's disease and eczema.

Availability
Asian stores stock fresh, frozen or dried whole rhizomes. Alternative/health stores offer dried whole rhizomes, and supermarkets sell ground turmeric.

How to Use in Juicing
Whole fresh root: Feed through tube along with other ingredients. Use ½- to 1-inch (1 to 2.5 cm) pieces for each 1 cup (250 mL) of juice. Leave peel on if organic.
Powder: Whisk 1 tsp (5 mL) powdered, dried root into 1 cup (250 mL) of juice or add to ingredients in blended drinks.
Infusion: In a teapot, pour ¼ cup (50 mL) boiling water over 1 tbsp (15 mL) freshly grated or 1 tsp (5 mL) dried turmeric. Steep for 10 minutes. Strain, discard herb, and add liquid to 1 cup (250 mL) of juice.

Valerian

Valeriana officinalis

A tall hardy perennial with strong-smelling white clustered flowers that grows wild in eastern Canada and the northeastern United States.

Parts Used
Root.

Healing Properties
Actions: Sedative, relaxant, antispasmodic.
Uses: High blood pressure, insomnia, anxiety, tension headaches, muscle cramps, migraines.

Caution
Some people experience adverse reactions to valerian.

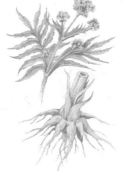

Availability
Roots can be harvested in late fall in the wild or in cultivated gardens. Dried roots and tinctures are available in alternative/health stores.

How to Use in Juicing
Whole fresh root: Because they're tiny and thin, fresh roots are difficult to feed through a juice machine. Instead, make a decoction, and add it to fresh juice.
Decoction: In a small saucepan, combine ¼ cup (50 mL) boiling water and 1 tbsp (15 mL) fresh chopped root or 1 tsp (5 mL) dried chopped root. Simmer with lid on 10 minutes. Steep 10 minutes. Strain, discard herb, and add liquid to 1 cup (250 mL) of juice.
Tincture: Add 20 to 40 drops to 1 cup (250 mL) of juice.

Vitex

(Chaste Tree) *Vitex agnus-castus*

A deciduous aromatic shrub or small tree, native to southern Europe. Grown in temperate climates (zones 7 to 10), chaste tree bears palmate leaves, and small, tubular, lilac, scented flowers and fleshy, red-black fruits.

Parts Used
Berries.

Healing Properties
Actions: Balances female sex hormones by acting on the anterior pituitary gland
Uses: Premenstrual symptoms, painful menstruation, menopausal symptoms

Caution
Not to be taken with progesterone drugs.

Availability
Dried berries are available in health/alternative stores. Also available as a tincture.

How to Use in Juicing
Infusion: In a teapot, pour ¼ cup (50 mL) boiling water over 1 tbsp (15 mL) fresh or 1 tsp (5 mL) dried, lightly crushed berries. Steep for 10 minutes. Strain, discard herb, and add liquid to 1 cup (250 mL) of juice.
Tincture: Add 10 to 20 drops to 1 cup (250 mL) of juice.

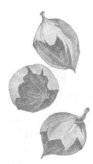

Wild Lettuce

Lactuca virosa

A tall biennial with lanceolate leaves and dandelion-like flowers that grows easily from seed.

Parts Used
Leaves and flowers.

Healing Properties
Actions: Nerve relaxant, mild sedative, mild pain reliever.
Uses: Anxiety, insomnia, hyperactivity in children.

Availability
Gather leaves in June and July, otherwise not widely available.

How to Use in Juicing
Infusion: Pour ¼ cup (50 mL) boiling water over 1 tsp (5 mL) dried cut or powdered leaf. Steep 10 minutes. Strain, discard herb, and add liquid to 1 cup (250 mL) of juice.

Yarrow

Achillea millefolium

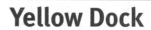

A one- to three-foot (30 to 90 cm) tall hardy perennial with feathery leaves and white (occasionally pink) flowers that grows wild in fields throughout North America and is easily grown in the garden.

Parts Used
Stem, leaves and flowers.

Healing Properties
Actions: Anti-inflammatory, bitter, promotes bile flow, diaphoretic, digestive, relaxant, promotes blood circulation, heals wounds.
Uses: High blood pressure, colds, fevers, influenza, varicose veins.

Caution
Large doses of yarrow are toxic if taken over a long period of time.

Availability
Harvest above-ground parts while flowering in the wild from June through September. Dried stems, leaves and flowers and tinctures are available in alternative/health stores.

How to Use in Juicing
Dried leaf, stems and flowers: Crush to a fine powder and whisk into fresh juice or add to ingredients in blended drinks. Use 1 tsp (5 mL) for each 1 cup (250 mL) of juice.
Infusion: In a teapot, pour ¼ cup (50 mL) boiling water over 1 tbsp (15 mL) fresh or 1 tsp (5 mL) dried flowerheads. Steep for 10 minutes. Strain, discard herb, and add liquid to 1 cup (250 mL) of juice.
Tincture: Add 40 drops to 1 cup (250 mL) of juice.

Yellow Dock

Rumex crispus

A large one- to five-foot (30 to 150 cm) tall perennial with small green-to-red flowers that grows in waste areas throughout North America.

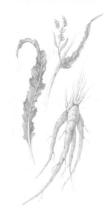

Parts Used
Root.

Healing Properties
Actions: Bitter, laxative, lymphatic, increases bile flow.
Uses: Fresh roots are rich in iron and can be used to treat iron-deficiency anemia. Yellow dock also helps cleanse the body by supporting liver function and eliminating toxins through the bile. It is an especially helpful cleanser for skin diseases, rheumatoid arthritis, swollen lymph glands and constipation.

Availability
The root can be harvested in the wild from September through November. Dried root is available in alternative/health stores.

How to Use in Juicing
Whole fresh root: Feed through tube along with other ingredients. Use 3- to 4-inch (7.5 to 10 cm) pieces for each 1 cup (250 mL) of juice. Leave peel on if organic.
Powder: Whisk 1 tsp (5 mL) powdered, dried root into 1 cup (250 mL) of juice.
Decoction: In a small saucepan, pour ¼ cup (50 mL) boiling water over 1 tbsp (15 mL) chopped fresh or 1 tsp (5 mL) chopped dried root. Simmer with lid on 10 minutes. Steep for 10 minutes. Strain, discard herb, and add liquid to 1 cup (250 mL) of juice.

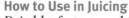

Other Ingredients

Blackstrap Molasses

Molasses is a thick syrup by-product of sugar refining, in which the sucrose (sugar) is separated from the liquid and nutrients from the raw cane plant. Several grades of molasses are available, but blackstrap contains the least sugar and the most nutrients: iron, six of the B vitamins, calcium, phosphorous and potassium.

For Juicing: Molasses has a strong flavor, so use sparingly, about 1 to 2 tsp (5 to 10 mL) per 1 cup (250 mL) in juice or tea that requires additional sweetening.

Carob

Ceratonia siliqua

Carob, which is powdered carob beans, is used as a substitute for cocoa and chocolate. Carob is healthier than chocolate because, unlike cocoa (from which chocolate is made), it has no caffeine, does not need extra sugar, is lower in fat and provides some calcium and phosphorus. It is available in baking chips, which can be used in hot drinks, as well as in powdered form, which can be blended into smoothies (see also Coconut/Carob Milk, page 328).

For Juicing: To add sweetness to juices; whisk up to 1 tbsp (15 mL) carob into 1 cup (250 mL) of juice.

For Pulping: Add up to 2 tbsp (25 mL) carob to ingredients before blending.

Cider Vinegar

Distilled white vinegar is a mixture of acetic acid and water. It is useful as a disinfectant and cleaning agent but is not valuable as a food. Naturally fermented vinegar made from wine or fruit juice, such as the cider vinegar widely available in grocery stores, contains some nutrients. However, the most nutritious cider vinegar is available at alternative/health stores. It is made from juice extracted from certified organic apples that is naturally fermented (without heat or the addition of clarifiers, enzymes or preservatives). This process yields a natural cider vinegar that contains some pectin and trace minerals, as well as beneficial bacteria and enzymes.

For Juicing: For overall health, add 1 tsp (5 mL) natural apple cider vinegar to juice and smoothie drinks.

Flax Seeds

Linum usitatissimum

Actions: Flax seed oil is the best vegetable source of essential omega-3 fatty acids, which help lubricate the joints and prevent absorption of toxins by stimulating digestion.

For Juicing: Whisk in 1 tbsp (15 mL) flax seed oil for up to 2 cups (500 mL) juice.

For Pulping: Add 1 tbsp (15 mL) whole flax seeds to other ingredients before blending.

Grains

Oats, wheat, rye, buckwheat, spelt, amaranth, quinoa

Whole grains are unrefined and therefore they retain all the nutritional value of the bran and germ. They also add fiber and complex carbohydrates to the diet. In all, whole grains offer protein, carbohydrates, phytate, vitamin E, fiber (including lignins), and some B vitamins (thiamin, riboflavin, niacin, folacin), iron, zinc and magnesium.

Actions: anti-cancer, antioxidant, fight heart disease, anti-obesity, lower blood sugar levels

For Pulping: Add 2 to 3 tbsp (25 to 45 mL) whole grain flakes to 1 cup (250 mL) blended drinks and milk shakes. Add to roots and nuts for roasted coffee-substitute blends.

Grasses

Wheat, barley

Wheat and barley grass is grown from the seeds (or "berries") of the wheat or barley plant. Harvested when 5 to 6 inches (12.5 to 15 cm) high, the grass is then eaten or juiced fresh or dried and used in powdered form or pressed into pills. High in chlorophyll (a powerful healing agent and infection fighter), beta carotene and vitamins C and E, these green foods are easily added to juices and blended drinks. They are also one of the best plant sources of protein, even better than soy and legumes.

Actions: antioxidant, anti-inflammatory, anticancer, antibiotic, blood cleanser, protects against radiation

For Juicing: Fresh wheat and barley grasses require a special juicer or attachment to extract their liquid. They have a strong flavor, so mix with water or vegetable juice, not fruit juices. Whisk 1 tbsp (15 mL) powdered wheat or barley grass with 1 to 2 cups (250 to 500 mL) vegetable juice or blended drinks.

Caution: Start with small amounts (no more than 2 tbsp/25 mL) wheatgrass juice daily. Large amounts may cause diarrhea and nausea.

Green Algae

Chlorella, spirulina

Rich in carotenoids and chlorophyll, these microscopic single-celled green algae have been shown to be effective in reducing the effects of radiation and may be helpful in treating HIV infections. Available in capsules or bulk loose powder.

Actions: Antioxidant, anticancer, boosts immunity, reduces heavy-metal toxicity, hypotensive.

For Juicing: Add 2 tsp (10 mL) to juice and blended drinks.

Hemp

Cannabis sativa

Hemp seeds are high in protein and contain about 30% oil, which is high in essential fatty acids — omega-3 and omega-6, as well as gamma linolenic acid (GLA). Hemp nuts, the hulled seeds of the hemp plant, can be used in nut butters, baked products, dips and spreads, and incorporated into blended drinks.

For Pulping: Add 2 to 3 tbsp (25 to 45 mL) hemp nuts to blended drinks.

Honey

Honey is almost as sweet as granulated white sugar. The difference is that honey has small amounts of

B vitamins, calcium, iron, zinc, potassium and phosphorous. It also acts as a potent bacteria killer. One tbsp (15 mL) contains just under 2% of the recommended daily intake of vitamins A and C, iron and calcium. Generally, the darker the honey the higher its antioxidant value.

Actions: Antioxidant, antibacterial, antimicrobial, calms nerves, antidiarrheal.

For Juicing: Use honey as a sweetener for bitter vegetable juices or add to hot toddies and cold remedies to soothe sore throats.

Caution: The National Honey Board, along with other health organizations, recommends that honey not be fed to infants under one year of age.

Honey-related products

Bee pollen is the male seeds of flower blossoms which collect on the legs of the bees as they work. The bees clean it off, mix it with nectar and their own enzymes. It contains proteins, vitamins A, B, C and E, calcium, magnesium, selenium, nucleic acids and lecithin and may be added to blended drinks. Use 1 tbsp (15 mL) bee pollen for up to 2 cups (500 mL) smoothie.

Propolis is a sticky resinous substance collected from coniferous trees, is supportive of the immune system and is used as a tonic. Propolis can be added to blended drinks, 1 tsp (5 mL) for each 1 cup (250 mL) of juice or smoothie.

Royal jelly is the milky product fed exclusively to the queen bee. It is known to be rich in the B complex vitamins, as well as vitamins A, C, D and E. Refrigerate fresh royal jelly or purchase freeze-dried for use in juices and blended drinks. Add 1 tbsp (15 mL) royal jelly for up to 2 cups (500 mL) juice or smoothie.

Maple Syrup

The sap from sugar maples (*Acer saccharum*), red maples (*A. rubrum*) and silver maples (*A. saccharinum*) is collected in the spring when it is flowing from the roots back into the aerial parts of the tree to provide energy for growth. The sap is 95 to 97% water, but when it is boiled down, a thick, sweet syrup composed of 65% sucrose is left behind. The syrup also contains organic acids, minerals (mainly potassium and calcium) and traces of amino acids and vitamins. One-quarter cup (50 mL) maple syrup provides 6% of the recommended daily intake of calcium and thiamin, and 2% of magnesium and riboflavin.

For Juicing: Stir 1 to 2 tbsp (15 to 25 mL) pure maple syrup (avoid "maple-flavored" syrup, which is primarily corn syrup with artificial flavor) into 1 to 2 cups (250 to 500 mL) juice if a sweetener is required.

Lecithin

Lecithin is one of the best sources of choline, which is known to improve memory by strengthening neurons in the brain's memory centers. Lecithin is available in alternative/health stores in capsule or granular form. Add two capsules or 1 tbsp (15 mL) lecithin granules to 1 to 2 cups (250 to 500 mL) of smoothie.

Nuts

All nuts — including peanuts, which are technically legumes — contain large amounts of protein, vitamin E, fiber and protease inhibitors, which are known to prevent cancer in laboratory animals. Although nuts are extremely high in fat, their oils are polyunsaturated and, as such, reduce blood cholesterol levels. Nuts also contain essential fatty acids, which are necessary for healthy skin, hair, glands, mucous membranes, nerves and arteries, as well as being helpful in preventing cardiovascular disease. Nuts allow a slow, steady rise in blood sugar and insulin, making them good foods for people with diabetes (see also Nut Milk, page 327).

Actions: Anticancer, lower blood cholesterol levels, regulate blood sugar level.

For Juicing: Use ground nuts as a garnish for juices.

For Pulping: Add up to 1/4 cup (50 mL) whole nuts or Nut Milk (see pages 327–28) for blending with other ingredients in smoothies and blended drinks.

Caution: Nuts can cause extreme allergic reactions in some people. Also, peanuts and peanut butter may be contaminated by aflatoxin mold, a carcinogen.

Protein Powder

Soy protein (the protein extracted from soybeans) is believed to help reduce the risk of cancers of the breast, endometrium and prostate if it contains isoflavones. Isoflavones mimic the action of estrogen and thus reduce the symptoms of menopause and help prevent the loss of calcium, which is linked to osteoporosis. Research has shown that soy protein reduces both the overall cholesterol level and the low-density lipoprotein (LDL), or "bad," cholesterol level. Choose raw soy protein powder made from soybeans that are water-washed (not washed in alcohol), organically grown and specifically tested for high isoflavone levels.

For Pulping: Add up to 3 tbsp (45 mL) to ingredients before blending.

Caution: There is growing concern over the prolonged use of soy (see Soy Products, page 155).

Psyllium Seeds

See page 144

Pumpkin Seeds

Pumpkin seeds are important to men because they contain high concentrations of amino acids that can reduce the symptoms of prostate enlargement.

For Pulping: Add 2 tbsp (25 mL) fresh hulled pumpkin seeds to ingredients for blending.

Ready-to-use Juices

Juice from fresh raw fruits, vegetables and herbs is the best source of nutrients and live energy. Canned or bottled juices have been processed at high heat and may contain added ingredients such as sugar, artificial flavorings, stabilizers, thickeners/thinners, and chemical preservatives. Should you wish to blend ready-to-use juices with fresh juice, choose pure juice with no sugar or additives.

Sea Herbs

Arame, dulse, nori, wakame, kelp

Their high concentrations of vitamin A, protein, calcium, iron and other minerals make sea herbs important to overall health.

Actions: Anticancer, diuretic, antibacterial, boost immune function.

For Juicing: Add the soaking water from sea herbs to fresh juices; the salty taste blends well in vegetable juices. Sprinkle powdered or finely cut sea herbs over juice as a garnish.

For Pulping: Add ¼ to ½ cup (50 to 125 mL) soaked, simmered sea herbs to other ingredients for smoothies or blended drinks.

Sesame Seeds

Sesamum indicum

High in calcium and a good source of incomplete protein, sesame seeds lend a light, nutty taste to juices and blended drinks. Sesame seed oil is exceptionally stable and is a source of vitamin E and coenzyme Q10, an essential coenzyme for metabolism, or the rate at which the body produces energy (or burns calories).

Actions: Emollient, laxative, antioxidant.

For Juicing: Sprinkle seeds over juices as a garnish or whisk 1 tsp (5 mL) sesame oil into juices.

For Pulping: Add 1 tbsp (15 mL) to other ingredients for blending.

Soy Products

High in calcium and a good source of incomplete protein, sesame seeds lend a light, nutty taste to juices and blended drinks. Sesame seed oil is exceptionally stable and is a source of vitamin E and coenzyme Q10, an essential coenzyme for metabolism, or the rate at which the body produces energy (or burns calories).

Actions: Emollient, laxative, antioxidant.

Caution: Due to new research and the effects of genetic modification and heavy chemical use on soybeans, buy only organic fresh or dried soybeans and soy products.

Availability: Available raw, dried or canned whole, or in paste (miso), soy milk, tofu and tempeh.

For Juicing or Pulping: Whisk ¼ cup (50 mL) into fresh juice or smoothies.

Caution: A large percentage of soybeans grown today are genetically modified and are produced using high amounts of pesticides. Fresh soybeans contain enzyme inhibitors that block protein digestion and may cause serious gastric distress

and organ damage. The inhibitors are not present in such high amounts in the fermented bean products of tofu, tempeh or soy sauce. The high amounts of phytic acid in soybeans and soy foods may block the uptake of essential minerals and cause deficiencies. Isoflavones, once thought to minimize cell damage from free radicals, block the damaging effects of hormonal or synthetic estrogens, and inhibit tumor cell growth, may in fact, be toxic.

Soybeans, and soy foods contain goitrogens, naturally occurring substances in certain foods that can interfere with the functioning of the thyroid gland. Individuals with already existing and untreated thyroid problems may want to avoid soy foods.

TVP (textured vegetable protein made from soybeans) is produced using chemicals and harmful techniques and is not considered a whole food.

Excessive soy intake should be avoided during pregnancy and soy-based baby formulas should not be used.

Tofu is a curd made from soybeans that is high in B vitamins, potassium and iron, as well as calcium, so long as that mineral has been used as the curdling agent (check the label). Tofu thickens and "smoothes" the taste of blended drinks. Silken tofu works best in smoothies. Add ¼ to ½ cup (50 to 125 mL) to any smoothie recipe.

Tempeh, a mild, firm cake made from fermented cooked soybeans, may also be used in smoothies. It is usually sold frozen. Add ¼ cup (50 mL) crumbled tempeh to any smoothie recipe.

Canned soybeans or cooked reconstituted dried soybeans are also good in smoothies and produce a thicker result. Add ½ cup (125 mL) canned or cooked soybeans per smoothie recipe.

Sprouts

A good source of B vitamins (except B12), sprouts also contain vitamins A and C, as well as bioflavonoids and enzymes. They add a green, living nutritional boost to juices and blended drinks. Alfalfa (and other grains), bean, pea and herb seeds are easy to sprout in a warm, moist environment and offer a concentrated blast of the nutrients found in the mature plants. Grow sprouts in the winter months, when fresh leafy greens are not at their best.

Caution: The safety of seed sprouts depends upon the quality of the water in which they are grown. Some sprouts have been linked with harmful bacteria, and water is the culprit in generating that bacteria. The best source for sprouts is to grow them from clean, organic seeds in water that has been boiled or that is known to be free of contaminants.

Buying and Storing: For reasons stated above, grow your own or purchase sprouts from reliable growers. Look for moist, crisp sprouts with no evidence of slime or wilting. Store in the refrigerator for up to one week.

For Juicing: Feed through tube interspersed with firm fruit or vegetables.

For Pulping: Add up to 1 cup (250 mL) to blended drinks.

Sunflower Seeds

Helianthus annus

A good source of vitamin E and zinc, sunflower seeds can be added to other ingredients before blending into smoothies.

For Pulping: Use 2 tbsp (25 mL) for up to 2 cups (500 mL) smoothies.

Tofu

See Soy Products

Wheat Germ

A good source of vitamin E and thiamin, wheat germ may be added to other ingredients before blending.

For Juicing or Pulping: Use 2 tbsp (25 mL) for up to 2 cups (500 mL) juice or smoothie.

Wheat Grass

See Grasses

Yogurt and Yogurt Products

Yogurt is produced from fermented milk. A beneficial type of bacteria (called lactobacilli) in yogurt restores and maintains a normal microbial balance in the intestinal tract. The acidophilus culture in yogurt helps protect against colon cancer. When buying, check the label to ensure that it "contains active cultures." Yogurt is usually safe for people with milk allergies and is essential to a vegetarian diet.

Actions: Antibacterial, anticancer, anti-ulcer, immune building, lowers blood cholesterol

For Juicing: Add up to 1 cup (250 mL) yogurt in blended drinks and stir up to ¼ cup (50 mL) into fruit or vegetable juices.

The Recipes

Juicing Guidelines

Taken as part of a healthy diet — and in amounts that are reasonable — juices round out our daily requirement for fresh fruits and vegetables. More importantly, they are the very best way to obtain the nutrients and phytochemicals those foods contribute to our health and well-being.

Taste

Juices should taste pleasant. When you begin to juice, unless you have already changed your diet to a whole foods way of eating, you may find that the taste of fresh, raw juice is "different" or too strong. But once your taste buds have adjusted, you will notice that both the juice and pulp from fresh, organic fruits and vegetables offer pure bursts of clear, true flavor. Fruit juices are intensely sweet and, depending on individual preferences, may need to be balanced with lemon or beet. Foods like sauces and soups cooked with the pulp are different from the bottled, canned and boxed tastes of convenience foods — they are the taste of health.

A rule of thumb for diluting stronger vegetable juices is to use the ratio of 3 mild ingredients (apples or carrots) to 1 strong ingredient (cabbage, broccoli, leafy dark vegetables).

When you begin juicing, purchase twice as many organic apples as any other single fruit or vegetable and use them in the above ratio. Gradually incorporate more variety and stronger-tasting vegetables such as cabbage, spinach and fresh herbs (leaves and roots). Start taking fresh raw juice slowly — one or two glasses a day for several days — to allow the body time to adjust. Minor discomfort may be experienced in the form of gas and slight abdominal pain. This transitory stage should be short. After that, drink as much raw juice as feels comfortable. It is impossible to overdose on raw juice if common sense is used. Sip slowly and savor each glass!

Juice fresh, drink immediately

Buy fresh, ripe organic fruits, vegetables and herbs. Juice immediately (or within one or two days) and drink right away. The nutrients in raw juice are highly volatile and will begin to deteriorate as soon as they are exposed to the air. Vitamin C — so important in preventing some types of cancer, cataracts in the eyes, heart disease, bleeding gums, high blood pressure and infertility — is extremely volatile, subject to deterioration by heat, exposure to air and storage. Consequently, when produce is picked, the vitamin C begins to dissipate. The very best way to ensure the maximum amount of vitamin C (and other critical enzymes and phytochemicals) from food is to take fresh, raw juice that has just been made.

Storing fresh juice

To maximize nutrients from the juice of fruits, vegetables and herbs, it is imperative to start with perfectly ripe produce and drink the raw juice immediately once it has been separated from the pulp. Should it be necessary to make juice in advance, keep the following in mind:
• Use glass containers, fill to the top and cap with a tight-fitting lid.
• Juices made at home are not pasteurized and have no "shelf-life." For this reason, they must be kept in the refrigerator and will stay mold- and bacteria-free for up to two days only. However, try to drink fresh juice within 1 to 2 hours.

Using pulp

Pulp is a natural by-product of juicing. While juices contain a concentrated amount of nutrients, the pulp retains the fiber and a substantial amount of nutrients as well. Pulp from fruits and vegetables can be saved for use in many recipes.

To use pulp for frozen desserts, soups, sauces, casseroles, vegetable stocks, dressings, baked goods, salads and many other dishes, cut out the core and seeds and peel the fruit or vegetable before juicing. For best results, blend pulp using blender or food processor before using. Measure 2 cups (500 mL) of the blended pulp and transfer to a freezer bag or covered container. Store in the refrigerator if the pulp will be used within a day, or label and freeze until needed. Versatile fruits or vegetables, such as apples, carrots and tomatoes, should be juiced first, the pulp collected and kept separate from other juice ingredients, making them easy to add to apple sauce, muffins, cakes or tomato sauces and salsas. For recipes that use pulp, see Frozen Treats (see page 342) and Roughies (see page 290).

Fruit and Vegetable Juices

Fruit Juices

Serves 1 or 2

Apple Beet Pear

2	apples	2
1	pear	1
3	beets, tops intact	3
½	lemon	½
1	½-inch (1 cm) piece gingerroot	1

1. Using a juicer, process apples, pear, beets, beet tops, lemon and ginger. Whisk and pour into 1 large or 2 smaller glasses.

Serves 1

Apple Fresh

3	apples	3
1 cup	red grapes	250 mL
½	lemon	½
½ tsp	powdered ginseng	2 mL

1. Using a juicer, process apples, grapes and lemon. Whisk together with ginseng and pour into a glass.

Serves 1

Apple Pear

2	apples	2
2	pears	2
1	½-inch (1 cm) piece gingerroot	1
½ cup	grapes	125 mL
½ tsp	ground cinnamon	2 mL

1. Using a juicer, process apples, pears, ginger and grapes. Whisk together with cinnamon and pour into a glass.

Serves 1

Apricot Peach

2	peaches, pitted	2
2	fresh apricots, pitted	2
½ cup	green grapes	125 mL
¼	fresh fennel bulb	¼

1. Using a juicer, process peaches, apricots, grapes and fennel. Whisk and pour into a glass.

Serves 1

Autumn Refresher

Tip

If using pulp for Basil-Pear Sherbet (see recipe, page 353), peel and seed pears and apple and remove white pith and seeds from the lime before juicing.

3	pears	3
2	peaches, pitted	2
1	apple	1
½	lime	½

1. Using a juicer, process pears, peaches, apple and lime. Whisk and pour into a glass.

Serves 1

Berry Best

1 cup	blueberries	250 mL
1 cup	pitted cherries	250 mL
½ cup	grapes	125 mL
¼	cantaloupe, cut in two	¼

1. Using a juicer, process blueberries, cherries, grapes and cantaloupe. Whisk and pour into a glass.

Serves 1	# Beta Blast	
3	carrots	3
2	fresh apricots, pitted	2
¼	cantaloupe, cut in two	¼

1. Using a juicer, process carrots, apricots and cantaloupe. Whisk and pour into a glass.

Serves 1	# Beta-Carro	
3	carrots	3
3	fresh apricots, pitted	3
3	peaches, pitted	3

1. Using a juicer, process carrots, apricots and peaches. Whisk and pour into a glass.

Serves 1	# Black Pineapple	
1 cup	blackberries	250 mL
3	sprigs fresh parsley (see Caution, left)	3
2	spears pineapple	2
½ cup	blueberries	125 mL
½ cup	raspberries	125 mL

Caution: Parsley should be avoided during pregnancy and in cases of kidney inflammation.

1. Using a juicer, process blackberries, parsley, pineapple, blueberries and raspberries. Whisk and pour into a glass.

Blueberry

1 cup	blueberries	250 mL
1 cup	pitted cherries	250 mL
½ cup	red grapes	125 mL
½ cup	raspberries	125 mL

1. Using a juicer, process blueberries, cherries, grapes and raspberries. Whisk and pour into a glass.

Blue Water

Tip
Use fresh or frozen whole cranberries in this antioxidant juice. Thaw frozen fruit slightly before attempting to juice.

1 cup	blueberries	250 mL
1	2-inch (5 cm) slice watermelon, cut to fit tube	1
¼ cup	whole cranberries	50 mL

1. Using a juicer, process blueberries, watermelon and cranberries. Whisk and pour into a glass.

Carrot Fennel Orange

Tip
If using pulp for Carrot, Fennel & Orange Frappé (see recipe, page 345), remove white pith and seeds from lemon and oranges before juicing.

4	oranges	4
3	carrots	3
1	lemon	1
¼	fresh fennel bulb	¼

1. Using a juicer, process oranges, carrots, lemon and fennel. Whisk and pour into 2 glasses.

Serves 1

C-Blend

Tip

If using pulp for Carrot, Fennel & Orange Frappé (see recipe, page 345), remove white pith and seeds from lemon and oranges before juicing.

2	oranges	2
1	grapefruit, cut to fit tube	1
1	lime	1
½ cup	whole cranberries, fresh or frozen	125 mL
1 tbsp	liquid honey, optional	15 mL

1. Using a juicer, process oranges, grapefruit, lime and cranberries. Whisk and pour into a glass. Whisk in honey, if desired.

Serves 1 or 2

C-Blitz

Tip

Parsley packs a whopping amount of vitamin C and is one of the few fresh herbs widely available throughout the year.

Caution: Parsley should be avoided during pregnancy and in cases of kidney inflammation.

1	grapefruit, cut to fit tube	1
2	oranges	2
6	sprigs fresh parsley (see Caution, left)	6
3	kiwifruits	3

1. Using a juicer, process grapefruit, oranges, parsley and kiwifruits. Whisk and pour into 1 large or 2 smaller glasses.

Serves 1

Cherry Juice

1 cup	pitted cherries	250 mL
¼	fresh fennel bulb	¼
1 cup	grapes	250 mL
½	lime	½

1. Using a juicer, process cherries, fennel, grapes and lime. Whisk and pour into a glass.

Cherry Sunrise

Tip

Served as a refreshing summer nightcap, 1 tsp (5 mL) of dried German chamomile may be used in place of the fresh herb.

1 cup	pitted cherries	250 mL
1	grapefruit, cut to fit tube	1
1	apple	1
1 tbsp	fresh chamomile flowers, optional	15 mL

1. Using a juicer, process cherries, grapefruit, apple and chamomile, if using. Whisk and pour into a glass.

Cran-Apple

¾ cup	whole cranberries, fresh or frozen	175 mL
3	carrots	3
2	apples	2

1. Using a juicer, process cranberries, carrots and apples. Whisk and pour into a glass.

Cranberries (*Vaccinium macrocarpon*)

Cranberries are native to North America, but were introduced to Europeans in 1677, when colonists sent King Charles II a gift from the New World consisting of 2 hogsheads of "samp" (Indian corn, broken and boiled), 3,000 codfish and 10 barrels of cranberries.

Cranberry vines grow in marshy ground or bogs, where they typically require 5 years to become established before harvesting. Once mature, like strawberry plants, they grow rapidly, with runners shooting out in all directions. An established plant should yield for more than 100 years.

Although mechanized harvesters are most common, some cranberries are still picked by hand, using a wooden scoop specially designed with wire tines forming a comb-like end that disengages the cranberries from the vines and funnels them into an attached box. Cranberries are sorted according to their bounce and packers have devised several ingenious devices to separate the berries with the most rubbery quality from their less energetic relations.

Serves 1		

Cranberry

1 cup	whole cranberries, fresh or frozen	250 mL
1 cup	grapes	250 mL
2	spears pineapple	2

1. Using a juicer, process cranberries, grapes and pineapple. Whisk and pour into a glass.

Serves 3		

Cranberry Juice

Cranberries may be (and often are) juiced and blended with sweeter juices, but this recipe provides the unmistakably tart, flavor of whole berries. The sugar content of this juice is much lower than that found in commercially prepared products.

Tips

Omit the cinnamon and nutmeg if you wish.

The astragalus adds immune-boosting properties to the juice.

4 cups	whole fresh cranberries	1 L
4 cups	water	1 L
2 cups	apple juice	500 mL
2	slices dried astragalus root, optional	2
2 tbsp	granulated sugar	25 mL
2 tsp	ground stevia	10 mL
½ tsp	ground cinnamon	2 mL
¼ tsp	ground nutmeg	1 mL

1. In a large saucepan, combine cranberries, water, apple juice, astragalus (if using), sugar and stevia. Bring to a boil over high heat. Reduce heat and let bubble gently for 15 minutes or until berries burst. Remove from heat, cool slightly and strain the mixture, pressing on solids to extract as much juice as possible.

2. When juice has drained through, discard astragalus (pulp may be used in another recipe) and whisk in cinnamon and nutmeg. Cool before drinking or blend with other juices for use in fruit punches or frozen treats.

3. *To store:* Pour juice into a clean glass container with lid. Keep in refrigerator and use within 2 days.

Eye Opener

2 cups	hulled fresh or frozen strawberries	500 mL
2	carrots	2
1	orange	1

1. Using a juicer, process strawberries, carrots and orange. Whisk and pour into a glass.

Gooseberry Berry

1 cup	gooseberries	250 mL
1 cup	blackberries	250 mL
1 cup	raspberries	250 mL
1	apple	1

1. Using a juicer, process gooseberries, blackberries, raspberries and apple. Whisk and pour into a glass.

Grapefruit

Tip

If using pulp for Grapefruit Frappé (see recipe, page 345), grate zest from orange and set aside to add to pulp. Remove white pith when peeling orange and remove the seeds.

1	orange	1
2	grapefruits, cut to fit tube	2
1	lemon	1
	Liquid honey, optional	

1. Using a juicer, process orange, grapefruits and lemon. Whisk together with honey to taste, if using, and pour into a glass.

Grape Power

Caution: Parsley should be avoided during pregnancy and in cases of kidney inflammation.

2 cups	green grapes	500 mL
1	green bell pepper, trimmed	1
3	sprigs fresh parsley (see Caution, left)	3
1	sprig fresh rosemary	1

1. Using a juicer, process grapes, pepper, parsley and rosemary. Whisk and pour into a glass.

Hangover Helper

2	star fruits	2
2	apples	2
1	½-inch (1 cm) piece gingerroot	1
½	lemon	½

1. Using a juicer, process star fruits, apples, ginger and lemon. Whisk and pour into a glass.

Hangover Remedy

4	apples	4
1	½-inch (1 cm) piece gingerroot	1
½	lemon	½
½ tsp	crushed lavender buds	2 mL

1. Using a juicer, process apples, ginger and lemon. Whisk in lavender and pour into a glass.

Lemon Aid

Serves 1

This juice is quite tart, but very refreshing, so taste before adding the honey.

Tip

Use pulp in Lemon Sauce (see recipe, page 295). Before juicing, be sure to remove white pith and seeds from lemons, and peel watermelon and cucumber.

2	lemons	2
1	2-inch (5 cm) slice watermelon, cut to fit tube	1
½	cucumber	½
1 tsp	liquid honey, optional	5 mL

1. Using a juicer, process lemons, watermelon and cucumber. Whisk and pour into a glass. If desired, whisk in honey.

Lemon Lime

Serves 1

Caution: Do not use licorice if you have high blood pressure.

1	orange	1
1	lime	1
1	lemon	1
1 tsp	powdered licorice (see Caution, left)	5 mL

1. Using a juicer, process orange, lime, and lemon. Whisk together with licorice and pour into a glass.

Mint Julep

Serves 2 or 3

Sweet and only a little minty, this juice is interesting if served in clear glasses so you can see the grape juice separate to the bottom. Use sprigs of mint for swizzle sticks.

Tip

If planning to use pulp in a frozen drink, remove and discard as many herb pieces as possible.

4	oranges	4
3 cups	red grapes	750 mL
¼ cup	fresh mint leaves	50 mL
6	sprigs fresh lemon balm	6
1	lemon	1

1. Using a juicer, process oranges, grapes, mint, lemon balm and lemon. Whisk and pour into glasses.

Orange Crush

Serves 1 or 2

3	oranges	3
1	carrot	1
½ cup	whole cranberries, fresh or frozen	125 mL
1 tsp	ground cinnamon	5 mL

1. Using a juicer, process oranges, carrot and cranberries. Whisk together with cinnamon and pour into 1 or 2 glasses.

Orange Pom

Serves 1

1	pomegranate, seeds only	1
2	oranges	2
1	apple	1
1	carrot	1

1. Using a juicer, process pomegranate seeds, oranges, apple and carrot. Whisk and pour into a glass.

Orange Star

Serves 1

2	star fruits	2
2	oranges	2
¼	cantaloupe, cut in two	¼
½	lemon	½

1. Using a juicer, process star fruits, oranges, cantaloupe and lemon. Whisk and pour into a glass.

Orange Zinger

1	orange	1
3	carrots	3
1	½-inch (1 cm) piece gingerroot	1
1	apple	1

1. Using a juicer, process orange, carrots, ginger and apple. Whisk and pour into a glass.

Pear Fennel

Caution: Do not use licorice if you have high blood pressure.

2	pears	2
¼	fresh fennel bulb	¼
2	apples	2
½ tsp	powdered licorice (see Caution, left)	2 mL

1. Using a juicer, process pears, fennel and apples. Whisk together with licorice and pour into a glass.

Pear Pineapple

2	pears	2
2	spears pineapple	2
1 cup	red or green grapes	250 mL
1	lemon	1

1. Using a juicer, process pears, pineapple, grapes and lemon. Whisk and pour into a glass.

Serves 1	# Pineapple Citrus	
½	pineapple, cut into spears	½
2	oranges	2
1	lime	1

1. Using a juicer, process pineapple, oranges and lime. Whisk and pour into a glass.

Serves 1	# Pine-Berry	
2	spears pineapple	2
1 cup	blueberries	250 mL
1 cup	pitted cherries	250 mL
½ cup	black currants	125 mL

Tip

Pulp from this juice may be used in Pineapple Sage Frappé (see recipe, page 346). Be sure to remove white pith and seeds from oranges and lime before juicing.

1. Using a juicer, process pineapple, blueberries, cherries and black currants. Whisk and pour into a glass.

Serves 1	# Pom Pom	
2	pomegranates, seeds only	2
1 cup	pitted cherries	250 mL
1	black plum, pitted	1
1	Red Delicious apple	1

1. Using a juicer, process pomegranate seeds, cherries, plum and apple. Whisk and pour into a glass.

Serves 1	# Raspberry Juice	
1 cup	raspberries	250 mL
1	apple	1
2	oranges	2

1. Using a juicer, process raspberries, apple and oranges. Whisk and pour into a glass.

Red Horizon

Serves 1

2	black plums, pitted	
1	pomegranate, seeds only	1
1	orange	1
1 cup	raspberries	250 mL

1. Using a juicer, process plums, pomegranate seeds, orange and raspberries. Whisk and pour into a glass.

Rhubarb

Serves 1

2	stalks fresh rhubarb, trimmed	2
1 cup	hulled fresh strawberries	250 mL
1	orange	1
1	½-inch (1 cm) piece gingerroot	1

1. Using a juicer, process rhubarb, strawberries, orange and ginger. Whisk and pour into a glass.

Roo-Berry Pie

Serves 2

2	stalks fresh rhubarb, trimmed	2
1 cup	raspberries	250 mL
1 cup	hulled fresh strawberries	250 mL
1 cup	blueberries	250 mL
1 cup	natural yogurt	250 mL

1. Using a juicer, process rhubarb, raspberries, strawberries and blueberries. Whisk together with yogurt and pour into glasses.

Sass in a Glass

2	star fruits	2
¼	cantaloupe, cut in two	¼
2	spears pineapple	2
1	lemon	1

1. Using a juicer, process star fruits, cantaloupe, pineapple and lemon. Whisk and pour into a glass.

Star Berry

2	star fruits	2
1 cup	blackberries	250 mL
½ cup	blueberries	125 mL
½ cup	raspberries	125 mL

1. Using a juicer, process star fruits, blackberries, blueberries and raspberries. Whisk and pour into a glass.

Strawberry-Orange Lemonade

1 cup	hulled fresh or frozen strawberries	250 mL
1	lemon	1
2	oranges	2
1 cup	sparkling mineral water	250 mL

1. Using a juicer, process strawberries, lemon and oranges. Whisk and pour into a pitcher. Whisk in mineral water.

Serves 2		

Summer Nectar

3	nectarines, pitted	3
2	fresh apricots, pitted	2
1 cup	blueberries	250 mL
2	peaches, pitted	2
2	plums, pitted	2

1. Using a juicer, process nectarines, apricots, blueberries, peaches and plums. Whisk and pour into glasses.

Serves 2		

Summer Swizzle

4	fresh apricots, pitted	4
1 cup	grapes	250 mL
4	peaches, pitted	4
1	2-inch (5 cm) slice watermelon, cut to fit tube	1

1. Using a juicer, process apricots, grapes, peaches and watermelon. Whisk and pour into glasses.

Serves 1		

Sunrise Supreme

1 cup	hulled fresh or frozen strawberries	250 mL
1 cup	red grapes	250 mL
1	orange	1

1. Using a juicer, process strawberries, grapes and orange. Whisk and pour into a glass.

Serves 1	**3PO**	
⅓	pineapple, cut into spears	⅓
1	red bell pepper, trimmed	1
2	black plums, pitted	2
1	orange	1

1. Using a juicer, process pineapple, red pepper, plums and orange. Whisk and pour into a glass.

Serves 1	**Watermelon Cooler**	
1	2-inch (5 cm) slice watermelon, cut to fit tube	1
½ cup	hulled fresh strawberries	125 mL
¼	fresh fennel bulb	¼
1	lemon	1

1. Using a juicer, process watermelon, strawberries, fennel and lemon. Whisk and pour into a glass.

Serves 1	**Watermelon Strawberry**	
1	2-inch (5 cm) slice watermelon, cut to fit tube	1
1 cup	hulled fresh strawberries	250 mL
½ cup	raspberries	125 mL
⅛ tsp	cinnamon	0.5 mL

1. Using a juicer, process watermelon, strawberries and raspberries. Whisk together with cinnamon and pour into a glass.

Vegetable Juices

Serves 1

ABC Juice

It's as easy as... well, A-B-C!

10	spears asparagus	10
1	apple	1
1	spear broccoli	1
2	carrots	2

1. Using a juicer, process asparagus, apple, broccoli and carrots. Whisk and pour into a glass.

Serves 1

Artichoke Carrot

In this immune-boosting combination, you can reduce or increase the amount of thyme according to taste.

1	handful Jerusalem artichoke roots	1
3	carrots	3
1 tbsp	fresh thyme or 1 tsp (5 mL) dried	15 mL
1	apple	1

1. Using a juicer, process artichokes, carrots, thyme and apple. Whisk and pour into a glass.

Artichoke Eight

Serves 2

1	handful Jerusalem artichoke roots	1
2	stalks celery	2
2	carrots	2
1	parsnip	1
¼	head cabbage, cut to fit tube	¼
1 cup	fresh spinach leaves	250 mL
1	apple	1
½	leek	½

1. Using a juicer, process artichokes, celery, carrots, parsnip, cabbage, spinach, apple and leek. Whisk and pour into glasses.

Beet

Serves 1 or 2

2	beets, tops intact	2
2	carrots	2
2	apples	2

1. Using a juicer, process beets, beet tops, carrots and apples. Whisk and pour into glasses.

Blazing Beets

Serves 1 or 2

This combination nourishes the immune system, is an excellent lymphatic cleanser and is believed to reduce tumors. Make it fresh each day. Take one serving daily for at least 5 days in one week.

3	beets, tops intact	3
1	½-inch (1 cm) piece gingerroot	1
1	fresh chile pepper	1
2	apples	2
1	clove garlic	1
2	stalks celery	2

1. Using a juicer, process beets, beet tops, ginger, chile, apples, garlic and celery. Whisk and pour into glasses.

Serves 1

Brocco-Artichoke

Caution: Parsley should be avoided during pregnancy and in cases of kidney inflammation.

1	spear broccoli	1
2	Jerusalem artichoke roots	2
3	sprigs fresh parsley (see Caution, left)	3
¼	fresh fennel bulb	¼

1. Using a juicer, process broccoli, artichoke roots, parsley and fennel. Whisk and pour into a glass.

Serves 1

Brocco-Carrot

1	spear broccoli	1
2	carrots	2
1	apple	1

1. Using a juicer, process broccoli, carrots and apple. Whisk and pour into a glass.

Serves 1

Cabbage Rose

Tip
Use the pulp from this juice as a salad. Be sure to peel, core and seed the apple before juicing.

⅛	cabbage	⅛
1	handful fresh spinach leaves	1
2	sprigs fresh rosemary or ½ tsp (2 mL) dried	2
2	carrots	2
1	apple	1

1. Using a juicer, process cabbage, spinach, rosemary, carrots and apple. Whisk and pour into a glass.

Chiles: the culinary firebrands

Chiles (*Capsicum* spp.), the pods that bite back, are a unique and diverse group of perennial shrubs (annual in northern climates) native to South and Central America and Mexico. The term "pepper" when appended to chile is misleading because the capsicum genus is not at all related to black pepper (*Piper nigrum*). The capsicum plant was mistakenly given the pepper moniker by early European spice seekers who confused their hot spiciness with the coveted and elusive pepper berries of India and the Spice Islands (Malaysia and Indonesia).

Ranging from fiery hot to sweet and mild, chiles are a study in contradiction. Well known by chefs for its ability to cause severe burns to the skin and eyes, the powerful element in all chiles — capsaicin — is the main ingredient in skin creams used to soothe the excruciating pain of arthritis and shingles. Chiles are often shunned by those who believe that they cause or irritate ulcers. Yet in Mexico, a long-standing remedy for stomach problems has been to consume a whole serrano or jalapeño chile.

And the confusion doesn't stop with their folk remedies. Chiles are a hotbed of conflicting species, varieties and pod types. The names change from region to region; just attempting to sort out the American/Mexican nomenclature is a huge challenge. Typically the fresh and dried version of the same chile bear different names, which are different again when the chile is smoked or green or ripe. Botanically, they are classified as berries. Horticulturally, they are fruits. We use them fresh as vegetables but when dried, they're a spice.

But that confusion aside, why is it that we love the palate-searing experience of eating chiles? Capsaicin irritates the pain receptors on the tongue that ignite the pain center in the brain, triggering a release of morphine-like natural pain killers — endorphins. They try to douse the fire by setting the body awash in a sense of well-being and we ride the wave of euphoria throughout the rest of the meal.

But that's not the only reason people are all fired up over chiles. In addition to their distinctive aroma and delicious taste, ¼ cup (50 mL) of the fresh, diced scorching orbs yields 4,031 IU of vitamin A, which becomes even more concentrated as the pod turns red and dries. Simply eating 1 tsp (5 mL) of red chili sauce supplies the body with the Recommended Dietary Allowance for vitamin A. The same ¼ cup (50 mL) of chopped fresh chile pepper delivers 91 mg of vitamin C — as compared to 66 mg in 1 orange. And while the vitamin C diminishes by more than half in the dried red pods, the effect is still more than a flash in the pan. See page 115 for more on the health actions of chiles.

Carrot Allium

Serves 1

3	carrots	3
1	handful fresh spinach leaves	1
1	clove garlic	1
½	lemon	½
Pinch	cayenne pepper	Pinch

1. Using a juicer, process carrots, spinach, garlic and lemon. Whisk together with cayenne and pour into a glass.

Carrot Apple

Serves 1

Caution: Parsley should be avoided during pregnancy and in cases of kidney inflammation.

4	carrots	4
2	stalks celery	2
1	apple	1
4	sprigs fresh parsley (see Caution, left)	4

1. Using a juicer, process carrots, celery, apple and parsley. Whisk and pour into a glass.

Carrot Head

Serves 1 or 2

3	carrots	3
2	pears	2
1	wedge green cabbage	1
¼	fresh fennel bulb	¼
2	cauliflower florets	2

1. Using a juicer, process carrots, pears, cabbage, fennel and cauliflower. Whisk and pour into glasses.

Cauli-Slaw

Tip

Use the pulp from this juice as a salad. Be sure to peel, core and seed the apple before juicing.

½	head cauliflower, cut to fit tube	½
⅛	head cabbage	⅛
2	carrots	2
2	stalks celery	2
¼	onion	¼
1	apple	1

1. Using a juicer, process cauliflower, cabbage, carrots, celery, onion and apple. Whisk and pour into glasses.

Celery

Tip

For more antioxidant power, add one clove of garlic.

4	stalks celery	4
2	carrots	2
¼	fresh fennel bulb	¼
½ tsp	ground cumin	2 mL

1. Using a juicer, process celery, carrots and fennel. Whisk and pour into a glass. Whisk in cumin.

C-Green

Caution: Parsley should be avoided during pregnancy and in cases of kidney inflammation.

3	sprigs fresh parsley (see Caution, left)	3
1	handful fresh spinach leaves	1
1	handful watercress	1
1	apple	1

1. Using a juicer, process parsley, spinach, watercress and apple. Whisk and pour into a glass.

The Chiller

Serves 1 or 2

1	carrot	1
2	stalks celery	2
1	apple	1
½	cucumber	½
½	zucchini	½
½	red bell pepper, trimmed	½

1. Using a juicer, process carrot, celery, apple, cucumber, zucchini and red pepper. Whisk and pour into glasses.

Cruciferous

Serves 1 or 2

The term *cruciferous* refers to the small cross formed when the flowers of particular plants are growing. Cruciferous vegetables include cabbage, broccoli, Brussels sprouts and cauliflower.

1	spear broccoli	1
¼	head cabbage, cut to fit tube	¼
¼	head cauliflower, cut to fit tube	¼
2	kale	2
½	lemon	½
2	apples	2

1. Using a juicer, process broccoli, cabbage, cauliflower, kale, lemon and apples. Whisk and pour into 1 large or 2 smaller glasses.

Cucumber Cooler

Serves 2

1	cucumber	1
2 cups	green grapes	500 mL
1	handful fresh borage leaves	1
1	handful fresh mint	1
2	apples	2
½	lemon	½

1. Using a juicer, process cucumber, grapes, borage, mint, apples and lemon. Whisk and pour into glasses.

Cucumber Fuzz

Serves 1

2	peaches, pitted	2
2	stalks celery	2
1	cucumber	1

1. Using a juicer, process peaches, celery and cucumber. Whisk and pour into a glass.

Dandelion Tonic

Serves 1

3	fresh young dandelions (roots and leaves)	3
2	radishes	2
1	handful watercress	1
1	apple	1
½	lemon	½
1	½-inch (1 cm) piece gingerroot	1

1. Using a juicer, process dandelions, radishes, watercress, apple, lemon and ginger. Whisk and pour into a glass.

Flaming Antibiotic

Serves 1

Tips

If you're unaccustomed to the heat of chiles, start with a small piece and add more once you become accustomed to the fire.

See page 189 for how to handle and use chiles for juices.

2	carrots	2
1	clove garlic	1
1	handful fresh thyme	1
1	chile pepper	1
½	cucumber	½
1	apple	1

1. Using a juicer, process carrots, garlic, thyme, chile, cucumber and apple. Whisk and pour into a glass.

Folic Plus

This juice is packed with folic acid, an essential nutrient for childbearing women.

2	oranges	2
3	kale	3
½ cup	fresh fresh spinach leaves	125 mL
5	stalks asparagus	5
1 tbsp	soy protein powder	15 mL

1. Using a juicer, process oranges, kale, spinach and asparagus. Whisk together with protein powder and pour into a glass.

Gallstone Solvent

As the name implies, this drink is used as a bitter tonic for treating gallstones.

Caution: Parsley should be avoided during pregnancy and in cases of kidney inflammation.

3	tomatoes	3
2	carrots	2
2	stalks celery	2
1	handful watercress	1
4	radishes	4
2	sprigs fresh parsley (see Caution, left)	2
½	lemon	½

1. Using a juicer, process tomatoes, carrots, celery, watercress, radishes, parsley and lemon. Whisk and pour into glasses.

Gingered Broccoli

2	spears broccoli	2
1	clove garlic	1
⅛	head cabbage	⅛
1	½-inch (1 cm) piece gingerroot	1

1. Using a juicer, process broccoli, garlic, cabbage and ginger. Whisk and pour into a glass.

Gout Buster Juice

Caution: Parsley should be avoided during pregnancy and in cases of kidney inflammation.

4	stalks celery	4
3	sprigs fresh parsley (see Caution, left)	3
1	carrot	1
1	clove garlic	1
1	handful kale	1
1	½-inch (1 cm) piece gingerroot	1

1. Using a juicer, process celery, parsley, carrot, garlic, kale and ginger. Whisk and pour into a glass.

Green Beet

Serves 1

½ cup	kelp or other sea herb	125 mL
1 cup	hot water	250 mL
1	beet, top intact	1
1 cup	fresh spinach leaves	250 mL
1	apple	1

1. In a medium bowl, pour water over kelp. Soak for 15 to 20 minutes or until kelp is soft. Drain soaking water, reserve for another use.

2. Using a juicer, process kelp, beet, beet top, spinach and apple. Whisk and pour into a glass.

Green Goddess

Serves 1

Caution: Parsley should be avoided during pregnancy and in cases of kidney inflammation.

1	spear broccoli	1
½	cucumber	½
½	green bell pepper	½
2	sprigs fresh parsley (see Caution, left)	2

1. Using a juicer, process broccoli, cucumber, parsley and pepper. Whisk and pour into a glass.

Trial by fire:
common chile peppers

There are five cultivated species of the *Capsicum* genus — *C. annuum*, *C. frutescens*, *C. chinense*, *C. baccatum* and *C. pubescens* — and over 20 wild varieties.

For juicing, use fresh chiles. Wash, remove stems and juice whole (or cut larger varieties in half). The hot, irritating component, capsaicin, is concentrated in the ribs of the flesh, not the seeds (as is commonly thought), so leave the seeds intact. When first using chile peppers for juicing, juice after all other ingredients have been put through the machine and keep the juice separate. Add it to vegetable juice blends by the teaspoon (5 mL) in order to gage the amount with which you are comfortable.

As an alternative to fresh chiles, whisk in a drop of hot or jerk sauce or ¼ tsp (1 mL) of powdered cayenne to juices and blended drinks. Adding yogurt to blended drinks helps to extinguish the fire. Dried or smoked chiles may be added to smoothies in small quantities. Remember to handle all chiles with care, washing hands thoroughly after touching.

Listed from mildest to hottest, the following are just a few of the hundreds of varieties enjoyed today.

New Mexican. Formerly called "Anaheim," the long green, mild chiles are available fresh, canned, roasted or left on the bush to turn red in the fall. Their taste is similar to mild bell peppers. They are used in most classic Tex-Mex dishes and are a good choice for novice chile users.

Poblano/Ancho. Poblano is the name of the fresh version of this big flat pepper, the widest of the hot peppers. Called ancho when dried, it acquires a nutty taste and raisin-like appearance and is the most commonly used variety in Mexico.

Jalapeño. Widely known, and at the halfway point on the Scoville Heat Unit Scale, they lend a meaty texture and rich flavor to dishes. Their thick flesh makes jalapeños an excellent juicing chile. When smoked and dried, jalapeños are called chipotles.

Serrano. More flavorful than jalapeño, the name serrano means "from the mountains." They are the most popular choice for fresh salsas, stews and moles.

Cayenne. Grown commercially in New Mexico, Africa, India, Japan and Mexico, the most common form is dried. A favorite in African and Cajun dishes, cayenne is a major ingredient in barbecue rubs and powders. See page 127 for health actions.

Habanero. Also known also as Scotch bonnet and rated a blazing 10+ on the Scoville Heat Unit Scale, this small, round chile really packs a punch in hot pepper and Caribbean jerk sauces, where it imparts a unique fruity, apricot-like aroma.

Visit www.nettally.com/saints/hotstuff.html or www.g6csy.net/chile/index.html for more information and links on chiles.

Green Magic

Serves 1

2	stalks celery	2
1	wedge cabbage	1
1	handful fresh spinach leaves	1
¼ cup	cubed pumpkin	50 mL
1 tsp	powdered ginkgo, optional	5 mL

1. Using a juicer, process celery, cabbage, spinach and pumpkin. Whisk together with ginkgo if using and pour into a glass.

Immunity

Serves 1

2	stalks celery	2
2	carrots	2
1	clove garlic	1
1	apple	1
1	½-inch (1 cm) piece gingerroot	1
½	lemon	½

1. Using a juicer, process celery, carrots, garlic, apple, ginger and lemon. Whisk and pour into a glass.

Kelp

Serves 1

6	kale	6
¼	fresh fennel bulb	¼
2	carrots	2
1 tsp	crumbled dried kelp	5 mL
Pinch	ground nutmeg	Pinch

1. Using a juicer, process kale, fennel and carrots. Whisk together with kelp and nutmeg and pour into a glass.

Leafy Greens

Serves 1

Tip
Substitute lettuce or cabbage leaves for any of the leaves in this recipe. Use the celery and apple to tap the leaves through the feed tube.

8	fresh spinach leaves	8
2	kale leaves	2
1	beet, top intact or turnip	1
2	stalks celery	2
1	apple	1

1. Using a juicer, process spinach, kale, beet, beet top, celery and apple. Whisk and pour into a glass.

Serves 1

Liquid Lunch

1	stalk celery	1
1	carrot	1
$\frac{1}{2}$	cucumber	$\frac{1}{2}$
1	sprig fresh dill	1
1	apple	1
1 tbsp	protein powder	15 mL

1. Using a juicer, process celery, carrot, cucumber, dill and apple. Whisk and pour into a glass. Whisk in protein powder.

Serves 1

Liquid Salsa

2	tomatoes	2
1	fresh jalapeño pepper	1
$\frac{1}{4}$	onion	$\frac{1}{4}$
6	sprigs fresh cilantro	6
$\frac{1}{2}$	lime	$\frac{1}{2}$

1. Using a juicer, process tomatoes, jalapeño pepper, onion, cilantro and lime. Whisk and pour into a glass.

Serves 1	# Moist & Juicy	
1	leek, white and tender green parts	1
2	kale leaves	2
2	carrots	2
2	apples	2
1 tsp	powdered ginkgo	5 mL

1. Using a juicer, process leek, kale, carrots and apples. Whisk together with ginkgo and pour into a glass.

Serves 1	# Nip of Goodness	
1	turnip	1
3	parsnips	3
1	apple	1
¼	fresh fennel bulb	¼

1. Using a juicer, process turnip, parsnips, apple and fennel. Whisk and pour into a glass.

Serves 1	# Peas and Carrots	
1 cup	fresh or frozen peas	250 mL
2	carrots	2
1	parsnip	1
¼	onion	¼
¼	fresh fennel bulb	¼

1. Using a juicer, process peas, carrots, parsnip, onion and fennel. Whisk and pour into a glass.

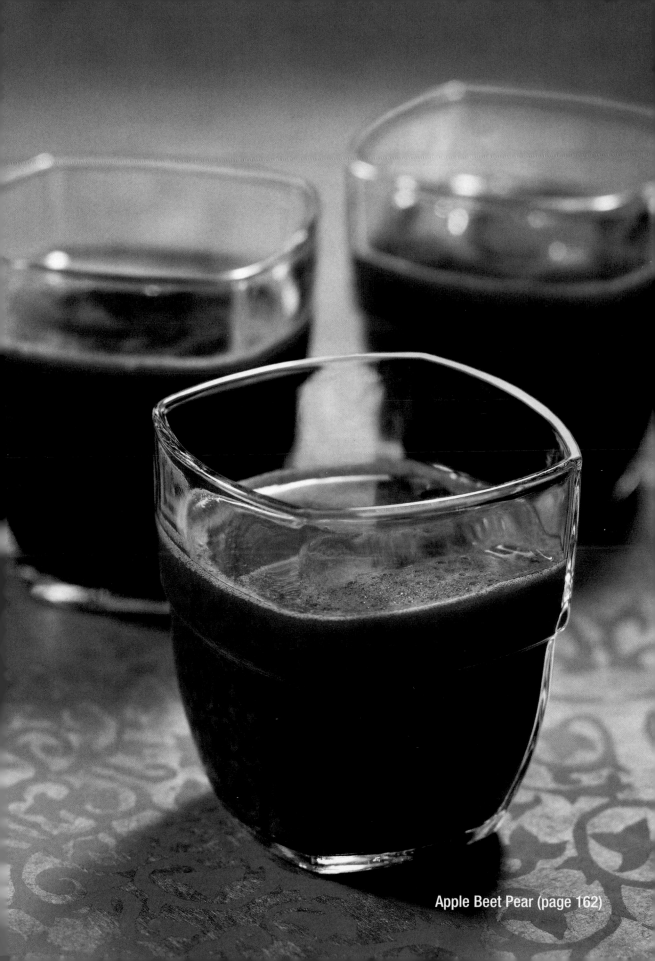

Apple Beet Pear (page 162)

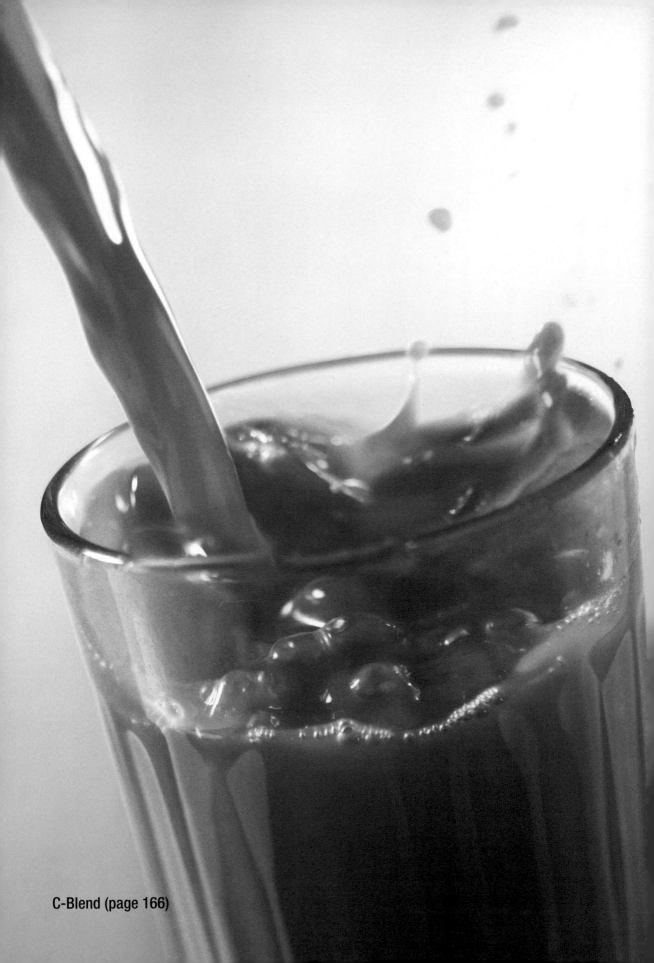

C-Blend (page 166)

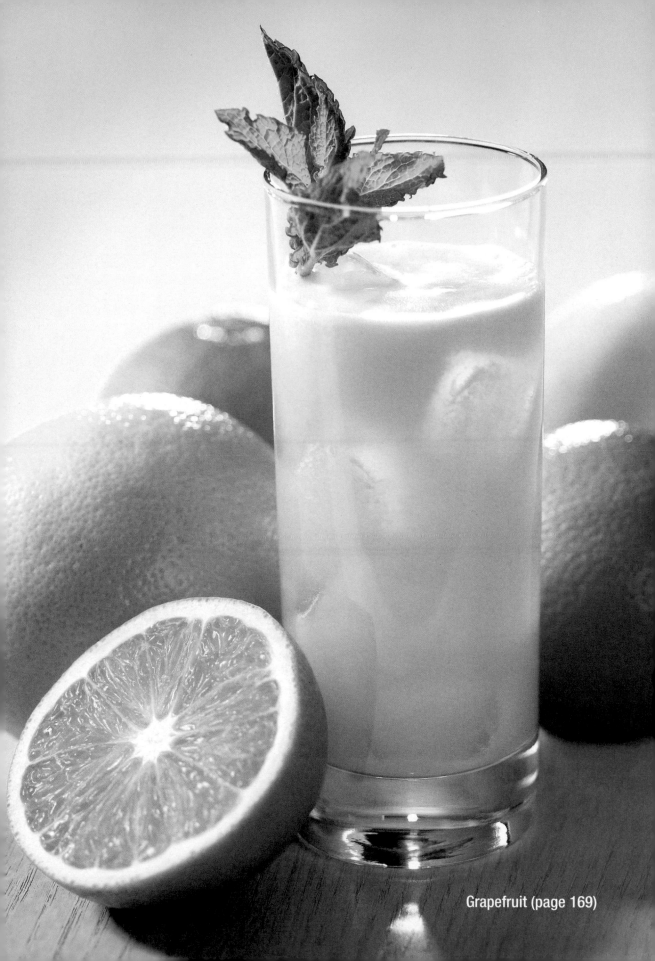

Grapefruit (page 169)

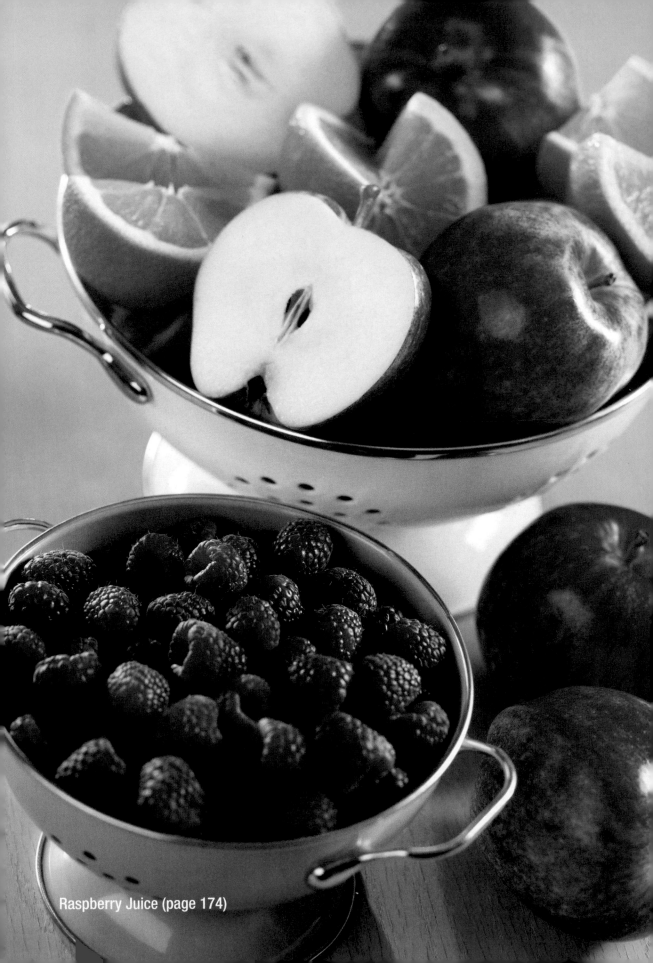
Raspberry Juice (page 174)

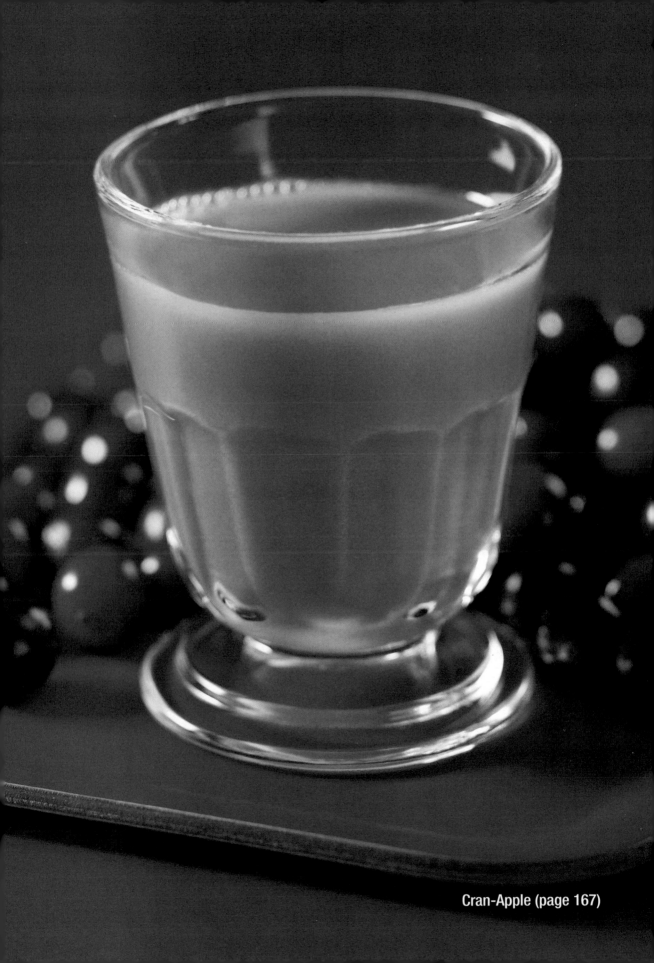

Cran-Apple (page 167)

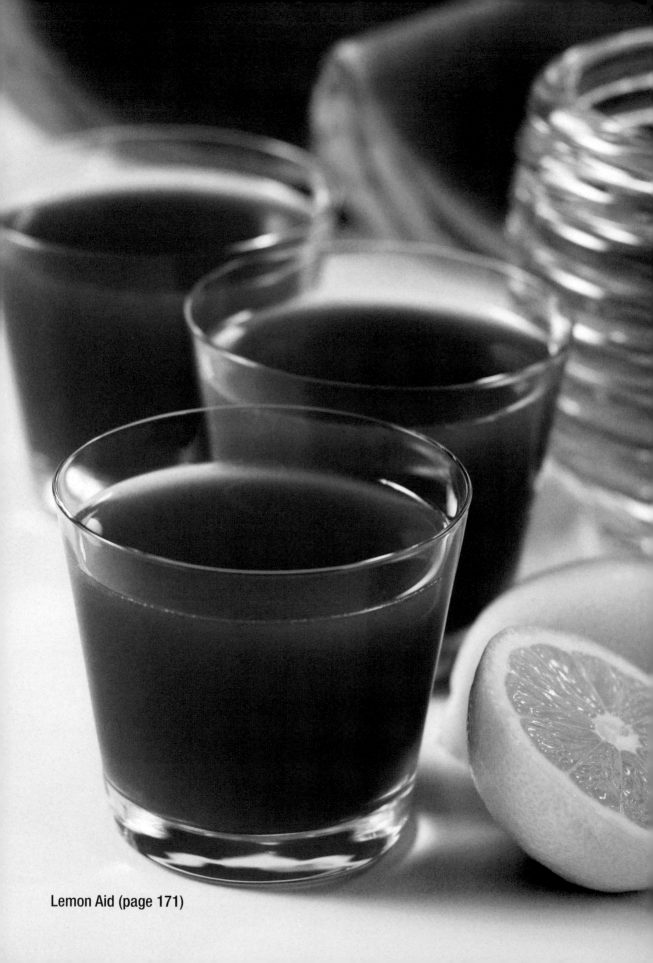

Lemon Aid (page 171)

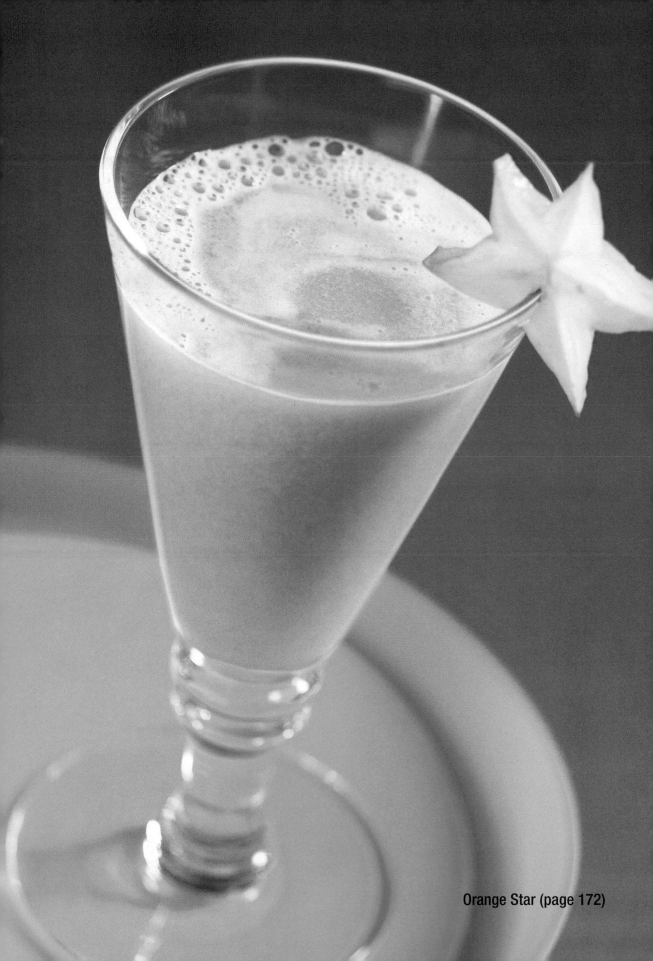

Orange Star (page 172)

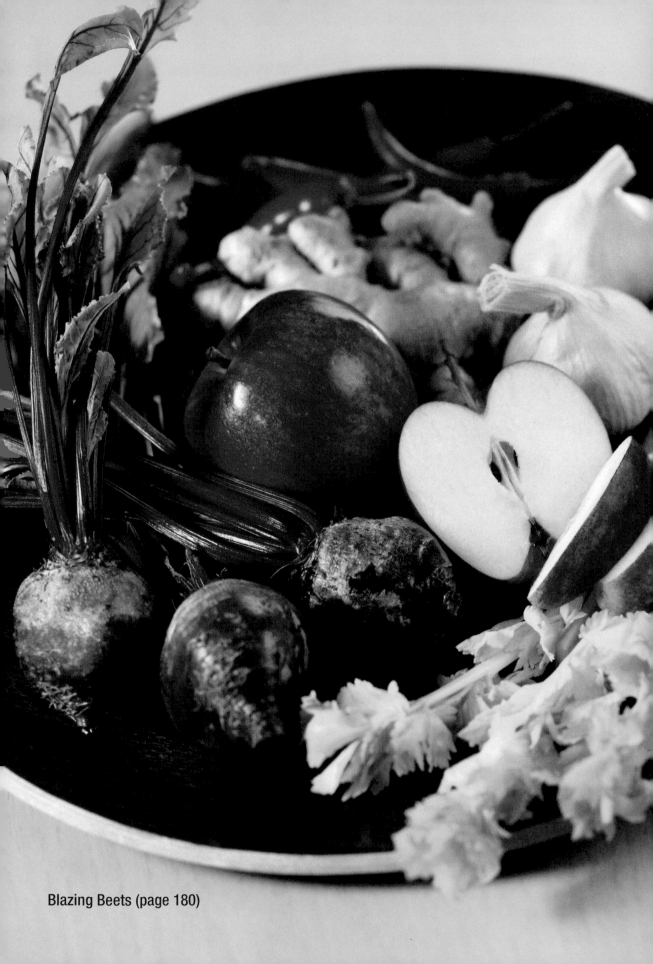

Blazing Beets (page 180)

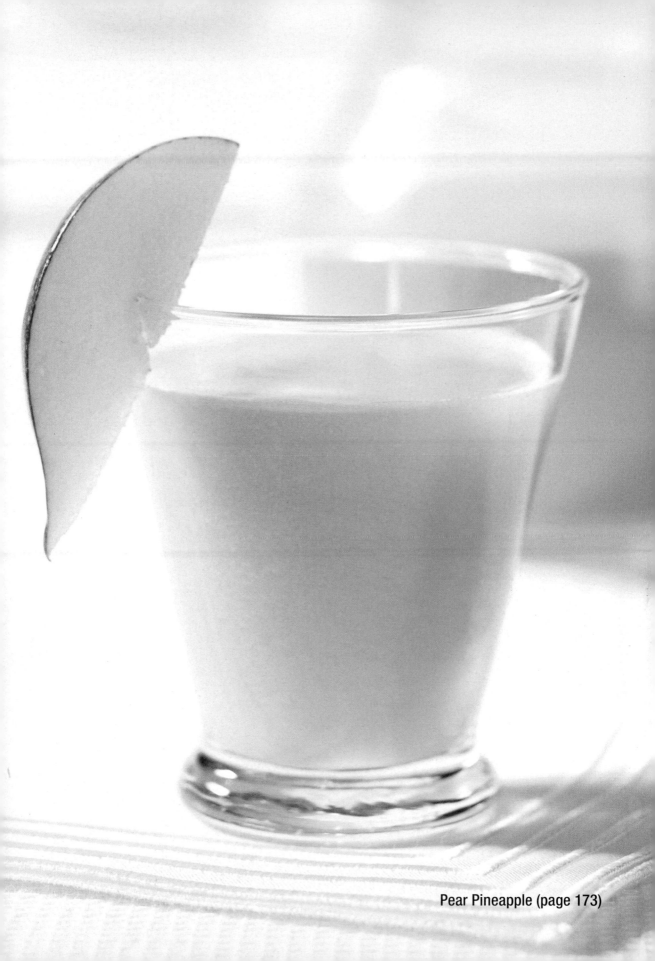

Pear Pineapple (page 173)

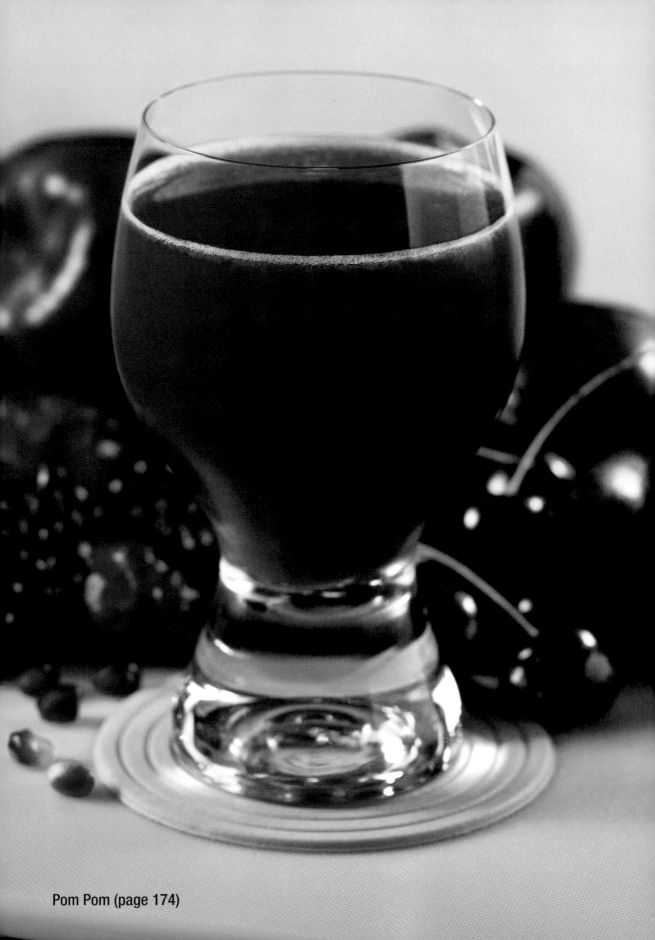

Pom Pom (page 174)

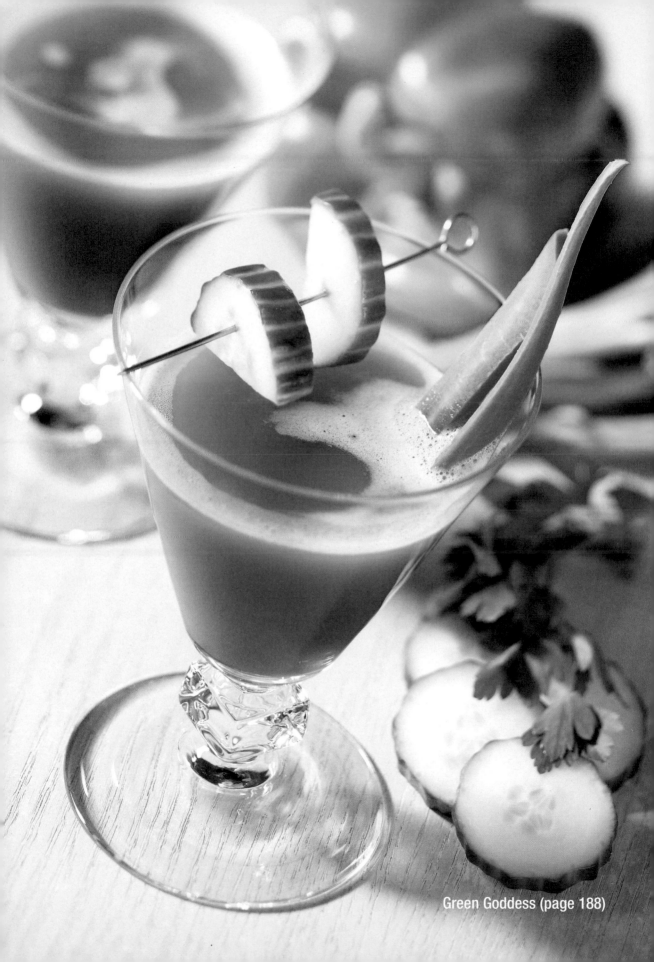

Green Goddess (page 188)

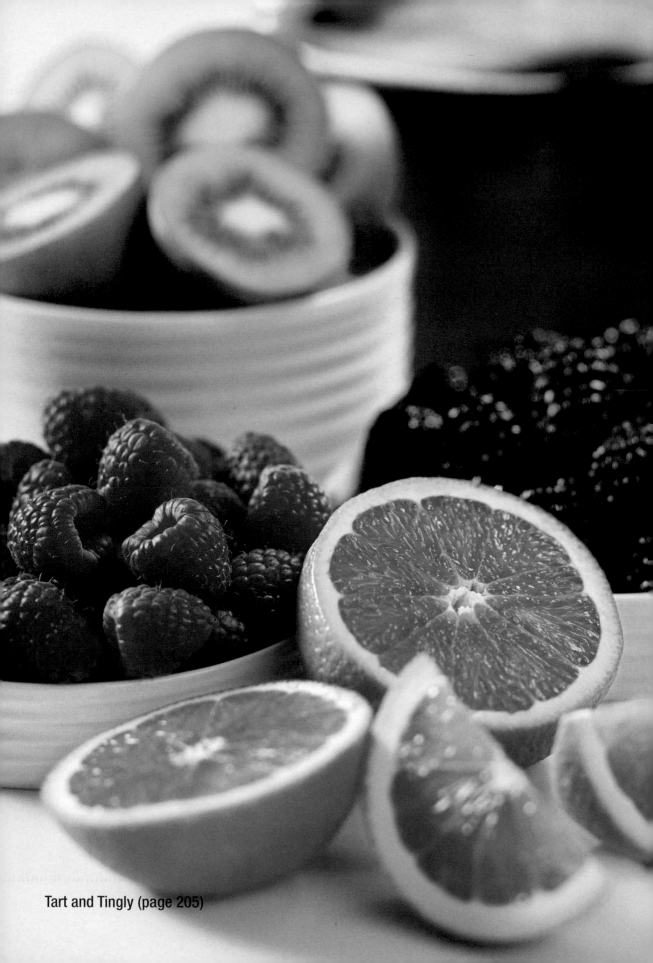

Tart and Tingly (page 205)

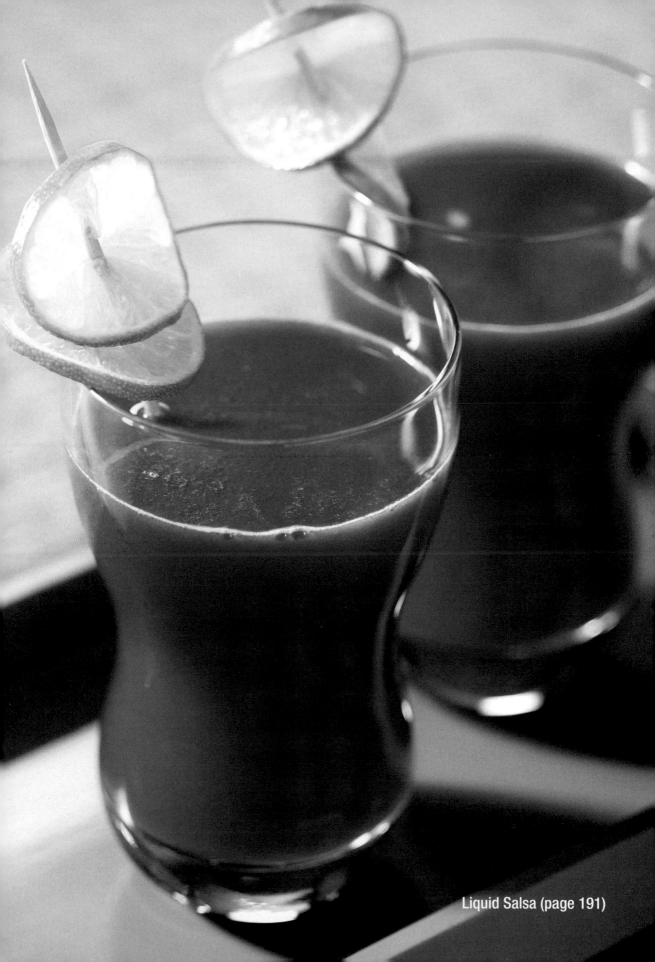

Liquid Salsa (page 191)

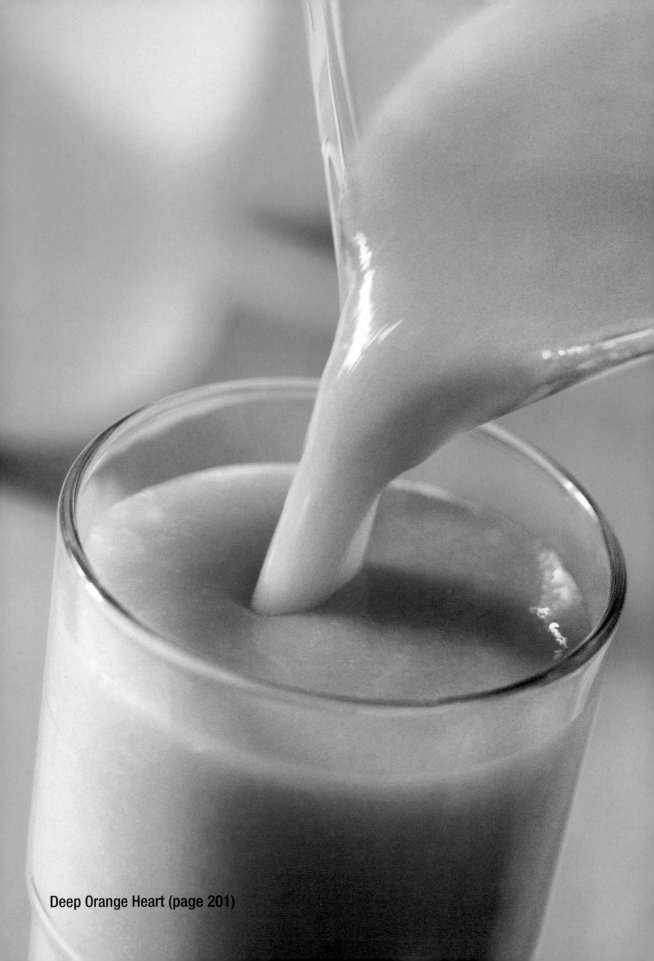

Deep Orange Heart (page 201)

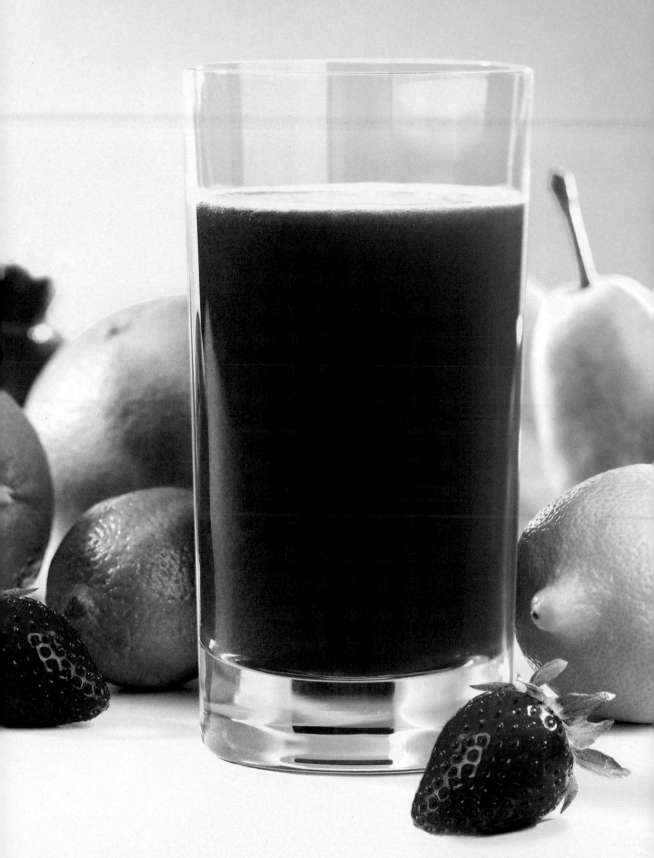

Deep Red Heart (page 202)

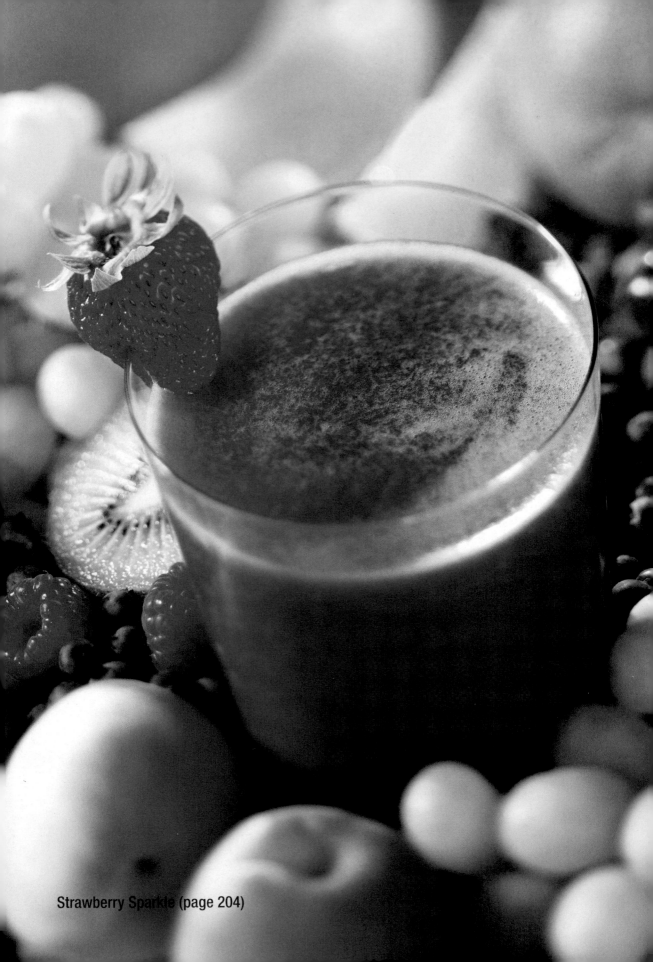

Strawberry Sparkle (page 204)

Peas Please

Serves 1

1 cup	fresh or frozen peas	250 mL
6	sprigs fresh parsley (see Caution, left)	6
2	carrots	2

1. Using a juicer, process peas, parsley and carrots. Whisk and pour into a glass.

Peppers Please

Serves 1

1	red bell pepper, trimmed	1
1	green pepper, trimmed	1
½	cucumber	½
1	carrot	1

1. Using a juicer, process red and green peppers, cucumber and carrot. Whisk and pour into a glass.

Red Devil

Serves 1

4	tomatoes	4
5	radishes	5
½	red bell pepper, trimmed	½
1	beet	1
Pinch	cayenne pepper	Pinch

1. Using a juicer, process tomatoes, radishes, pepper and beet. Whisk together with cayenne and pour into a glass.

Root Combo

Serves 1

1	parsnip	1
2	carrots	2
1	beet	1
1	apple	1

1. Using a juicer, process parsnip, carrots, beet and apple. Whisk and pour into a glass.

Sea Herb Surprise

Serves 1

Tip
Wakame, nori or kelp can be substituted for the dulse.

3	stalks celery	3
2	carrots	2
1 cup	cubed squash	250 mL
1 tsp	extra-virgin olive oil or hemp oil	5 mL
1 tsp	crumbled dried dulse	5 mL

1. Using a juicer, process celery, carrots and squash. Whisk together with oil and dulse and pour into a glass.

Slippery Beet

Serves 2

2	beets	2
1	clove garlic	1
1	apple	1
1 tbsp	powdered slippery elm, optional	15 mL

1. Using a juicer, process beets, garlic and apple. Whisk together with slippery elm, if using, and pour into a glass.

Soft Salad

Serves 1

½	head bok choy	½
1	carrot	1
2	stalks celery	2
¼ cup	bean sprouts	50 mL
1	wedge pineapple	1

1. Using a juicer, process bok choy, carrot, celery, bean sprouts and pineapple. Whisk and pour into a glass.

Spiced Carrot

Serves 1

3	carrots	3
1	spear broccoli	1
½ cup	fresh spinach leaves	125 mL
1	½-inch (1 cm) piece gingerroot	1
½ tsp	ground cinnamon	2 mL
⅛ tsp	cayenne pepper, or to taste	0.5 mL

1. Using a juicer, process carrots, broccoli, spinach and ginger. Whisk together with cinnamon and cayenne and pour into a glass.

Spring Celebration

Serves 1

10	spears asparagus	10
2	beets, tops intact	2
6	fresh spinach leaves	6
1	handful watercress or dandelion leaves	1
1	apple	1
2 tbsp	maple sap, optional	25 mL

1. Using a juicer, process asparagus, beets, beet tops, spinach, watercress and apple. Whisk together with maple sap, if using, and pour into a glass.

Serves 1	# Squash Special	
1	sweet potato	1
1 cup	cubed squash	250 mL
½ tsp	cayenne pepper	2 mL
½ tsp	dried dill	2 mL
½ tsp	ground cumin	2 mL

1. Using a juicer, process sweet potato. Set aside. Using another container, process squash. Whisk in cayenne, dill and cumin.

2. When starch from sweet potato has settled on the bottom of the first container, pour the clarified sweet potato juice carefully into squash juice, leaving starch behind. Discard starch. Whisk and pour into a glass.

Serves 1	# Thorny Pear	
2	pears	2
1	red bell pepper, trimmed	1
1	cucumber	1
1 tsp	powdered hawthorn	5 mL

1. Using a juicer, process pears, red pepper and cucumber. Whisk together with hawthorn and pour into a glass.

Tomato Tang

Serves 1

2	tomatoes	2
2	carrots	2
1	beet	1
¼ cup	whole cranberries, fresh or frozen	50 mL

1. Using a juicer, process tomatoes, carrots, beet and cranberries. Whisk and pour into a glass.

Watercress

Serves 1

3	handfuls fresh watercress	3
2	stalks celery	2
2	sprigs fresh basil	2
1	parsnip	1
½	green bell pepper, trimmed	½

1. Using a juicer, process watercress, celery, basil, parsnip and green pepper. Whisk and pour into a glass.

Zippy Tomato

Serves 1

Caution: Parsley should be avoided during pregnancy and in cases of kidney inflammation.

1	tomato	1
1	½-inch (1 cm) piece gingerroot	1
4	sprigs fresh parsley, (see Caution, left)	4
½	lemon	½

1. Using a juicer, process tomatoes, ginger, parsley and lemon. Whisk and pour into a glass.

Juices for Healthy Bodies

Heart-Healthy Tonics

Best Heart-Healthy Juice Ingredients

Fruits: apples, apricots, blueberries, blackberries, citrus fruits*, cranberries, kiwifruits, mangos, melons, papayas, plums, pomegranates, raspberries, red grapes, strawberries
Vegetables: asparagus, carrots, celery, dark leafy green vegetables, garlic, onions, squash, tomatoes
Herbs: cayenne, chicory root, dandelion leaf and root**, fenugreek seeds, garlic, ginger, hawthorne, linden flowers, parsley***, rosemary, stinging nettles, turmeric

*   Avoid grapefruit if you are using calcium channel blocker medication.
**   People who are allergic to ragweed are sometimes also allergic to herbs in the same botanical family (compositae or daisy). Some of the herbs in this family include burdock, calendula, chamomile, chicory, dandelion, echinacea, feverfew, milk thistle and yarrow (avoid yarrow if you are pregnant).
***   If you are pregnant, limit your intake of parsley to ½ tsp (2 mL) dried or one sprig fresh per day. Do not take parsley if you are suffering from kidney inflammation.

Serves 1 or 2	**Cabbage Patch**	

¼	red or green cabbage	¼
4	stalks fresh asparagus	4
2	apples	2
1	carrot	1
½ cup	hulled fresh or frozen strawberries	125 mL

1. Using a juicer, process cabbage, asparagus, apples, carrot and strawberries. Whisk and pour into glasses.

Serves 1		

Deep Green Heart

Any dark green leafy vegetable such as spinach, Swiss chard or beet tops may be used in this nourishing drink.

2 cups	dark leafy greens	500 mL
2	apples	2
1	carrot	1
¼	lime	¼

1. Using a juicer, process greens, apples, carrot and lime. Whisk and pour into a glass.

Serves 1 or 2		

Deep Orange Heart

1	mango, pitted	1
1	wedge cantaloupe	1
2	fresh apricots, pitted	2
1	orange	1

1. Using a juicer, process mango, cantaloupe, apricots and orange. Whisk and pour into glasses.

Serves 1 or 2		

Deep Purple Heart

¾ cup	red grapes	175 mL
½ cup	blueberries	125 mL
½ cup	black cherries, pitted	125 mL
1	red or black plum, pitted	1
½ cup	cranberry juice	125 mL

1. Using a juicer, process grapes, blueberries, cherries and plum. Whisk together with cranberry juice and pour into glasses.

Deep Red Heart

Serves 1

Tip
During the winter months, thaw and use frozen raspberries and strawberries for this drink.

2	red or black plums, pitted	2
½ cup	raspberries	125 mL
½ cup	hulled fresh strawberries	125 mL
½ cup	cranberry juice	125 mL

1. Using a juicer, process plums, raspberries and strawberries. Whisk together with cranberry juice and pour into a glass.

De-Vine Fruits

Serves 1 or 2

4	tomatoes, quartered	4
1 cup	hulled fresh strawberries	250 mL
1	wedge honeydew melon	1
¼	lime	¼

1. Using a juicer, process tomatoes, strawberries, honeydew melon and lime. Whisk and pour into glasses.

Grape Heart

Serves 1

Tip
Use pulp in Grapefruit Frappé (see recipe, page 345). Be sure to remove white pith and seeds before juicing.

2 cups	red grapes	500 mL
1	grapefruit, cut in thirds	1
1 tsp	powdered dried linden flowers	5 mL

1. Using a juicer, process grapes and grapefruit. Whisk and pour into a glass. Whisk in linden flowers.

Heart Beet

Serves 1 or 2

2	beets, tops intact	2
2	carrots	2
2	stalks celery	2
1	apple	1
½	Vidalia onion	½

1. Using a juicer, process beets, beet tops, carrots, celery, apple and onion. Whisk and pour into glasses.

Melon Mania

Serves 1 or 2

¼	cantaloupe	¼
¼	honeydew melon	¼
1	2-inch (5 cm) slice watermelon, cut to fit tube	1
1	orange	1

1. Using a juicer, process cantaloupe, honeydew melon, watermelon and orange. Whisk and pour into a glass.

Orange Sunrise

Serves 1 or 2

2	oranges	2
2	kiwifruits	2
1	papaya, seeded	1
1	carrot	1

1. Using a juicer, process oranges, kiwifruits, papaya and carrot. Whisk and pour into glasses.

Serves 1	# Pomegranate Plus	
1	pomegranate, seeds only	1
2	red or black plums, pitted	2
½ cup	black cherries, pitted	125 mL
½ cup	hulled fresh strawberries	125 mL

1. Using a juicer, process pomegranate, plums, cherries and strawberries. Whisk and pour into a glass.

Serves 1	# Pumpkin Heart	
¼	acorn or butternut squash, cut to fit tube	¼
2	carrots	2
1	apple	1
1	clove garlic	1

1. Using a juicer, process squash, carrots, apple and garlic. Whisk and pour into a glass.

Serves 1 or 2	# Strawberry Sparkle	
1 cup	hulled fresh strawberries	250 mL
1	pomegranate, seeds only	1
½ cup	raspberries	125 mL
1	½-inch (1 cm) piece gingerroot	1
½ cup	cranberry juice	125 mL

1. Using a juicer, process strawberries, pomegranate, raspberries and ginger. Whisk together with cranberry juice and pour into glasses.

Tart and Tingly

Serves 1

3	kiwifruits	3
1	orange	1
½ cup	blackberries or raspberries	125 mL
½ cup	cranberry juice	125 mL

1. Using a juicer, process kiwifruits, orange and blackberries. Whisk together with cranberry juice and pour into a glass.

Tomato Tango

Serves 2

6	tomatoes	6
2	carrots	2
2	spring onions	2
¼	lime	¼
¼ tsp	cayenne pepper	1 mL

1. Using a juicer, process tomatoes, carrots, onions and lime. Whisk together with cayenne and pour into glasses.

Wake Up and Shine

Serves 1 or 2

2	oranges	2
1	grapefruit, cut to fit tube	1
1	pomegranate, seeds only	1
½ cup	hulled fresh strawberries	125 mL
1 tsp	blue-green algae	5 mL

1. Using a juicer, process oranges, grapefruit, pomegranate and strawberries. Whisk together with algae and pour into glasses.

Aperitifs and Digestives

Aperitifs

"The old pharmacopoeias recognized major bitters (roots of parsley, fennel, asparagus and butcher's broom) and minor bitters (roots of maidenhair fern, couchgrass, thistle, rest-harrow and strawberry-plant). The term as used today only applies to stimulants of appetite.

"Aperitifs served in cafés are drinks of a greater or lesser degree of bitterness, variously flavored, which are drunk neat or diluted with water. They generally have a strong alcoholic content, because the essences of which they are composed are not soluble except in strong alcohol (which is why they go cloudy when mixed with water) and this alcohol content to a great extent nullifies the beneficial action of the bitters.

"But through sheer force of habit (or perhaps through imagination), some people think that they have no appetite unless they have their daily aperitif (or aperitifs). It is this fact, which has led to the coining of the phrase that if an aperitif can open the appetite, it does so with a skeleton key. Be this as it may, the aperitif was, and still is, a traditional rite in certain circles."

The New Larousse Gastronomique. P. Montagné. New York: Crown Publishers, Inc., 1977.

Digestives

Digestive problems, or indigestion, is the inability to digest food and absorb the nutrients from it. Gas and bloating are often the result. These problems may mask more serious medical conditions that should always be attended to by a medical practitioner. Age often plays a major role in the decline of the body's digestive abilities; indigestion can be alleviated with foods or herbs. In many cases, eating foods in a specific order or following guidelines for food combining (see page 15) reduces gas, bloating, flatulence and burping.

The recipes in this section are to be prepared fresh, just before or after dinner. They are particularly useful in overcoming a feeling of fullness, and are sophisticated enough to accompany even the most elegant meal.

Best Digestive Juice Ingredients

Fruits: apples, blueberries, blackberries, grapes, kiwifruits, lemons, papayas, pineapples
Vegetables: bitter greens (page 218), cabbages, fennel, onions, red bell peppers
Herbs: basil, cardamom, cayenne, German chamomile, cinnamon, cloves, coriander, cumin, dill, fennel seeds, garlic, ginger, mustard seed, peppermint, thyme
Other: see Natural Aids to Digestion, page 213

Before Dinner Mint

This aperitif is naturally sweet, with just a hint of mint. Take it before eating to help stimulate liver and gall bladder function by increasing bile flow to the liver and intestines.

Tip

If fresh mint is not available, whisk 1 tbsp (15 mL) powdered dried peppermint into juice

3	kiwifruits	3
8	sprigs fresh peppermint	8
1	apple	1
	Ice, optional	

1. Using a juicer, process kiwifruits, peppermint and apple. Pour into a large glass over ice, if using.

Creamy Pineapple

½	pineapple, sliced	½
1	mango, pitted	1
1 cup	blueberries	250 mL
½ cup	natural yogurt	125 mL

1. Using a juicer, process pineapple, mango and blueberries. Whisk together with yogurt and pour into glasses.

Fennel Fantasy

Using both fresh fennel bulb and dried seeds, this drink has a strong anise flavor.

½	fresh fennel bulb, cut in half	½
2	apples	2
½ cup	red grapes	125 mL
¼ tsp	ground cinnamon	1 mL
Pinch	ground fennel, optional	Pinch

1. Using a juicer, process fennel, apples and grapes. Whisk together with cinnamon and ground fennel, if using, and pour into a glass.

Kiwi Kick

3	kiwifruits	3
1	wedge pineapple	1
½	lemon	½
¼ tsp	cayenne pepper or ground mustard seed	1 mL

1. Using a juicer, process kiwifruits, pineapple and lemon. Whisk together with cayenne and pour into a glass.

Papaya Punch

1	papaya, seeded	1
2	kiwifruits	2
1	apple	1
1	1-inch (2 cm) piece gingerroot	1

1. Using a juicer, process papaya, kiwifruits, apple and ginger. Whisk and pour into a glass.

Tropical Twister

1	papaya, seeded	1
¼	pineapple, cut in wedges	¼
¼	lemon	¼
2	fresh peppermint sprigs, optional	2

1. Using a juicer, process papaya, pineapple, lemon and peppermint, if using. Whisk and pour into a glass.

After Dinner Cocktail Smoothie

⅔ cup	mineral water	150 mL
2	papayas, seeded	2
½ cup	natural yogurt	125 mL
½	pineapple, sliced	½
1	½-inch (1 cm) piece gingerroot	1
	Ice, optional	

1. Using a Vita-Mix or a blender, process mineral water, papayas, yogurt, pineapple and ginger. Pour into cocktail glasses over ice, if using.

Berry Fine

Serves 1

1 cup	red grapes	250 mL
½ cup	blueberries	125 mL
½ cup	blackberries	125 mL
½	lemon	½

1. Using a juicer, process grapes, blueberries, blackberries and lemon. Whisk and pour into a glass.

Cabbage Head

Serves 2

½	head cabbage, cut to fit tube	½
1	handful fresh basil	1
2	carrots	2
1	apple	1
¼ tsp	crushed dill seeds	1 mL

1. Using a juicer, process cabbage, basil, carrots and apple. Whisk together with dill seeds and pour into glasses.

Dandelion Slam Dunk

½ cup	fresh dandelion leaves	125 mL
¼	cabbage, cut to fit tube	¼
2	apples	2
1	1-inch (2.5 cm) piece fresh dandelion root	1

1. Using a juicer, process dandelion leaves, cabbage, apples and dandelion root. Whisk and pour into a glass.

Digestive Cocktail Juice

This powerful drink will really get the digestive juices flowing. For a milder version, omit the garlic.

Tip
Serve before or after dinner in small glasses over ice and, for an extra kick, add a dash of cayenne.

2	tomatoes	2
2	carrots	2
¼	fresh fennel bulb	¼
1	clove garlic	1
4	fresh basil leaves	4
4	sprigs fresh dill	4
2	sprigs fresh thyme	2
2	stalks celery	2
1	beet	1
½ tsp	ground turmeric	2 mL
¼ tsp	powdered mustard	1 mL
¼ tsp	ground cumin	1 mL
Pinch	ground cloves, optional	Pinch

1. Using a juicer, process tomatoes, carrots, fennel, garlic, basil, dill, thyme, celery and beet. Pour into a pitcher and whisk in turmeric, mustard, cumin and cloves if using.

Digestive (Gripe) Water

Fennel seeds are calming and antiflatulent and have been safely given to babies to treat colic for centuries. This water is also effective as a digestive for adults and especially recommended after eating oily fish or fried foods.

Tip

To store: Pour into a clean (or sterile) jar. Cover tightly and keep in refrigerator for up to 2 days.

1 tsp	fennel seeds	5 mL
3	fresh stevia leaves or 1 tsp (5 mL) dried, optional	3
1¼ cups	boiling water	300 mL

1. With a mortar and pestle, crush fennel and stevia if using. Transfer to a non-reactive teapot.

2. Pour boiling water over crushed herbs. Cover and steep for 20 minutes. Strain, discarding solids.

For adults: Sip 1 serving, warm or cold, after eating.
For babies: Make sure all solids are strained out. Dilute ¼ cup (50 mL) gripe water with ½ cup (125 mL) warm water or chamomile tea. Fill the baby's bottle with the warm mixture for drinking

Digestive Seed Tea

Tea blend

Anise seeds (*Pimpinella anisum*) or star anise (*Illicium anisatum*) can be used in this recipe. Both have digestive properties.

1 part	anise seed	1 part
1 part	dill seed	1 part
1 part	fennel seed	1 part

1. In a medium bowl, combine anise, dill and fennel. Transfer to a clean jar with lid and label. Store in a cool, dry dark place.

2. *To make tea:* Into a mortar or small electric grinder, measure 1 tsp (5 mL) blended seeds for every 1 cup (250 mL) to be made. Lightly crush seeds (with pestle or grinder.) Place crushed seeds in a non-reactive teapot and cover with boiling water. Steep for 15 minutes. Strain and drink warm.

Serves 2	**Granate Berry**	
1	pomegranate, seeds only	1
1 cup	raspberries	250 mL
1 cup	cherries or blueberries	250 mL
½ cup	natural yogurt	125 mL
¼ tsp	ground cinnamon	1 mL

1. Using a juicer, process pomegranate seeds, raspberries and cherries. Whisk together with yogurt and cinnamon and pour into glasses.

Serves 1	**Great Grape**	
1 cup	grapes	250 mL
¼	pineapple, sliced	¼
2	apples	2
½	lime	½

1. Using a juicer, process grapes, pineapple, apples and lime. Whisk and pour a glass.

Beans and the digestive system

Dried beans are rich in oligosaccharides — complex sugars that can't be broken down by human digestive enzymes. When you eat legumes, the oligosaccharides enter the lower intestine, where they are met by bacteria that eat the starches and, in the process, create gas. To combat this effect, some cultures combine savory (*Satureja*) with beans, peas and lentils. Drinking carminative herbs (cayenne, chamomile, cinnamon, clove, lavender, peppermint, parsley, rosemary) in teas is helpful as well.

Natural Aids to Digestion

Acidophilus (see Yogurt, page 156). *Lactobacillus acidophilus* is a "friendly" type of bacteria used to ferment milk into yogurt. It replaces the intestinal bacteria necessary for digestion which are destroyed by antibiotics.

Calendula (*Calendula officinalis*, see page 126). Stimulates bile production and in this way aids digestion. Calendula may be included in aperitifs and makes an attractive garnish for drinks.

Cinnamon (*Cinnamomum zeylanicum*, see page 128). A warming carminative used to promote digestion, cinnamon adds a pleasant taste to aperitif and digestive drinks.

Dandelion root (*Taraxacum officinale*, see page 130). Easily obtained, fairly mild but bitter laxative that stimulates the liver and gall bladder and increases the flow of bile to aid digestion. Dandelion leaves act as a diuretic.

Fennel (*Foeniculum vulgare*, see pages 116 and 132). Juice the bulb or make tea from the seeds to aid digestion and soothe discomfort from heartburn and indigestion.

Fiber (see page 363). Insoluble fiber in fruits, vegetables and whole grains helps prevent constipation and digestive diseases such as diverticulosis and colon cancer.

German chamomile (*Matricaria recutita*, see page 133). As Peter Rabbit's mother knew, chamomile soothes upset tummies and inflammations and reduces flatulence and pain caused by gas.

Ginger (*Zingeber officinalis*, see page 134). Ginger is used to stimulate blood flow to the digestive system and to increase absorption of nutrients. It increases the action of the gallbladder while protecting the liver against toxins.

Kiwifruits (*Actinidia chinensis*, see page 103). Enzymes in kiwifruits help digestion.

Licorice (*Glycyrrhiza glabra*, see page 139). Soothes gastric mucus membranes and eases spasms of the large intestine. Should be avoided in cases of high blood pressure.

Papayas (*Carica papaya*, see page 105). Papaya is a traditional remedy for indigestion. It contains an enzyme called papain, which is similar to pepsin, an enzyme that helps digestion of protein.

Peppermint (*Mentha piperita*, see page 143). Peppermint contains flavonoids that stimulate the liver and gallbladder and increases the flow of bile. Its antispasmodic effect on the smooth muscles of the digestive tract make it a good choice in after-dinner drinks.

Pineapples (*Ananas comosus*, see page 106). Pineapple is rich in the antibacterial enzyme bromelain, which is anti-inflammatory and helps in the digestive process.

Turmeric (*Curcuma longa*, see page 149). Increases bile production and bile flow.

James Duke's Carminatea

Makes ¼ cup (50 mL) tea blend

The world's foremost authority on healing herbs and the healing traditions of different cultures, James Duke has written several books on the practical use of herbs for medicinal purposes. Here is a recipe for deflating flatus, based on his recipe for Carminatea from his book, *The Green Pharmacy*.

Caution: Do not use licorice if you have high blood pressure.

2 tbsp	peppermint	25 mL
1 tbsp	German chamomile	15 mL
1 tbsp	lemon balm	15 mL
2 tsp	dill seeds	10 mL
1 tsp	fennel seeds	5 mL
1 tsp	powdered licorice (see Caution, left)	5 mL

1. In a medium bowl, combine peppermint, chamomile, lemon balm, dill, fennel and licorice. Transfer to a clean jar with a lid and label. Store in a cool, dry dark place.

2. For each 1 cup (250 mL) tea, lightly crush 1 tsp (5 mL) blended herbs with a mortar and pestle or small food grinder. Add to a non-reactive warmed teapot and pour in boiling water. Steep for 15 minutes. Strain and drink warm.

Peppered Fruit

Serves 1

2	apples	2
2	red bell peppers, trimmed	2
1 cup	grapes	250 mL
¼ tsp	cayenne pepper	1 mL

1. Using a juicer, process apples, red peppers and grapes. Whisk together with cayenne and pour into a glass.

Peppery Cabbage

1	red bell pepper, trimmed	1
1	green bell pepper, trimmed	1
1	wedge red or green cabbage	1
1	apple	1
1	clove garlic	1

1. Using a juicer, process red pepper, green pepper, cabbage, apple and garlic. Whisk and pour into glasses.

Rosy Peppermint Tea

Take this digestive tea after meals. Be sure to use organic herbs and rose petals that have not been exposed to pesticides. Roses from floral shops must not be used for food or drinks.

1 tbsp	fresh peppermint leaves or 1 tsp (5 mL) dried	15 mL
1 tbsp	fresh rose petals or 1 tsp (5 mL) dried	15 mL
2 cups	boiling water	500 ml
2	slices kiwifruit, optional	2

1. In a mortar, lightly bruise peppermint and rose petals. Place in a non-reactive teapot and pour boiling water over. Cover and steep for 10 minutes.

2. Strain the tea into mugs and garnish with kiwifruit slices, if using.

Spiced Cabbage

¼	cabbage, cut to fit tube	¼
¼	fresh fennel bulb	¼
1	apple	1
1	½-inch (1 cm) piece gingerroot	1
⅛ tsp	cinnamon	1 mL

1. Using a juicer, process cabbage, fennel, apple and ginger. Whisk together with cinnamon and pour into a glass.

Serves 1 or 2

Spiced Papaya Tea

Sweet enough to enjoy on its own, this tea also brings a fine meal to a satisfying conclusion.

2 tbsp	chopped dried papaya	25 mL
½ tsp	slippery elm bark powder	2 mL
½ tsp	lightly crushed coriander seeds	2 mL
¼ tsp	ground cinnamon	1 mL
¼ tsp	ground cumin	1 mL
¼ tsp	ground turmeric	1 mL
2 cups	boiling water	500 mL

1. In a non-reactive teapot, combine papaya, slippery elm bark, coriander, cinnamon, cumin and turmeric. Pour boiling water over herbs. Cover and steep for 15 minutes. Strain the tea into cups and drink warm.

Serves 1

Vidalia Vigor

¼	cabbage, cut to fit tube	¼
½	red bell pepper, trimmed	½
½	Vidalia onion	½
¼	fresh fennel bulb	¼
Pinch	ground fennel seeds	Pinch

1. Using a juicer, process cabbage, red pepper, onion and fennel. Whisk together with ground fennel seeds and pour into a glass.

Bitters

Herbalists agree that bitters support the heart, small intestines and liver, as well as reduce fever. The astringent taste of greens such as endive, chicory, sheep sorrel, radicchio, dandelion and yellow dock awakens the palate and makes it more receptive to appreciate other flavors. The digestive tonic action promotes the secretion of hydrochloric acid that aids digestion. A glass of bitter juice is an excellent tool for whetting the appetite, but may take some getting used to.

In Chinese medicine, bitters are cool and drying, and therefore used to reduce fevers and dry excess body fluids. In the Ayurvedic model, bitter foods have a similar function: to stimulate the digestion to absorb phlegm and to treat fevers or skin disease.

Scientists say we have about 10,000 taste buds, with each one living not much longer than a week before it is shed and regenerated. Taste buds are clusters of cells in the tongue and in the mouth that relay the four tastes —sweet, salty, bitter and sour — to the brain. Some herbalists and ancient traditions link the four tastes to effects on the mind. For example, a balanced intake of bitter flavors could be thought to encourage honesty, integrity, optimism and a loving heart.

To start enjoying the medicinal effects of bitters, it might be helpful to begin with a combination of bitter and slightly sweet juices, then gradually eliminate the sweeter juices until you are taking the bitters on their own. Keep in mind that the bitter taste must be present in order to realize the medicinal effects; to sweeten them is to cancel their effect.

Use any or all of the bitter herbs and vegetables listed here to blend your own bitters. Try to use them fresh in juices, teas and salads — all of them are easily grown, most are available fresh in supermarkets and some may be wildcrafted.

Bitter Greens

Dandelion leaf (*Taraxacum officinale*, see page 130). Leaves may be dried for bitter tea blends.
Chicory (*Cichorium intybus*). Use fresh or dried root or leaves for bitter teas.
Endive (*Cichorium endivia*). Good for salads to start or end to a meal.
Radicchio (*Cichorium endivia*). A red version of Belgium endive.
Rapini (*Brassica rapa*, *Ruvo*). Flowering stems and leaves have a mildly bitter flavor. Often found in European markets.
Sheep sorrel (*Rumex acetoselia*). A close relative to French sorrel (*Rumex scutatus*). Use either in bitters. Traditionally used for fevers, inflammation, diarrhea, excessive menstruation and cancer (sheep sorrel is one of the four ingredients of the Essiac anti-cancer remedy).
Watercress (*Nasturtium officinale*, see page 121). A sharp, peppery, but not unpleasant taste makes watercress a welcome addition to salads and sandwiches.
Yellow dock (*Rumex crispus*, see page 151). Leaves have a distinctive, sour flavor that combines well with dandelion leaves, chickweed, chicory and the milder lettuces. Wash dock leaves before eating raw: the chrysophanic acid irritates the mouth and can cause a numbing sensation of the tongue and lips for several hours.

Bitter Bite

Serves 2

Serve this in a small glass just before eating.

1	bunch endive	1
1	handful fresh spinach	1
2	carrots	2
¼ tsp	ground cardamom	1 mL

1. Using a juicer, process endive, spinach and carrots. Whisk together with cardamom and pour into glasses.

Dandelion Bitters

Serves 1 or 2

As your taste for bitters increases, the apple can be gradually withdrawn from this drink. Drink ¼ cup (50 mL) at noon and/or just before dinner.

1	4-inch (10 cm) piece fresh dandelion root	1
2	carrots	2
1	apple	1

1. Using a juicer, process dandelion, carrots and apple. Whisk and pour into 1 large or 2 smaller glasses.

Dandelion Delight

1 tbsp	chopped dried dandelion root	15 mL
2 cups	water	500 mL
1 tbsp	fresh German chamomile flowers or 1 tsp (5 mL) dried	15 mL
1 tsp	fennel seeds	5 mL

1. In a non-reactive saucepan over medium heat, bring dandelion root and water to a slow simmer. Cover pot, reduce heat and simmer for 20 minutes.

2. Place chamomile and fennel seeds in a ceramic teapot. Pour hot dandelion water over herbs, straining out dandelion and steep for 5 minutes. Drink hot or cool to room temperature.

Spring Green Bitters

Use this drink sparingly. Make the recipe once in the spring and take daily for as long as it lasts (maximum 2 to 3 days). If desired repeat once again in the fall.

Tip

Sorrel leaves have a high oxalic acid content, so eat when young and tender in the spring, in small amounts.

6	yellow dock leaves with stems	6
4	endive leaves	4
4	sprigs sheep sorrel	4
4	stalks celery	4
	Liquid honey, optional	

1. Using juicer, process yellow dock, endive, sheep sorrel and celery. Whisk in honey to taste, if using. Take 1 or 2 tbsp (15 or 25 mL) before the main meal of the day.

Endocrine Elixirs

Best Endocrine Juice Ingredients

Fruits: apples, blueberries, citrus fruits, pears
Vegetables: cruciferous vegetables (broccoli, cauliflower, kale, Brussels sprouts, bok choy), onions, sea vegetables, spinach
Herbs: cinnamon, cloves, coriander, dandelion root and leaf, evening primrose oil, fenugreek seeds, garlic, ginger, ginkgo, linden flower, stevia, turmeric, yarrow*

*   Avoid yarrow if you are pregnant.

Tea blend

Adrenal Support Tea

Tip
Use dried herbs for tea blends.

Caution: Do not use licorice if you have high blood pressure.

2 parts	borage leaves	2 parts
2 parts	stinging nettle leaves	2 parts
2 parts	oat straw	2 parts
1 part	basil	1 part
1 part	gotu kola	1 part
½ part	chopped gingerroot or ¼ part ground	½ part
½ part	chopped licorice or ¼ part powdered (see Caution, left)	½ part

1. In an airtight tin or dark-colored jar, blend together borage, stinging nettle, oat straw, basil, gotu kola, ginger and licorice. Store in a cool, dry, dark place.

2. *To make tea:* Crush a small amount of blend to a fine powder and measure 1 tsp (5 mL) per 1 cup (250 mL) water. Place in a warmed ceramic teapot, add 1 tsp (5 mL) "for the pot" and pour boiling water over herbs. Cover the pot and put a cork in the spout. Steep for about 15 minutes and strain into cups.

Serves 1 or 2

Cruciferous Chiller

1	cauliflower florets	4
4	broccoli florets	4
1 cup	torn kale, spinach or bok choy leaves	250 mL
½	Vidalia onion	½
	Ice, optional	

1. Using a juicer, process cauliflower, broccoli, kale and onion. Whisk and pour over ice, if using.

Serves 1

Diabetic Breakfast

Tip

Use a citrus press if you have one for this perfectly balanced drink. A regular juicer may be used for peeled, whole citrus fruit and the result is a creamier juice.

2	oranges, halved	2
1	grapefruit, halved	1
½	lemon, halved	½
½	lime	½
1 tsp	ground flax seeds	5 mL
½ tsp	ground cinnamon, optional	2 mL

1. Using a citrus press, squeeze oranges, grapefruit, lemon and lime. Whisk together with ground flax seeds and cinnamon if using and pour into a glass.

Serves 1

Endo-Cran

1 cup	whole cranberries, fresh or frozen	250 mL
1	orange	1
1	grapefruit, cut to fit tube	1
10	drops stinging nettle tincture	10
Pinch	powdered turmeric	Pinch

1. Using a juicer, process cranberries, orange and grapefruit. Whisk together with stinging nettle tincture and turmeric and pour into a glass.

Hormone Balancing Tea

This tea nourishes the reproductive system.

Caution: Do not take this tea if pregnant.

3 parts	red raspberry leaves	3 parts
2 parts	chaste berries	2 parts
2 parts	lemon balm	2 parts
1 part	stinging nettle	1 part
1 part	yarrow, aerial parts	1 part
1 part	red clover flowers	1 part
1 part	chopped gingerroot or ½ part ground	1 part
1 part	German chamomile flowers	1 part
1 part	rosemary	1 part

1. In an airtight tin or dark-colored jar, blend together raspberry, chaste berries, lemon balm, stinging nettle, yarrow, red clover, ginger, chamomile and rosemary. Store in a cool, dark, dry place.

2. *To make tea:* Crush a small amount of blend to a fine powder and measure 1 tsp (5 mL) per 1 cup (250 mL) water. Place in a warmed ceramic teapot, add 1 tsp (5 mL) "for the pot" and pour boiling water over herbs. Cover the pot and put a cork in the spout. Steep for about 15 minutes and strain into cups.

Cramp cure

High-bush cranberry (*Viburnum opulus*), also called cramp bark, is a completely different plant from the popular cranberry, but one that is highly regarded by the Catawba, Penobscot, Meskawaki and Menominee, who still use the bark to treat cramps, muscle tension, swollen glands, colic and diarrhea.

A simple tea to relieve menstrual cramps: 1 cup (250 mL) boiling water poured over 1 tbsp (15 mL) dried cramp bark and allowed to steep for 15 minutes. Sip often throughout the day as long as the pains are present.

Hormone Healthy

1 cup	fresh spinach	250 mL
3	stalks celery	3
3	carrots	3
½	red bell pepper, trimmed	½
1 tsp	powdered dulse or kale	5 mL

1. Using a juicer, process spinach, celery, carrots and red pepper. Whisk together with dulse and pour into a glass.

Hypo-Health

2	carrots	2
1	beet	1
1	spear broccoli	1
1 tsp	spirulina	5 mL
½ tsp	ground ginseng	2 mL

1. Using a juicer, process carrots, beet and broccoli. Whisk together with spirulina and ginseng and pour into a glass.

Mandarin Orange

Tip
Use navel oranges when blood oranges are not available.

1	can (12 oz/341 mL) mandarin orange sections drained, juice reserved	1
2	blood oranges	2
1	grapefruit, cut to fit tube	1
½ cup	blackberries	125 mL
½	lemon	½

1. Using a juicer, process mandarin orange segments, blood oranges, grapefruit, blackberries and lemon. Whisk together with reserved mandarin juice and pour into glasses.

Serves 1	# Orange Yogurt	
2	oranges	2
2	fresh apricots, pitted	2
½	grapefruit, cut to fit tube	½
¼ cup	natural yogurt	50 mL
¼ tsp	ground fenugreek	1 mL

1. Using a juicer, process oranges, apricots and grapefruit. Whisk together with yogurt and fenugreek and pour into a glass.

Serves 1	# Pear-Pom	
2	pears	2
1	pomegranate, seeds only	1
1	orange	1
Pinch	ground cloves	Pinch

1. Using a juicer, process pears, pomegranate seeds and orange. Whisk together with ground cloves and pour into a glass.

Serves 1

Seedy Kiwi

3	kiwifruits	3
1	orange	1
1	grapefruit, cut to fit tube	1
½	lime	½
1 tsp	ground flax seeds	5 mL

1. Using a juicer, process kiwifruits, orange, grapefruit and lime. Whisk together with flax seeds and pour into a glass.

Serves 1

Strawberry Citrus

1 cup	hulled fresh strawberries	250 mL
2	fresh apricots, pitted	2
1	orange	1
1	can (12 oz/341 mL) mandarin orange sections drained, juice reserved	1
½	lemon	½

1. Using a juicer, process strawberries, apricots, orange, mandarin orange segments and lemon. Whisk together with reserved mandarin juice and pour into a glass.

Immune Boosters

Best Immune Juice Ingredients

Fruits: antioxidant fruits (see page 110), citrus fruits, black plums, red and purple grapes

Vegetables: antioxidant vegetables (see page page 122), avocados, cruciferous vegetables (broccoli, cauliflower, kale, Brussels sprouts, bok choy), shiitake mushrooms, tomatoes

Herbs: astragalus, burdock (leaf, root and seeds)*, cayenne, cloves, echinacea*, elderflower and elderberries, garlic, ginseng, green tea, licorice**, parsley***, red clover, rosemary, sage, St. John's wort, thyme, turmeric, yarrow*

Other: flax seed oil, green tea

*   People who are allergic to ragweed are sometimes also allergic to herbs in the same botanical family (compositae, or daisy). Some of the herbs in this family include burdock, calendula, chamomile, chicory, dandelion, echinacea, feverfew, milk thistle and yarrow (avoid yarrow if you are pregnant).

**   Avoid licorice if you have high blood pressure. The prolonged use of licorice is not recommended under any circumstances.

*** If you are pregnant, limit your intake of parsley to ½ tsp (2 mL) dried or one sprig fresh per day. Do not take parsley if you are suffering from kidney inflammation.

The power of garlic

Garlic provides strong antioxidant action to protect cell membranes against free-radical formation. Some studies show that even in low doses, garlic stimulates the immune system, increasing the activity of natural "killer cells" to ward off pathogens.

Garlic also has strong antibiotic properties. It kills intestinal parasites and worms, as well as gram-negative bacteria. In recent studies, researchers using fresh and powdered garlic solutions discovered that garlic inhibited many bacteria, including *Staphylococcus auras*, *E. coli*, *Proteus vulgaris*, *Salmonella enteritidis*, *Klebsiella pneumonia* and many others.

And when compared to antibiotics such as penicillin, tetracycline, erythromycin and others commonly prescribed, garlic proved to be as effective. One medium-size garlic clove delivers the antibacterial equivalent of about 100,000 units of penicillin (typical oral penicillin doses range from 600,000 units to 900,000 units). Therefore a dose of 6 to 9 garlic cloves has roughly the same effect as a shot of penicillin.

Aller-free Tea

2 parts	stinging nettle	2 parts
2 parts	elderflowers	2 parts
2 parts	rose hips	2 parts
2 parts	crushed cinnamon stick or 1 part ground cinnamon	2 parts
1 part	thyme	1 part
½ part	chopped gingerroot or ¼ part ground	½ part
½ part	peppermint	½ part

1. In an airtight tin or dark-colored jar, blend together stinging nettle, elderflowers, rose hips, cinnamon, thyme, ginger and peppermint. Store in a cool, dry, dark place.

2. *To make tea:* Crush a small amount of blend to a fine powder and measure 1 tsp (5 mL) per 1 cup (250 mL) water. Place in a warmed ceramic teapot, add 1 tsp (5 mL) "for the pot" and pour boiling water over herbs. Cover the pot and put a cork in the spout. Steep for about 15 minutes and strain into cups.

Allium Antioxidant

3	stalks celery	3
½	onion	½
1	clove garlic	1
1	spear broccoli	1
1	apple	1

1. Using a juicer, process celery, onion, garlic, broccoli and apple. Whisk and pour into a glass.

Antibiotic Toddy

Serves 2

Tip

For a heartier drink that retains the goodness of the roots, do not strain mixture after it has simmered. Use a Vita-Mix to liquefy and blend all ingredients before pouring into mugs and topping with orange or lemon slices. If the blended mixture is too thick, dilute it with boiled water.

2 cups	apple cider	500 mL
2 cups	orange juice	500 mL
½ cup	elderberries or cranberries, fresh or dried	125 mL
1	3-inch (7.5 cm) piece echinacea root	1
1	3-inch (7.5 cm) piece ginseng root	1
1	3-inch (7.5 cm) piece cinnamon stick	1
2 tbsp	finely chopped gingerroot	25 mL
3	whole cloves	3
3	allspice berries	3
1 tbsp	stevia leaves	15 mL
1 tbsp	liquid honey	15 mL
1 tbsp	apple cider vinegar	15 mL
1	lemon, juiced	1
2	orange or lemon slices, optional	2

1. In a saucepan over medium heat, combine apple cider, orange juice, elderberries, echinacea root, ginseng root, cinnamon stick, ginger, cloves, allspice berries and stevia leaves. Bring to just under a boil on high heat. Cover, reduce heat and simmer for 10 minutes.

2. Strain mixture through a sieve, pressing on solids to extract all liquid. Stir in honey, vinegar and lemon juice. Pour into glasses and serve hot with orange or lemon slices, if using.

Tea blend

Antioxi-T

Scottish researchers have found that among the 75 chemicals found in thyme extract, 25% of them have antioxidant properties.

2 parts	thyme	2 parts
1 part	peppermint	1 part
1 part	rosemary	1 part
½ part	sage	½ part

1. In an airtight tin or dark-colored jar, blend together thyme, peppermint, rosemary and sage. Store in a cool, dry, dark place.

2. *To make tea:* Crush a small amount of blend to a fine powder and measure 1 tsp (5 mL) per 1 cup (250 mL) water. Place in a warmed ceramic teapot, add 1 tsp (5 mL) "for the pot" and pour boiling water over herbs. Cover the pot and put a cork in the spout. Steep for about 15 minutes and strain into cups.

Serves 2

Berry Young

Approximate ORAC Value*
12,000–14,000 per serving

1 cup	blueberries	250 mL
1 cup	blackberries	250 mL
1 cup	raspberries	250 mL
1 cup	hulled fresh strawberries	250 mL

1. Using a juicer, process blueberries, blackberries, raspberries and strawberries. Whisk and pour into glasses.

Serves 1

Blue Star

Approximate ORAC Value*
22,000–24,000

*Source: USDA data on foods with high levels of antioxidants.

3	star fruits	3
1 cup	blueberries	250 mL
1 cup	blackberries	250 mL
1	black plum, pitted	1

1. Using a juicer, process star fruits, blueberries, blackberries and plum. Whisk and pour into a glass.

Serves 2

Approximate ORAC Value*
15,000–17,000 per serving

*Source: USDA data on
foods with high levels of
antioxidants.

Tip
Use ¼ cup (50 mL) liquid
açai or açai blend in place
of the frozen pulp.

Brazilian Berry Smoothie

½ cup	orange juice	125 mL
1	banana, cut into pieces	1
1	mango, pitted and cut into pieces	1
1	packet slightly thawed açai berry pulp	1

1. Using a blender, process orange juice, banana, mango and açai berry pulp until smooth.

Serves 1

Burdock and Melon

¼	cantaloupe	¼
2	fresh apricots, pitted	2
2	carrots	2
1 tsp	ground burdock seeds or ½ tsp (2 mL) burdock tincture	5 mL

1. Using a juicer, process cantaloupe, apricots and carrots. Whisk together with burdock seeds and pour into a glass.

Cold and Flu-T

Makes 4 cups (1 L) tea

Powerfully antibiotic and antiviral, this tea fights colds and flu. Garlic is one of the key ingredients in this blend and it must be taken fresh because the powdered form has little medicinal value. For this reason, make up in small quantities and use when cold and flu symptoms first appear.

Caution: Do not use licorice if you have high blood pressure.

2 tsp	fresh thyme or 1 tsp (5 mL) dried thyme	10 mL
1 tsp	chopped fresh lemon balm or ½ tsp (2 mL) dried lemon balm	5 mL
1	clove garlic, finely chopped	1
1 tsp	ground echinacea or astragalus	5 mL
½ tsp	finely grated gingerroot or ¼ tsp (1 mL) ground	2 mL
½ tsp	chopped dried licorice or ¼ tsp (1 mL) powdered licorice (see Caution, left)	2 mL
4 cups	boiling water	1 L

1. In a non-reactive teapot, combine thyme, lemon balm, garlic, echinacea, ginger and licorice. Cover with boiling water and steep for 15 minutes. Strain into a clean jar, cover with a lid. Store in refrigerator for up to 2 days. Drink ½ to 1 cup (125 mL to 250 mL) four times per day.

Cran Attack

Serves 2

This juice really wages war on toxins.

Approximate ORAC Value* 17,000–19,000 per serving

*Source: USDA data on foods with high levels of antioxidants.

1 cup	whole cranberries, fresh or frozen	250 mL
1 cup	raspberries	250 mL
1 cup	hulled fresh strawberries	250 mL
½ cup	açai berries, thawed	125 mL

1. Using a juicer, process cranberries, raspberries, strawberries and açai berries. Whisk and pour into glasses.

Fruit of Life

Serves 1

Approximate ORAC Value*
30,000–35,000

½ cup	açai berries, thawed	125 mL
1	pomegranate, seeds only	1
1	cup blueberries	250 mL

1. Using a juicer, process açai berries, pomegranate seeds and blueberries. Whisk and pour into a glass.

The Green Diablo

Serves 4

Garnished with slices of lime, this green devil is an excellent antioxidant tea.

Caution: Parsley should be avoided during pregnancy and in cases of kidney inflammation.

2 tsp	green tea leaves	10 mL
1 tsp	parsley (see Caution, left)	5 mL
1 tsp	citrus peel	5 mL
1 tsp	ground cayenne pepper	5 mL
½ tsp	stevia leaves	2 mL
5 cups	boiling water	1.25 L
4	slices lime, optional	4

1. In a non-reactive teapot, combine green tea, parsley, citrus peel, cayenne and stevia. Pour in boiling water and steep, covered, for 15 minutes. Strain the tea into cups and garnish with lime slices, if using.

Green Gift

Serves 2

Approximate ORAC Value*
7,000–9,000

*Source: USDA data on foods with high levels of antioxidants.

Caution: Parsley should be avoided during pregnancy and in cases of kidney inflammation.

1 cup	chopped kale	250 mL
1 cup	broccoli florets	250 mL
4	sprigs fresh parsley (see Caution, left)	4
1 cup	green grapes	250 mL
1 cup	green tea	250 mL

1. Using a juicer, process kale, broccoli, parsley and grapes. Whisk together with green tea and pour into glasses.

Green Tea and Blueberries

Serves 2

Approximate ORAC Value*
14,000–15,000 per serving

Source: USDA data on foods with high levels of antioxidants.

1 cup	blueberries	250 mL
1 cup	blackberries	250 mL
2	black plums, pitted	2
½ cup	green tea, steeped and chilled	125 mL

1. Using a juicer, process blueberries, blackberries, prunes and plums. Whisk together with green tea and pour into glasses.

Herp-eze Tea

Tea blend

Nerve nourishing, immune system supporting, and antiviral to the *Herpes* virus, these herbs work to relieve and protect from infection.

Caution: Omit St. John's wort if you are taking prescription drugs.

2 parts	chopped echinacea root or 1 part powdered	2 parts
2 parts	lemon balm	2 parts
1 part	St. John's wort flowers (see Caution, left)	1 part
1 part	calendula petals	1 part
1 part	red raspberry leaves	1 part
1 part	burdock leaf or chopped root	1 part
½ part	peppermint	½ part

1. In an airtight tin or dark-colored jar, blend together echinacea, lemon balm, St. John's wort, calendula, raspberry, burdock and peppermint. Store in a cool, dark, dry place.

2. *To make tea:* Crush a small amount of blend to a fine powder and measure 1 tsp (5 mL) per 1 cup (250 mL) water. Place in a warmed ceramic teapot, add 1 tsp (5 mL) "for the pot" and pour boiling water over herbs. Cover the pot and put a cork in the spout. Steep for about 15 minutes and strain into cups.

Tea blend

Immune Regulator Tea

These are excellent herbs for supporting the immune system.

Caution: Do not use licorice if you have high blood pressure.

2 parts	lemon balm	2 parts
2 parts	rose hips	2 parts
1 part	German chamomile flowers	1 part
1 part	red clover flowers	1 part
1 part	thyme	1 part
½ part	chopped licorice (see Caution, left)	½ part
½ part	chopped gingerroot	½ part

1. In an airtight tin or dark-colored jar, blend together lemon balm, rose hips, German chamomile, red clover, thyme, licorice and ginger. Store in a cool, dark, dry place.

2. *To make tea:* Crush a small amount of blend to a fine powder and measure 1 tsp (5 mL) per 1 cup (250 mL) water. Place in a warmed ceramic teapot, add 1 tsp (5 mL) "for the pot" and pour boiling water over herbs. Cover the pot and put a cork in the spout. Steep for about 15 minutes and strain into cups.

Immune Tea Blend

Makes 1¾ cups (425 mL) root blend

A good all-round blend of herbs that will serve as a general tonic and keep the immune system healthy. Use fresh roots if available.

Caution: Do not use licorice if you have high blood pressure.

- Preheat oven to 300°F (150°C)
- Large baking sheet, ungreased

½ cup	chopped burdock root	125 mL
½ cup	chopped ginseng	125 mL
¼ cup	chopped astragalus	50 mL
¼ cup	chopped licorice (see Caution, left)	50 mL
¼ cup	barley or oat flakes	50 mL

1. Spread burdock, ginseng, astragalus, licorice and barley flakes on baking sheet. Bake in preheated oven, stirring once, for 20 minutes or until golden. Cool, mix well and transfer to an airtight jar to store.

2. *To make tea:* Grind a small amount of the blend to a fine powder and measure 2 tsp (10 mL) per 1 cup (250 mL) water. Place in a warmed ceramic teapot, add 1 tsp (5 mL) "for the pot" and pour boiling water over herbs. Cover the pot and put a cork in the spout. Steep for about 5 minutes and strain into cups.

Live Young

Serves 1

Approximate ORAC Value* 8,000–10,000

*Source: USDA data on foods with high levels of antioxidants.

1 cup	coarsely chopped kale	250 mL
½ cup	broccoli florets	125 mL
2	carrots	2
1	Red Delicious apple	1

1. Using a juicer, process kale, broccoli, carrots and apple. Whisk and pour into a glass.

Plum Immune

Serves 1

Approximate ORAC* Value
20,000–30,000

1 cup	blueberries	250 mL
2	black plums, pitted	2
½ cup	pitted stewed prunes	125 mL
½ cup	cranberry juice	125 mL
1 tsp	flax seed oil, optional	5 mL

1. Using a juicer, process blueberries, plums and prunes. Whisk together with cranberry juice and flax seed oil, if using, and pour into a glass.

Razz-Man-Flax

Serves 2

Approximate ORAC Value*
10,000–12,000 per serving

1	can (12 oz/341 mL) mandarin orange sections drained, juice reserved	1
1 cup	blueberries	250 mL
1 cup	raspberries	250 mL
½ cup	pitted stewed prunes or raisins	125 mL
1 tsp	flax seed oil	5 mL

1. Using a juicer, process mandarin orange segments, blueberries, raspberries and prunes. Whisk together with reserved mandarin juice and flax seed oil and pour into glasses.

Razzy Orange

Serves 2

Approximate ORAC Value*
10,000–12,000 per serving

*Source: USDA data on foods with high levels of antioxidants.

2	oranges	2
1 cup	raspberries	250 mL
1 cup	red grapes	250 mL
½ cup	raisins	125 mL

1. Using a juicer, process oranges, raspberries, grapes and raisins. Whisk and pour into a glass.

Serves 2

Approximate ORAC Value*
10,000–15,000 per serving

Razzy Strawberry

1 cup	hulled fresh strawberries	250 mL
1 cup	raspberries	250 mL
1 cup	purple grapes	250 mL
2	black plums, pitted	2

1. Using a juicer, process strawberries, raspberries, grapes and plums. Whisk and pour into glasses.

Serves 1

Red Pepper

1	red bell pepper, trimmed	1
2	carrots	2
1	apple	1
1	spear broccoli	1
½ tsp	cayenne pepper	2 mL

1. Using a juicer, process red pepper, carrots, apple and broccoli. Whisk together with cayenne and pour into a glass.

Serves 2

Approximate ORAC Value*
14,000–15,000

*Source: USDA data on foods with high levels of antioxidants.

The Rio Thing

½ cup	cranberry juice	125 mL
½ cup	raspberries	125 mL
1	packet slightly thawed açai berry pulp	1

1. Using a blender, process cranberry juice, raspberries and açai berry pulp until smooth.

Rust Proofer #1

In simple terms, aging is the process whereby our cells are damaged by oxidation. In truth, we are rusting from the inside out. Antioxidant herbs and vitamins help prevent the damage to cells by oxidizing agents, which makes them a kind of rust proofer!

$\frac{1}{2}$	sweet potato	$\frac{1}{2}$
4	sprigs fresh peppermint	4
3	carrots	3
1	spear broccoli	1

1. Using a juicer, process sweet potato. Set aside. Using another container, process the peppermint, carrots and broccoli.

2. When white starch has settled on the bottom of the first container, pour sweet potato juice carefully into carrot juice mixture, being careful to leave starch behind. Discard starch. Whisk and pour into a glass.

Rust Proofer #2

Tip

Try $\frac{1}{2}$ tsp (5 mL) curry powder or turmeric whisked into this drink.

Caution: Parsley should be avoided during pregnancy and in cases of kidney inflammation.

1	apple	1
3	sprigs fresh parsley (see Caution, left)	3
1	handful fresh thyme	1
1	carrot	1
2	tomatoes	2

1. Using a juicer, process apple, parsley, thyme, carrot and tomatoes. Whisk and pour into a glass.

Tea blend

Tonic T

This tea feeds the cells of the body and boosts the immune system. It can be used every day by the young and old. The quantities are easily doubled for a bigger batch. Once the tea is made, store in a clean jar with a lid for up to 2 days. Take 1 cup (250 mL) daily. To cook with Tonic T, add 1 cup (250 mL) to soups and stocks and use in place of other liquids in cooking. This tonic may be used by cancer patients before, during and after treatment.

Caution: Parsley should be avoided during pregnancy and in cases of kidney inflammation.

1 part	chopped astragalus root	1 part
1 part	parsley (see Caution, left)	1 part
1 part	alfalfa, aerial parts	1 part

1. In an airtight tin or dark-colored jar, combine astragalus, parsley and alfalfa. Store in a cool, dark, dry place.

2. *To make tonic:* Crush a small amount of the blend to a fine powder and measure 1 tsp (5 mL) per 1 cup (250 mL) water. Place in a warmed ceramic teapot, add 1 tsp (5 mL) "for the pot" and pour boiling water over herbs. Cover the pot and put a cork in the spout. Steep for about 5 minutes and strain into cups.

Muscle Powers

Best Muscle and Bone-Building Juice Ingredients

Fruits: all raw fruits including citrus fruits, kiwifruits, strawberries and purple fruits
Note: for Osteoporosis, avoid acid-forming fruits such as cranberries, plums and prunes
Vegetables:
For calcium: broccoli, cabbage, leafy greens, sea vegetables
For magnesium: beans, dark green vegetables
For boron: raisins, prunes, almonds
For manganese: leafy greens, beet tops, pineapple
Herbs: alfalfa, dandelion leaf, German chamomile, oat straw, parsley*, plantain, stinging nettle
Other: almonds, blackstrap molasses, dried fruits, tofu, soymilk, cod liver oil, spirulina, yogurt with active bacterial cultures

*   If you are pregnant, limit your intake of parsley to $\frac{1}{2}$ tsp (2 mL) dried or one sprig fresh per day. Do not take parsley if you are suffering from kidney inflammation.

Serves 1 or 2

Berry Yogurt Flip

Tips
Use Cranberry Juice, page 168 or commercial juice in this recipe.

Using frozen açai berries in smoothies thickens the drink.

$\frac{1}{2}$ cup	cran-raspberry juice	125 mL
1 cup	blueberries	250 mL
$\frac{1}{2}$ cup	açai berries	125 mL
6	almonds	6
$\frac{1}{2}$ cup	natural yogurt	125 mL

1. In a blender, combine cran-raspberry juice, blueberries, açai berries and almonds. Place lid on blender and blend on low for 30 seconds. Add yogurt and blend on high for 30 seconds or until smooth.

Bone Blend Tea

This tea nourishes bone tissue and speeds repair. Horsetail (*Equisetum arvense*) is high in silica and, if used internally, should only be gathered from the wild early in the season (before June). Horsetail is usually available from alternative/health stores.

Caution: Do not use licorice if you have high blood pressure.

2 parts	horsetail	2 parts
2 parts	stinging nettle	2 parts
2 parts	oat straw	2 parts
1 part	red clover flowers	1 part
1 part	sage	1 part
½ part	chopped licorice or ¼ part powdered (see Caution, left)	½ part

1. In an airtight tin or dark-colored jar, blend together horsetail, stinging nettle, oat straw, red clover, sage and licorice. Store in a cool, dark, dry place.

2. *To make tea:* Crush a small amount of blend to a fine powder and measure 1 tsp (5 mL) per 1 cup (250 mL) water. Place in a warmed ceramic teapot, add 1 tsp (5 mL) "for the pot" and pour boiling water over herbs. Cover the pot and put a cork in the spout. Steep for about 15 minutes and strain into cups.

Bone Builder

The calcium, boron and magnesium delivered by the ingredients in this drink make it good for bones.

Caution: Parsley should be avoided during pregnancy or in cases of kidney inflammation.

½ cup	kelp or other sea herb	125 mL
1 cup	hot water	250 mL
2	spears broccoli	2
2	kale	2
2	stalks celery	2
½	green bell pepper	½
4	sprigs fresh parsley (see Caution, left)	4
1	apple	1

1. In a medium bowl, pour water over kelp. Soak kelp for 15 to 20 minutes, or until reconstituted. Drain soaking water and reserve for another use.

2. Using a juicer, process kelp, broccoli, kale, celery, green pepper, parsley and apple. Whisk and pour into glasses.

The Cool Down

Serves 1

The natural calming effect of lemon balm and the potassium-rich banana refresh the body after any type of activity.

½ cup	carrot juice	125 mL
2	pineapple spears, cut in chunks	2
1	banana, cut in chunks	1
1	sprig fresh lemon balm	1

1. Using a blender, process carrot juice, pineapple, banana and lemon balm until smooth. Pour into a glass.

Cream of Broccoli Smoothie

Serves 1

Tip

Blanching vegetables makes them easier to blend for drinks. To blanch vegetables, immerse in boiling water for 1 to 2 minutes. Remove and plunge into cold water. Drain well.

¼ cup	soymilk or coconut milk	50 mL
2	spears broccoli, blanched	2
1 cup	cauliflower florets, blanched	250 mL
1 cup	spinach	250 mL
3 tbsp	crumbled feta cheese	45 mL
3 tbsp	natural yogurt	45 mL

1. In a blender, combine soymilk, broccoli, cauliflower and spinach. Place lid on blender and blend on low for 30 seconds. Stop and add feta cheese and yogurt. Replace lid and increase speed to high. Blend until smooth.

The Curl

1 cup	coarsely chopped kale leaves	250 mL
1	apple	1
2	celery stalks	2
3	sprigs fresh parsley (see Caution, left)	3
½	lemon	½

1. Using a juicer, process kale, celery, parsley and lemon. Whisk and pour into a glass.

Gold Star

3	star fruits	3
2	oranges	2
1	mango, pitted	1
¼ tsp	ground turmeric	1 mL
¼ tsp	ground ginger	1 mL

1. Using a juicer, process star fruits, oranges and mango. Whisk together with turmeric and ginger and pour into a glass.

Green Bean

1	handful green beans	1
1	handful fresh alfalfa or 1 tbsp (15 mL) dried	1
1 cup	spinach	250 mL
¼	cabbage, cut to fit tube	¼
½	lemon	½

1. Using a juicer, process green beans, alfalfa, spinach, cabbage and lemon. Whisk and pour into a glass.

Iron Builder Tea

Serves 2 or 3

Young people experiencing puberty require extra iron to help them cope with the rapid changes within their bodies.

6	sprigs fresh peppermint	6
4	fresh stinging nettle tops	4
1	fresh yellow dock root	1
1	small fresh burdock leaf, chopped	1
½ cup	chopped fresh sweet cicely	125 mL
3 cups	boiling water	750 mL

1. In a non-reactive teapot or heatproof jar, combine peppermint, stinging nettle, yellow dock, burdock and sweet cicely. Pour boiling water over herbs and steep, covered, for at least 12 hours (the longer steeping time is necessary to extract the minerals from the herbs). Strain and drink ½ cup (125 mL) twice daily. Store tonic in a clean jar with a lid in the refrigerator for up to 3 days.

Iron Ice

Serves 2

Caution: Parsley should be avoided during pregnancy and in cases of kidney inflammation.

1	handful spinach	1
1	handful fresh parsley (see Caution, left)	1
½ cup	coarsely chopped kale	125 mL
2	carrots	2
1	stalk celery	1
1	avocado, pitted	1
½	lemon	½
	Ice, optional	

1. Using a juicer, process spinach, parsley, kale, carrots, celery, avocado and lemon. Whisk and pour over ice, if using.

Serves 1

Lofty Leaves

1 cup	coarsely chopped Swiss chard	250 mL
1 cup	coarsely chopped kale	250 mL
1	wedge pineapple	1
1	handful fresh stinging nettle or 1 tsp (5 mL) dried	1

1. Using a juicer, process Swiss chard, kale, pineapple and stinging nettle. Whisk and pour into a glass.

Serves 1

Mighty Mineral Smoothie

½ cup	kelp or dulse	125 mL
½ cup	chopped leafy vegetable	125 mL
½ cup	soymilk	125 mL
6	almonds	6
½ tsp	green algae	2 mL

1. In a medium bowl, pour water over kelp. Soak kelp for 15 to 20 minutes, or until reconstituted. Drain soaking water and reserve for another use.

2. In blender, combine kelp, leafy vegetable, soymilk, almonds and algae. Place lid on blender and blend on low for 30 seconds. Gradually increase speed to high and blend until smooth.

Popeye's Power

2	kale leaves	2
6	spinach leaves	6
1	beet, top intact	1
1	fresh dandelion root	1
2 tsp	blackstrap molasses	10 mL

1. Using a juicer, process kale, spinach, beet, beet top and dandelion root. Whisk together with molasses and pour into a glass.

Pump It Up

With its natural sugar carbohydrates, and potassium from the banana, this drink helps to prepare the body for intensive activity. Drink it before exercising, walking or any strenuous work. If using a nut milk, omit the almonds.

1 cup	soymilk or nut milk	250 mL
1	banana, cut in chunks	1
½ cup	pitted cherries	125 mL
¼ cup	blueberries, fresh or frozen	50 mL
1 tbsp	organic protein powder	15 mL
2 tbsp	ground almonds	25 mL

1. Using a blender, process soymilk, banana, cherries, blueberries and protein powder until smooth. Pour into glasses and garnish with ground almonds.

Purple Power

Serves 1

2	plums, pitted	2
1 cup	purple grapes	250 mL
1 cup	blackberries	250 mL
1 tsp	cod liver oil	5 mL

1. Using a juicer, process plums, grapes and blackberries. Whisk together with cod liver oil and pour into a glass.

Spin Doctor

Serves 1

1 cup	fresh spinach	250 mL
2	carrots	2
1	apple	1
1	tomato	1
½ tsp	turmeric	2 mL

1. Using a juicer, process spinach, carrots, apple and tomato. Whisk together with turmeric and pour into a glass.

Nerve Nourishers

Best Nerve Juice Ingredients

Fruits and vegetables: all fruits and vegetables nourish the nerves, so juice and eat a wide variety daily

Herbs: alfalfa, borage, dandelion greens, garlic, German chamomile, kava kava, lavender, lemon balm, parsley*, St. John's wort**, skullcap, valerian

Other: almonds, cashews, walnuts, sesame seeds, sunflower seeds, pumpkin seeds, flax seed oil, spirulina, sea vegetables

*   If you are pregnant, limit your intake of parsley to ½ tsp (2 mL) dried or one sprig fresh per day. Do not take parsley if you are suffering from kidney inflammation.

**   Omit St. John's wort if taking prescription drugs

Serves 1		

Apple Chamomile

2	apples	2
1 cup	grapes	250 mL
2 tbsp	fresh German chamomile flowers or 1 tsp (5 mL) dried	10 mL
½ tsp	skullcap	2 mL

1. Using a juicer, process apples, grapes and chamomile. Whisk together with skullcap and pour into a glass.

Purchase vanilla custard or vanilla pudding for this delicious drink.

Cherry Custard Smoothie

¼ cup	soymilk	50 mL
2 cups	cherries, pitted	500 mL
½ cup	vanilla custard	125 mL
1 tbsp	rolled oats	15 mL
¼ tsp	ground nutmeg	1 mL

1. In a blender, combine soymilk, cherries, custard and oats. Blend until smooth, pour into glasses and garnish with nutmeg.

This tea stimulates blood circulation, enhancing the nourishment to all body cells. Make up 1 cup (250 mL) of this tea, strain and combine with the same amount of fresh carrot or beet juice for extra healing power.

Circulation Tea

3 parts	ginkgo	3 parts
2 parts	stinging nettle	2 parts
2 parts	rosemary	2 parts
1 part	chopped gingerroot or ½ part ground	1 part
1 part	ground cinnamon	1 part
1 part	yarrow, aerial parts	1 part
¼ part	cardamom seeds	¼ part

1. In an airtight tin or dark-colored jar, blend together ginkgo, stinging nettle, rosemary, ginger, cinnamon, yarrow and cardamom. Store in a cool, dark, dry place.

2. *To make tea:* Crush a small amount of blend to a fine powder and measure 1 tsp (5 mL) per 1 cup (250 mL) water. Place in a warmed ceramic teapot, add 1 tsp (5 mL) "for the pot" and pour boiling water over herbs. Cover the pot and put a cork in the spout. Steep for about 15 minutes and strain into cups.

Tea blend	# Nerve Nourisher	

Caution: Do not use licorice if you have high blood pressure. Omit St. John's wort if you are taking prescription drugs.

2 parts	oat straw	2 parts
2 parts	lemon balm	2 parts
1 part	German chamomile flowers	1 part
1 part	chopped licorice or $\frac{1}{2}$ part powdered (see Caution, left)	1 part
1 part	rosemary	1 part
1 part	vervain	1 part
1 part	skullcap	1 part
1 part	St. John's wort flowers (see Caution, left)	1 part

1. In an airtight tin or dark-colored jar, blend together oat straw, lemon balm, chamomile, licorice, rosemary, vervain, skullcap and St. John's wort. Store in a cool, dark, dry place.

2. *To make tea:* Crush a small amount of the blend to a fine powder and measure 1 tsp (5 mL) per 1 cup (250 mL) water. Place in a warmed ceramic teapot, add 1 tsp (5 mL) "for the pot" and pour boiling water over herbs. Cover the pot and put a cork in the spout. Steep for about 15 minutes and strain into cups.

Tea blend

Nerve Support

Caution: Omit St. John's wort if you are taking prescription drugs.

1 part	German chamomile flowers	1 part
1 part	lemon balm	1 part
1 part	linden flowers	1 part
1 part	St. John's wort flowers (see Caution, left)	1 part

1. In an airtight tin or dark-colored jar, blend together chamomile, lemon balm, linden flowers and St. John's wort. Store in a cool, dark, dry place.

2. *To make tea:* Crush a small amount of blend to a fine powder and measure 1 tsp (5 mL) per 1 cup (250 mL) water. Place in a warmed ceramic teapot, add 1 tsp (5 mL) "for the pot" and pour boiling water over herbs. Cover the pot and put a cork in the spout. Steep for about 5 minutes and strain into cups.

Serves 1 or 2

Pinea-Colada

½	pineapple, cut in wedges	½
1	handful fresh lemon balm	1
½	lemon	½
½ cup	coconut milk	125 mL
½ tsp	flax seed oil	2 mL

1. Using a juicer, process pineapple, lemon balm and lemon. Whisk together with coconut milk and flax seed oil and pour into glasses.

Pretty Nervy

1 cup	raspberries	250 mL
1	handful fresh lemon balm or 1 tsp (5 mL) dried	1
4	fresh borage sprigs or 1 tsp (5 mL) dried	4
1	apple	1
½	red bell pepper, trimmed	½

1. Using a juicer, process raspberries, lemon balm, borage apple and red pepper. Whisk and pour into a glass.

Sea Vitamins

1 cup	kelp or dulse	250 mL
1 cup	spinach	250 mL
1	apple	1
1 tsp	spirulina	5 mL

1. In a medium bowl, pour water over kelp. Soak kelp for 15 to 20 minutes, or until reconstituted. Drain soaking water and reserve for another use.

2. Using a juicer, process kelp, spinach and apple. Whisk together with spirulina and pour into a glass.

Spirit Raising Tea

This pleasant-tasting tea can shift the blues.

Caution: Omit St. John's wort if you are taking prescription drugs.

2 parts	linden flowers	2 parts
2 parts	lemon verbena	2 parts
2 parts	St. John's wort flowers (see Caution, left)	2 parts
1 part	rosemary	1 part
1 part	lavender flowers	1 part
1 part	vervain	1 part
1 part	thyme	1 part

1. In an airtight tin or dark-colored jar, blend together linden flowers, lemon verbena, St. John's wort, rosemary, lavender, vervain and thyme. Store in a cool, dark, dry place.

2. *To make tea:* Crush a small amount of blend to a fine powder and measure 1 tsp (5 mL) per 1 cup (250 mL) water. Place in a warmed ceramic teapot, add 1 tsp (5 mL) "for the pot" and pour boiling water over herbs. Cover the pot and put a cork in the spout. Steep for about 15 minutes and strain into cups.

Serves 1

Stinging Bs

½	cantaloupe, cut to fit tube	½
2	carrots	2
1 cup	red grapes	250 mL
1 tsp	dried stinging nettles	5 mL
1 tsp	flax seed oil	5 mL

1. Using a juicer, process cantaloupe, carrots and grapes. Whisk together with stinging nettles and flax seed oil and pour into a glass.

Serves 1	# Swiss Knife	
¼ cup	dulse or kelp	50 mL
1 cup	coarsely chopped Swiss chard	250 mL
1 cup	grapes	250 mL
1 tsp	spirulina	5 mL

1. In a medium bowl, pour water over dulse. Soak dulse for 15 to 20 minutes, or until reconstituted. Drain soaking water and reserve for another use.

2. Using a juicer, process dulse, Swiss chard and grapes. Whisk together with spirulina and pour into a glass.

Respiratory Juices

Best Respiratory Juice Ingredients

Fruits and vegetables: antioxidant-rich fruits and vegetables (see pages 110 and 122), cruciferous vegetables (broccoli, cauliflower, Brussels sprouts), yellow and red onions,
Herbs: garlic, ginger, oregano, pumpkin seeds, thyme
Other: herbal teas, homemade vegetable broths, flax seeds, flax seed oil, borage oil, evening primrose oil, sprouted seeds and grains, fish oils

---

Serves 2

Brazilians have used Açai berries for centuries and they have become a staple food, as important as bread, rice and milk.

Tip
You can substitute green tea for the Lung Relief Tea.

Açai Berry Combo

¼ cup	Lung Relief Tea (see recipe, page 257)	50 mL
1 cup	açai berries	250 mL
½ cup	blueberries	125 mL
½ cup	raspberries or pitted cherries	125 mL
1 tbsp	fresh thyme leaves	15 mL

1. In a blender, combine Lung Relief Tea, açai berries, blueberries, raspberries and thyme. Process on high for 1 minute or until smooth.

Serves 1

Tip
You can substitute green tea for the Lung Relief Tea.

Breathe-Ease

2	carrots	2
1	beet	1
1	apple	1
1	½-inch (2 cm) piece fresh gingerroot	1
¼ cup	Lung Relief Tea (see recipe, page 257)	50 mL

1. Using a juicer, process carrots, beet, apple and ginger. Whisk together with Lung Relief Tea and pour into a glass.

Breath of Autumn

2	apples	2
2	pears	2
2	carrots	2
¼ cup	Lung Relief Tea (see recipe, page 257)	50 mL
1 tsp	borage or evening primrose oil	5 mL

1. Using a juicer, process apples, pears and carrots. Whisk together with Lung Relief Tea and borage oil and pour into a glass.

Cream of the Crop

3 tbsp	natural yogurt	45 mL
1	spear broccoli, cooked	1
1	cauliflower floweret, cooked	1
2	cooked carrots	2
1	stalk celery	1
1	green onion	1
1 tsp	fresh thyme leaves	5 mL

1. In a blender, combine yogurt, broccoli, cauliflower, carrots, celery, green onion and thyme. Process on high for 1 minutes or until smooth.

Ginger Smoothie

¼ cup	vegetable broth	50 mL
1	cooked beet	1
¼	fresh fennel bulb	¼
½	avocado, cut into chunks	½
1	½-inch (2 cm) piece gingerroot	1

1. In a blender, combine broth, beet, fennel, avocado and ginger. Process on high for 1 minute or until smooth.

Lung Relief Tea

This tea is expectorant, antibacterial and soothing to the lungs. Make up 1 cup (250 mL) of this tea, strain and combine with the same amount of fresh carrot or beet juice for extra healing power (see Breathe-Ease, page 255).

Caution: Do not use licorice if you have high blood pressure.

1 part	marshmallow leaves or root	1 part
1 part	hyssop	1 part
1 part	thyme	1 part
½ part	chopped licorice or ¼ part powdered (see Caution, left)	½ part

1. In an airtight tin or dark-colored jar, blend together marshmallow, hyssop, thyme and licorice. Store in a cool, dark, dry place.

2. *To make tea:* Crush a small amount of blend to a fine powder and measure 1 tsp (5 mL) per 1 cup (250 mL) water. Place in a warmed ceramic teapot, add 1 tsp (5 mL) "for the pot" and pour boiling water over herbs. Cover the pot and put a cork in the spout. Steep for about 15 minutes and strain into cups.

Oaty Orange

Tip
You can substitute green tea for the Lung Relief Tea.

2	carrots	2
1	orange	1
1	mango, pitted	1
¼ cup	Lung Relief Tea (see recipe, above)	50 mL
1 tbsp	finely ground oatmeal	15 mL

1. Using a juicer, process carrots, orange and mango. Whisk together with Lung Relief Tea and oatmeal and pour into a glass.

Orange Slushie

Serves 2

¼ cup	natural yogurt	50 mL
3	fresh apricots, pitted	3
1	orange, sectioned	1
¼ cup	frozen strawberries	50 mL
¼ cup	frozen açai berries	50 mL
1 tbsp	pumpkin seeds	15 mL

1. In a blender, combine yogurt, apricots, orange, strawberries, açai berries and pumpkin seeds. Process on high for 1 minutes or until smooth.

Stress Busters

Stress increases adrenal gland hormones and causes white blood cells to be inhibited, which leads to a significant suppression of immune function. In addition, our immune system is balanced and repaired during sleep, and stress often interrupts our ability to benefit from sleep, further compromising our immune functions. See pages 226 to 239 for Immune Boosters.

Stress may be one of the contributing factors in many diseases, and it is essential that we learn methods of coping with and reducing stress. Positive mental attitude, daily exercise, meditation or relaxation activities are all tools to help cope with busy, stressful lives.

Stress-Easing Herbs

Albizia flower (*Albizia julibrissin*). A legume plant, native to Asia (called He Huan Hua) that produces fragrant flowers with a cluster of stamens in place of petals. Considered a tonic herb, Albizia flowers are carminative and digestive. They are used to treat insomnia, irritability, breathlessness and poor memory.

German chamomile (*Matricaria recutita*, see page 133). The tryptophan acts like a sedative and relaxant in the body to induce sleep.

Hops (*Humulus lupulus*). Hops flowers relax and strengthen the nerves, thus relaxing tension and relieving anxiety. Hops also ease headaches, produce restful sleep and act as a digestive stimulant.

Lemon balm (*Melissa officinalis*, see page 138). A lemon-flavored tea herb that eases anxiety, depression, stress, flatulence, indigestion and insomnia.

Linden flower (*Tilia* x *europaea*, see page 139). A pleasant-tasting, relaxing remedy for stress, anxiety, tension headache and insomnia.

Passionflower (*Passiflora incarnata*, see page 143). In cases of worry, over-tiredness, emotional upset or hysteria, passionflower is used to reduce tension.

Polygala root (*Polygala tenuifolia*). An Asian tonic herb (called Yuan Zhi) believed to have powerful mind and spirit developing powers. Used to relax the mind, calm the emotions and to ease sleep. Whisk 1 tsp (5 mL) polygala root power into any of the drinks in this section.

Skullcap (*Scutellaria laterifolia*, see page 146). With its deep action on the nervous system, skullcap helps ease many nervous disorders, such as neuralgia, aches and pains.

St. John's wort (*Hypericum perforatum*, see page 148). A sedative and nervous system tonic, St. John's wort is effective in treating some forms of depression.

Valerian (*Valeriana officinalis*, see page 150). A nervine that quiets, soothes and heals nerves, valerian is a gentle sleep aid.

Beet Retreat

Tip
You can substitute chamomile tea for the Calming Cuppa Tea.

4	carrots	4
2	beets	2
½	cucumber	½
1	stalk celery	1
¼ cup	Calming Cuppa Tea (see recipe, page 261)	50 mL

1. Using a juicer, process carrots, beets, cucumber and celery. Whisk together with Calming Cuppa Tea and pour into a glass.

Calming Chamomile Juice

Make a pot of chamomile tea using fresh German chamomile flowers or a commercial chamomile tea. Use some of the tea hot or cooled in this juice. Store the remaining tea in a covered glass container in the refrigerator for 1 or 2 days.

2	apples	2
1	stalk celery	1
¼ cup	chamomile tea	50 ml

1. Using a juicer, process apples and celery. Whisk together with chamomile tea and pour into a glass.

Calming Cuppa Tea

Have a calming "cuppa" to ease stress any time of day, and to induce sleep at night. Make up a pot of tea and whisk ¼ cup (50 mL) into any juice recipe (see Serenity Berry, page 266).

2 parts	lemon balm	2 parts
2 parts	skullcap	2 parts
1 part	lemon verbena	1 part
1 part	linden flowers	1 part
1 part	lavender flowers	1 part
1 part	passionflower	1 part

1. In an airtight tin or dark-colored jar, blend together lemon balm, skullcap, lemon verbena, linden flowers, lavender flowers and passionflower. Store in a cool, dark, dry place.

2. *To make tea:* Crush a small amount of blend to a fine powder and measure 1 tsp (5 mL) per 1 cup (250 mL) water. Place in a warmed ceramic teapot, add 1 tsp (5 mL) "for the pot" and pour boiling water over herbs. Cover the pot and put a cork in the spout. Steep for about 15 minutes and strain into cups.

Serves 1 or 2

Chamomile-Licorice-Ginger Tea

A calming, digestive and liver-supportive tea.

Caution: Do not use licorice if you have high blood pressure.

1 tbsp	German chamomile flowers	15 mL
1 tsp	powdered licorice (see Caution, left)	5 mL
½ tsp	powdered ginger	2 mL
3 cups	boiling water	750 mL

1. In a non-reactive teapot, combine chamomile, licorice and ginger. Cover with boiling water and steep for 15 minutes. Strain into cups and serve.

Digestive Stress Soother

A tasty, mucilage-rich tea to soothe digestive tract inflammation. This tea can be taken after meals for indigestion and before bed to protect the digestive tract from acid damage at night. Make 1 cup (250 mL) of this tea, strain and combine with the same amount of fresh carrot or beet juice for extra healing power.

Caution: Do not use licorice if you have high blood pressure.

1 part	slippery elm bark powder	1 part
1 part	marshmallow leaf or chopped marshmallow root	1 part
1 part	German chamomile flowers	1 part
½ part	chopped licorice or ¼ part powdered licorice (see Caution, left)	½ part
½ part	fennel seeds	½ part

1. In an airtight tin or dark-colored jar, blend together elm bark, marshmallow, chamomile, licorice and fennel seeds. Store in a cool, dark, dry place.

2. *To make tea:* Crush a small amount of blend into a fine powder and measure 1 tsp (5 mL) per 1 cup (250 mL) water. Place in a warmed ceramic teapot, add 1 tsp (5 mL) "for the pot" and pour boiling water over herbs. Cover the pot and put a cork in the spout. Steep for about 15 minutes and strain into cups.

Serves 1

Green Peace

Caution: Parsley should be avoided during pregnancy and in cases of kidney inflammation.

1	handful spinach leaves	1
1	handful fresh parsley (see Caution, left)	1
½ cup	coarsely chopped Swiss chard	125 mL
1	celery stalk	1
1	apple	1
1 tsp	spirulina	5 mL

1. Using a juicer, process spinach, parsley, Swiss chard, celery and apple. Whisk together with spirulina and pour into a glass.

Hot Spiced Carrots

Serves 1

4	carrots	4
1	handful spinach leaves	1
1	Granny Smith apple	1
1	½-inch (2 cm) piece fresh gingerroot	1
¼ tsp	ground cinnamon	1 mL
¼ tsp	ground cardamom seeds	1 mL

1. Using a juicer, process carrots, spinach, apple and ginger. Whisk together with cinnamon and cardamom and pour into a glass.

Lights Out

Serves 1

1 cup	chopped kale	250 mL
1	beet, top intact	1
2	celery stalks, leaves intact	2
1	apple	1
1 tsp	passionflower	5 mL

1. Using a juicer, process kale, beet, beet top, celery and apple. Whisk together with passionflower and pour into a glass.

Melon Nightcap

Serves 2

1	wedge cantaloupe	1
1	wedge Crenshaw melon	1
1	2-inch (5 cm) slice watermelon, cut to fit tube	1
1	nectarine, pitted	1
1 cup	hulled fresh strawberries	250 mL
¼ cup	Nightcap Tea (see recipe, below)	50 mL

1. Using a juicer, process cantaloupe, Crenshaw melon, watermelon, nectarine and strawberries. Whisk together with Nightcap Tea and pour into a glass.

Nightcap Tea

Serves 1

Sweet cicely is a popular tea herb because it adds a sweet flavor to tea blends. It may be found in alternative/health stores. Take this tea just before retiring for bed.

1 tsp	German chamomile flowers	5 mL
1 tsp	sweet cicely	5 mL
½ tsp	ground valerian	2 mL
1 tsp	honey, optional	5 mL
1 cup	boiling water	250 mL

1. Add chamomile, sweet cicely, valerian and honey if using to a ceramic teapot. Pour boiling water over herbs. Cover the pot and put a cork in the spout. Steep for about 15 minutes and strain into a cup.

Raspberry Relaxer

Serves 1

1 cup	raspberries	250 mL
1 cup	açai berries	250 mL
½	lemon	½
¼ cup	Raspberry Tea (see recipe, page 265)	50 mL

1. Using a juicer, process raspberries, açai berries and lemon. Whisk together with Raspberry Tea and pour into a glass.

Serves 1 or 2

Raspberry Tea

This tea calms the muscles and nerves.

¼ cup	raspberries, fresh or frozen	50 mL
1 tsp	raspberry leaves	5 mL
1 tsp	lemon balm	5 mL
2 cups	boiling water	500 mL

1. In a non-reactive teapot, combine raspberries, raspberry leaves and lemon balm. Cover with boiling water and steep for 15 minutes. Strain into cups and drink warm.

Tea blend

Relax Tea

2 parts	skullcap	2 parts
2 parts	linden flower	2 parts
2 parts	lemon balm	2 parts
1 part	cramp bark	1 part
1 part	lemon verbena	1 part
1 part	passionflower	1 part
1 part	lavender flowers	1 part

1. In an airtight tin or dark-colored jar, blend together skullcap, linden flower, lemon balm, cramp bark, lemon verbena, passionflower and lavender. Store in a cool, dark, dry place.

2. *To make tea:* Crush a small amount of blend to a fine powder and measure 1 tsp (5 mL) per 1 cup (250 mL) water. Place in a warmed ceramic teapot, add 1 tsp (5 mL) "for the pot" and pour boiling water over herbs. Cover the pot and put a cork in the spout. Steep for about 15 minutes and strain into cups.

Serenity Berry

1 cup	raspberries	250 mL
½ cup	pitted cherries	125 mL
¼ cup	Calming Cuppa Tea (see recipe, page 261)	50 mL

1. Using a juicer, process raspberries and cherries. Whisk together with Calming Cuppa Tea and pour into a glass.

Suite Vegetables

Use crushed linden flower tea from a commercial tea bag for this soothing drink.

2	tomatoes	2
2	stalks celery	2
1	apple	1
1	carrot	1
½	red bell pepper, trimmed	½
½	cucumber	½
1 tsp	linden flowers	5 mL

1. Using a juicer, process tomatoes, celery, apple, carrot, red pepper and cucumber. Whisk together with linden flowers and pour into a glass.

Tonics

By definition, a tonic is an infusion of herbs that invigorates or strengthens the system. Often tonics act as stimulants and alteratives. Taken either hot or cold, tonics restore tone, purify the blood and act as nutritive builders. Tonic water is a vestige of earlier practices: in the 1500s, Europeans learned of chinchona bark (*Chinchona officinalis*), which contains quinine (a tonic effective against maleria) and have used it ever since. Throughout history, and even as late as the twentieth century, spring tonics have been used in North America to cleanse the system after a long winter of preserved meats with no fresh fruit or vegetables. Spring tonics and fasts helped to prepare the body for the shock of astringent spring greens, and were even used as a kind of personal extension of the traditional household "spring cleaning."

Tonic herbs support the body's systems in maintaining health. Depending on what herbs are used, they can support the whole body or specific systems or organs. They are able to do this because they contain opposing groups of constituents that can lower (or raise), stimulate (or depress), increase (or decrease) individual biological processes. Tonics increase the tone of the body tissues, imparting strength and vitality by promoting the digestive process, improving blood circulation and increasing the supply of oxygen to the tissues.

Tonic herbs are safe to use daily except during pregnancy. Following is a list of tonic herbs.

Alfalfa (*Medicago sativa*, see page 123). A nutritive tonic for the musculoskeletal system.
Astragalus (*Astragalus membranaceus*, see page 124). Promotes tissue regeneration, and is a heart tonic as well as a powerful immune system stimulator for virtually every phase of immune system activity.
Dandelion (*Taraxacum officinale*, see page 130). A liver and digestive tonic.
Devil's claw (*Harpagophytum procumbens*). A liver tonic.
Echinacea (*Echinacea angustifolia* or *E. purpurea*, see page 131). An immune system tonic.
Ginseng (*Panex cinquefolium*, see page 134). An adaptogen used to relieve stress.
Licorice (*Glycyrrhiza glabra*, see page 139). Licorice root is considered to be one of the best tonic herbs because it provides nutrients to almost all body systems.
Parsley (*Petroselinum crispum*, see page 142). Acts as a general tonic.

Adaptogen

1 part	chopped ginseng	1 part
1 part	chopped astragalus	1 part
½ part	parsley (see Caution, left)	½ part
½ part	alfalfa, aerial parts	½ part
¼ part	chopped licorice (see Caution, left)	¼ part

1. In an airtight tin or dark-colored jar, blend together ginseng, astragalus, parsley, alfalfa and licorice. Store in a cool, dark, dry place.

2. *To make tonic:* Crush a small amount of blend to a fine powder and measure 1 tsp (5 mL) per 1 cup (250 mL) of water. Place in a warmed ceramic teapot, add 1 tsp (5 mL) "for the pot" and pour boiling water over the herbs. Cover the pot and put a cork in the spout. Steep for about 5 minutes and strain into cups.

Makes 3 cups (750 mL)

Barley Water

¼ cup	Scotch barley or spelt flakes	50 mL
1 cup	filtered water	250 mL
1 tbsp	lemon juice	15 mL
2 cups	mineral water	500 mL
Pinch	ground nutmeg	Pinch

1. In a saucepan over medium-high heat, combine barley and water and bring to a boil. Reduce heat and simmer gently, stirring often, for 10 minutes.

2. Turn off heat and allow mixture to cool sitting on the element. Stir in lemon juice, mineral water and nutmeg. Pour into a clean jar with a lid. Store in refrigerator for up to 3 days.

For the Field or Workshop, Nourishing, as well as Allaying Thirst...

"Make oatmeal into a thin gruel; then add a little salt and sugar to taste, with a little grated nutmeg and 1 well-beaten egg to each gallon, well stirred in while yet warm. This was first suggested by the Church of England leaflets, put out among the farmers and others, to discourage them from carrying whiskey into the field.

"If the above plan is too much trouble, although it is, indeed, very nourishing and satisfactory, take the Scotch plan of stirring raw oatmeal into the bucket of cold water, and stir when dipped up to drink. I drank of this at the building of the New York and Brooklyn Bridge, which I visited with my son, while in New York, in the Centennial year of 1876, on our way from Philadelphia, and we were highly pleased with it. As near as I could judge, $\frac{1}{2}$ to 1 pint was stirred into a common 12-quart pail. The workmen drank freely, preferring it to plain water very much."

From Dr. Chase's *New Receipt Book or Information for Everybody*. Toronto: G.M. Rose & Sons Co. Limited, Date unknown.

Tea blend

This tea feeds the cells of the body and boosts the immune system. It can be used every day by the young and old. Make it up in larger quantity and store in a clean jar with a lid for up to 2 days. Add 1 cup (250 mL) to soups and stocks and use in place of other liquids in cooking. This tonic may be used by cancer patients before, during and after treatment.

Caution: Parsley should be avoided during pregnancy and in cases of kidney inflammation.

General Tonic

1 part	chopped astragalus root	1 part
1 part	parsley (see Caution, left)	1 part
1 part	alfalfa, aerial parts	1 part

1. In an airtight tin or dark-colored jar, blend together astragalus, parsley and alfalfa. Store in a cool, dark, dry place.

2. *To make tonic:* Crush a small amount of blend to a fine powder, then measure 1 tsp (5 mL) per 1 cup (250 mL) water. Place in a warmed ceramic teapot, add 1 tsp (5 mL) "for the pot" and pour boiling water over herbs. Cover the pot and put a cork in the spout. Steep for about 5 minutes and strain into cups.

Iron Builder

Makes 3 cups (750 mL)

Young people experiencing puberty require extra iron to help them cope with the rapid changes within their bodies.

6	sprigs fresh peppermint	6
4	fresh stinging nettle tops	4
1	fresh yellow dock root	1
1	fresh burdock leaf, chopped	1
½ cup	chopped fresh sweet cicely	125 mL
3 cups	boiling water	750 mL

1. In a non-reactive teapot or heatproof jar, combine peppermint, stinging nettle, yellow dock, burdock and sweet cicely. Pour in boiling water and steep, covered, for at least 12 hours (the longer steeping time is necessary to extract the minerals from the herbs). Strain and drink ½ cup (125 mL) twice daily. Store tonic in a clean jar with a lid in the refrigerator for up to 3 days.

Spring Tonic

Makes 3 cups (750 mL)

Caution: Parsley should be avoided during pregnancy and in cases of kidney inflammation.

3 cups	filtered water	750 mL
1	2-inch (5 cm) piece fresh ginseng, chopped	1
1	2-inch (5 cm) piece fresh dandelion root, chopped	1
1	2-inch (5 cm) piece fresh burdock root, chopped	1
1 tbsp	chopped fresh parsley (see Caution, left)	15 mL
2	fresh stinging nettle tops	10 mL
¼ cup	maple sap	50 mL

1. In a non-reactive saucepan over medium heat, pour water over ginseng, dandelion and burdock. Cover and bring to a boil. Turn off heat and steep, covered, for 5 minutes.

2. Stir in parsley and nettle. Steep, covered, for another 10 minutes. Strain into a clean jar. Stir in maple sap. Use immediately or cover tightly and keep in refrigerator for up to 2 days.

Cleansers

People in central Europe began to juice cabbages, potatoes and beetroot to treat ulcers, cancer and leukemia in the late 1800s. But the practice of pressing the water from fruits and vegetables for health reasons is centuries old, being rooted in many religious faiths and indigenous cultures. Modern science is pointing to the fact that the future of health care in today's stressful and toxic environments will have as its core a whole food diet and regular, safe cleansing or detoxification of the body.

The goal of cleansing, detoxifying or fasting is to release and eliminate toxins stored in the colon and fat cells of the body. Those toxins re-enter the bloodstream where they recirculate in the body. That is why at the beginning of a cleansing, fasting or detoxifying program, diarrhea, headaches, irritability and catarrh can occur. As toxins are released, they are able to unleash their damage again. So it is important to ensure that they are eliminated. After a 5- to 10-day cleanse, a 3- to 5-day fast, or a supervised detoxifying program, most people feel calmer, with a sense of well-being, clear-headed and energetic.

A cleansing regime can consist of a restricted diet of vegetable soups, raw fresh salads, whole grains and other high-fiber foods, limited fruit juices, vegetable and herb juices, blended drinks and herbal teas. While cleansing, it is important to drink 8 to 10 glasses of pure water and eat only organic fruits, vegetables, herbs and grains while abstaining from fats (especially fried foods, red meats and milk products), alcohol, soft drinks, caffeine, refined foods and sugar or other sweeteners.

Fasting involves avoiding solid food for a prescribed period of time and should be undertaken with the help of a health practitioner. You should first define the purpose of the fast, whether to address a specific condition, to relieve and regenerate internal organs, or to simply lose weight. Then, with the help of a medical herbalist or other natural health practitioner, you can determine which of the five systems (digestion, circulation, elimination, respiration or nervous) or combinations of the five systems require support.

Fasting is always approached with a cleansing diet as described above for a minimum of 2 days preceding and following the actual fasting period. Fasts in the true sense call for water only, or water and clear juices only. However, juice "fasts" have come into popular use, allowing all types of fruit or vegetable juices along with herbal teas. These fasts are simple and safe for everyone in general good health (except anyone with a chronic degenerative disease or those who suffer from hyperthyroidism or anemia and pregnant or lactating women).

To promote proper elimination of the released toxins, whether cleansing or fasting, the main organs of elimination — liver, kidney, respiratory and lymph systems and skin — must be supported. Fresh, raw juice is a natural choice for cleansing. The concentrated nutrients are assimilated quickly without putting stress on the organs of digestion or elimination. Also, many fruits, vegetables and herbs are high in antioxidants, which are necessary for the elimination of toxins and free radicals. Only fresh, organic fruit, vegetable and herb juices are used in cleanses or fasts. Some experts recommend using only vegetable juices; others claim that both fruit and vegetable juices may be used. If using both, take fruit juices in the morning and at lunch and take only vegetable juices from mid-afternoon onward. Organ-supporting herbal teas and tonics, light to moderate exercise (sweating is one of the body's primary mechanisms for getting rid of toxic wastes) and saunas or baths, along with dry brushing, assist in the process of elimination. Psyllium seeds and a minimum of 10 glasses of pure, filtered water also help to remove toxins.

Short-term cleanses and juice fasts work best when part of a healthy lifestyle that includes a whole food diet, regular exercise, and a strong commitment to inner growth and spiritual nurturing.

The herbs listed below provide support for cells, organs and the process of elimination and cleansing. Juice fresh herbs when available or whisk up to 1 tsp (5 mL) dried herbs into juices and blended drinks or add to supportive cleansing teas.

Astragalus root (*Astragalus membranacus*, see page 124). A tonic and immune-enhancing herb that can be used in vegetable soups and whisked into juices. Use dried astragalus in tea blends.

Burdock root (*Arctium lappa*, see page 126). A skin and blood cleanser, burdock stimulates urine flow and sweating while supporting the liver, lymphatic glands and digestive system. Use fresh root or leaves in juices or vegetable soups. Make teas from dried burdock.

Cayenne (*Capsicum*, see page 127). Stimulates blood circulation, purifies the blood, expels mucus and promotes fluid elimination and sweat. Juice fresh chile peppers with other cleansing fruits, vegetables and herbs or use dried in teas.

Dandelion root (*Taraxacum officinale*, see page 130). A common herb, dandelion cleans the liver and blood, filters toxins, acts as a mild laxative, and increases the flow of urine. Best blended with fruits or vegetables, juice the fresh root or leaves or use dried root in coffee substitutes and teas.

Echinacea root (*Echinacea angustifolia* or *E. purpurea*, see page 131). Available in dried whole or cut form, and fresh from growers in the fall, echinacea helps stimulate the immune system while cleansing the lymph system.

Elderberry (*Sambucus nigra*, see page 102). Supports detoxification by promoting bowel movements, urination, sweating, and secretion of mucus.

Gingerroot (*Zingeber officinalis*, see page 134). Ginger helps elimination of toxins by stimulating circulation and sweating. Widely available, it is used in healing juices and grated into supportive teas and coffee substitutes.

Licorice (*Glycyrrhiza glabra*, see page 139). With its gentle laxative effect, licorice is often included in cleansing supportive teas.

Milk thistle (*Silybum marianus*, see page 140). Containing some of the most potent liver cleansing and protecting compounds known, 1 tbsp (15 mL) milk thistle seed is an excellent addition to pulped drinks and cleansing supportive teas.

Yellow dock root (*Rumex crispus*, see page 151). A cleansing herb that supports the liver, lymphatic glands and digestive system, dock is a strong laxative. It can be blended with other herbs when used for detoxifying.

Cell Support Juice

While the cleansing effects of juicing are taking place, this drink supports and nourishes the cells.

Caution: Parsley should be avoided during pregnancy and in cases of kidney inflammation.

3	apples	3
1	handful fresh parsley (see Caution, left)	1
1	handful fresh alfalfa tops or 1 tbsp (15 mL) dried	1

1. Using juicer, process apples, parsley and, if using fresh, the alfalfa. Whisk together and pour into a large glass. If using dried alfalfa, whisk into juice.

Cleansing Tea

Tea blend

This mineral-rich tea stimulates the bowel, liver, kidneys and lymphatic glands. It also aids cleansing and hormone balancing.

Caution: Do not use licorice if you have high blood pressure.

1 part	chopped burdock root	1 part
1 part	chopped dandelion root	1 part
1 part	chopped yellow dock root	1 part
1 part	stinging nettle	1 part
1 part	plantain	1 part
1 part	red clover flowers	1 part
½ part	chopped gingerroot or ¼ part ground	½ part
½ part	chopped licorice or ¼ part powdered (see Caution, left)	½ part
½ part	fennel seeds	½ part

1. In an airtight tin or dark-colored jar, blend together burdock, dandelion, yellow dock, stinging nettle, plantain, red clover, ginger, licorice and fennel seeds. Store in a cool, dark, dry place.

2. For each cup of tea, in a medium saucepan, combine 1 tsp (5 mL) of the lightly crushed herb mix with 1 cup (250 mL) water. Cover saucepan tightly and simmer for 15 minutes. Strain tea and serve. Drink ½ to 1 cup (125 to 250 mL) three times daily. To store, strain into a clean jar. Cover tightly and refrigerate for up to 2 days.

Crimson Cleanser Juice

The brilliant red color of beets signals a high beta carotene content. Coupled with the toxin-clearing ability of dandelion, it provides a pleasant internal wash.

1	apple	1
1	handful fresh dandelion leaves,	1
1	beet	1
2 tsp	maple syrup or to taste	10 mL

1. Using a juicer, process apple, dandelion and beet. Whisk together and pour into a glass. Whisk in maple syrup to taste.

Lemon Cleanser Juice

It is generally believed that lemon has "solvent properties," which makes this drink important when treating gallstones.

Tip
Substitute ¼ tsp (1 mL) powdered stevia for maple syrup, if desired.

2	lemons	2
1	apple	1
2 tsp	maple syrup	10 mL
¼ tsp	cayenne pepper	1 mL

1. Using juicer, process lemons and apple. Whisk together with maple syrup and cayenne and pour into a glass.

Root Decoction

Caution: Do not use licorice if you have high blood pressure.

1 tbsp	chopped dandelion root	15 mL
1 tsp	chopped licorice (see Caution, left)	5 mL
2 tsp	chopped ginseng	10 mL
4 cups	water	1 L

1. In a saucepan over medium-high heat, combine dandelion, licorice, ginseng and water; bring to a light boil. Cover pan, reduce heat and lightly simmer for 15 minutes. Remove from heat and steep for 5 minutes. Strain into cups and serve.

Healing Teas

Second only to water as the world's leading beverage, tea has been cultivated and harvested for at least 1,700 years. During that time, green and black teas, along with herbs, have been used to aid digestion, lift the spirits, calm nerves and stomach upsets, induce sleep and stimulate the system. Herb teas are gaining in popularity now because of the health benefits of the active ingredients and the gentle, caffeine-free flavor.

Herb teas are effective as a therapeutic tool because when boiling water is poured over the herbs and then allowed to steep, the cell walls are broken, releasing soluble organic compounds and essences into the water.

While fresh herbs can be used to make nutritive teas, most medicinal tea recipes call for dried herbs because dried herbs are easiest to store, transport and use. In the following recipes, amounts given are for dried herbs unless otherwise stated. Fresh herbs cannot be substituted for dried in tea blends since they will mildew during storage.

Tea blends

Just as commercial tea producers blend several tea leaves for each kind of tea, so herbalists have learned that combining different herb leaves, flowers and seeds, adding spices and sometimes citrus peel, produces a richer tasting tea. Sweet cicely (see page 324) and stevia (see page 148) are often added to herbal tea blends because of their ability to sweeten more bitter herbs. (See Tea Herbs, page 324.)

To make herb blends: Dry herbs for teas by hanging upside down in a dark, hot, dry place until they are crackling-dry. Strip leaves from the stems, but try to keep the leaves whole for storage. Blend the dried leaves according to your creative whim or use the following recipes for more specific effects. Store herb blends in a labeled airtight tin or dark-colored jar in a dark, cool, dry cupboard.

How to use tea as a gargle: Some herb teas, such as Throat Saver Tea Blend (see recipe, page 287), are excellent when used as a gargle for sore throats and to act as an antibiotic swab. Brew the tea following the directions given for the recipe. After steeping the tea, strain into a clean jar with a lid. Cool to room temperature with the lid on, store in the refrigerator. Gargle $1/4$ to $1/2$ cup (50 to 125 mL) at a time, every 1 to 2 hours or as needed.

Tea blend		

Energizer

Basil leaves are difficult to dry at home. Use commercially dried basil found in alternative/health stores.

1 part	sage	1 part
1 part	rosemary	1 part
1 part	thyme	1 part
1 part	basil	1 part
½ part	chopped gingerroot or ¼ part ground	½ part
½ part	lightly crushed cinnamon stick or ¼ part ground	½ part

1. In an airtight tin or dark-colored jar, combine sage, rosemary, thyme, basil, gingerroot and cinnamon. Store in a cool, dark, dry place.

2. *To make tea:* Crush a small amount of blend to a fine powder and measure 1 tsp (5 mL) per 1 cup (250 mL) water. Place in a warmed ceramic teapot, add 1 tsp (5 mL) "for the pot" and pour boiling water over herbs. Cover the pot and put a cork in the spout. Steep for about 15 minutes and strain into cups.

How to brew the perfect cup of tea

Bring fresh cold filtered water to the boil. Rinse a teapot with some of the boiling water, and pour off. (Do not use metal teapots and keep a teapot strictly for medicinal teas.) Measure 1 tsp (5 mL) crushed herbs per 1 cup (250 mL) water into the warmed pot. If making more than 2 cups of tea, add an extra 1 tsp (5 mL) dried herbs "for the pot." Pour boiling filtered water over; put a lid on the pot and a stopper in the spout. Steep 15 minutes before straining into cups. Herb teas should be consumed as soon as they are brewed. Otherwise, the volatile oils evaporate and the taste and medicinal benefit can be dispersed in the steam.

Flu Fighter

This tea promotes sweating to relieve symptoms of a cold or flu and helps speed recovery.

Tip
Use papaya or mango in place of the pineapple.

2 parts	chopped dried pineapple	2 parts
1 part	chopped gingerroot (or ½ part ground)	1 part
½ part	chopped echinacea root or ¼ part powdered	½ part
½ part	dried elderberries	½ part
¼ part	powdered boneset	¼ part
⅛ part	cayenne pepper	⅛ part

1. In an airtight tin or dark-colored jar, combine pineapple, gingerroot, echinacea, elderberries, boneset and cayenne. Store in a cool, dark, dry place.

2. *To make tea:* Crush a small amount of blend to a fine powder and measure 1 tsp (5 mL) per 1 cup (250 mL) water. Place in a warmed ceramic teapot, add 1 tsp (5 mL) "for the pot" and pour boiling water over herbs. Cover the pot and put a cork in the spout. Steep for about 15 minutes and strain into cups.

Free Flow Tea

This tea is diuretic, anti-inflammatory, soothing and antiseptic to the urinary tract.

2 parts	marshmallow leaf	2 parts
1 part	yarrow	1 part
1 part	plantain	1 part
1 part	stinging nettle tops	1 part
1 part	goldenrod, aerial parts	1 part
½ part	ground cinnamon	½ part

1. In an airtight tin or dark-colored jar, combine marshmallow, yarrow, plantain, stinging nettle, goldenrod and cinnamon. Store in a cool, dark, dry place.

2. *To make tea:* Crush a small amount of blend to a fine powder and measure 1 tsp (5 mL) per 1 cup (250 mL) water. Place in a warmed ceramic teapot, add 1 tsp (5 mL) "for the pot" and pour boiling water over herbs. Cover the pot and put a cork in the spout. Steep for about 15 minutes and strain into cups.

Ginger Tea

1 part	chopped gingerroot	1 part
⅓ part	fennel seeds	⅓ part
⅓ part	lemon balm	⅓ part

1. In an airtight tin or dark-colored jar, combine ginger, fennel and lemon balm. Store in a cool, dark, dry place.

2. *To make tea:* Crush a small amount of blend to a fine powder and measure 1 tsp (5 mL) per 1 cup (250 mL) water. Place in a warmed ceramic teapot, add 1 tsp (5 mL) "for the pot" and pour boiling water over herbs. Cover the pot and put a cork in the spout. Steep for about 15 minutes and strain into cups.

Ginseng

This tea stimulates circulation, digestion and energy.

1 part	powdered ginseng	1 part
1 part	fennel seeds	1 part
1 part	stinging nettle	1 part
½ part	ground gingerroot	½ part
¼ part	powdered stevia	¼ part

1. In an airtight tin or dark-colored jar, combine ginseng, fennel, stinging nettle, gingerroot and stevia. Store in a cool, dark, dry place.

2. *To make tea:* Crush a small amount of blend to a fine powder and measure 1 tsp (5 mL) per 1 cup (250 mL) water. Place in a warmed ceramic teapot, add 1 tsp (5 mL) "for the pot" and pour boiling water over herbs. Cover the pot and put a cork in the spout. Steep for about 15 minutes and strain into cups.

Gout Buster Tea

This tea stimulates elimination of wastes, including excess uric acid.

Caution: Do not use licorice if you have high blood pressure.

2 parts	stinging nettle	2 parts
1 part	burdock seed	1 part
1 part	celery seed	1 part
½ part	powdered licorice (see Caution, left)	½ part

1. In an airtight tin or dark-colored jar, combine stinging nettle, burdock, celery seed and licorice. Store in a cool, dark, dry place.

2. *To make tea:* Crush a small amount of blend to a fine powder and measure 1 tsp (5 mL) per 1 cup (250 mL) water. Place in a warmed ceramic teapot, add 1 tsp (5 mL) "for the pot" and pour boiling water over herbs. Cover the pot and put a cork in the spout. Steep for about 15 minutes and strain into cups.

Green Giant Tea Blend

2 parts	ginkgo	2 parts
1 part	German chamomile flowers	1 part
1 part	green tea	1 part
½ part	sweet cicely, aerial parts	½ part
¼ part	sage	¼ part

1. In an airtight tin or dark-colored jar, combine ginkgo, chamomile, green tea, sweet cicely and sage. Store in a cool, dark, dry place.

2. *To make tea:* Crush a small amount of blend to a fine powder and measure 1 tsp (5 mL) per 1 cup (250 mL) water. Place in a warmed ceramic teapot, add 1 tsp (5 mL) "for the pot" and pour boiling water over herbs. Cover the pot and put a cork in the spout. Steep for about 15 minute sand strain into cups.

Hangover Rescue Tea

2 parts	German chamomile flowers	2 parts
1 part	meadowsweet	1 part
½ part	ground gingerroot	½ part
¼ part	lavender buds	¼ part

1. In an airtight tin or dark-colored jar, combine chamomile, meadowsweet, gingerroot and lavender. Store in a cool, dark, dry place.

2. *To make tea:* Crush a small amount of blend to a fine powder and measure 1 tsp (5 mL) per 1 cup (250 mL) water. Place in a warmed ceramic teapot, add 1 tsp (5 mL) "for the pot" and pour boiling water over herbs. Cover the pot and put a cork in the spout. Steep for about 15 minutes and strain into cups.

Lavender Tea

This antioxidant tea stimulates circulation and digestion. It is also relaxing and liver supportive.

2 parts	lemon balm	2 parts
1 part	lavender flowers	1 part
1 part	German chamomile flowers	1 part
1 part	passionflower	1 part

1. In an airtight tin or dark-colored jar, combine lemon balm, lavender, chamomile and passionflower. Store in a cool, dark, dry place.

2. *To make tea:* Crush a small amount of blend to a fine powder and measure 1 tsp (5 mL) per 1 cup (250 mL) water. Place in a warmed ceramic teapot, add 1 tsp (5 mL) "for the pot" and pour boiling water over herbs. Cover the pot and put a cork in the spout. Steep for about 15 minutes and strain into cups.

Tea blend

Memory Booster Tea Blend

1 part	ginkgo	1 part
1 part	crushed dandelion root	1 part
$\frac{1}{4}$ part	rosemary	$\frac{1}{4}$ part
$\frac{1}{4}$ part	sage	$\frac{1}{4}$ part
$\frac{1}{4}$ part	chopped gingerroot or $\frac{1}{8}$ part powdered	$\frac{1}{4}$ part
$\frac{1}{4}$ part	stevia leaves or $\frac{1}{8}$ part powdered	$\frac{1}{4}$ part

1. In an airtight tin or dark-colored jar, combine ginkgo, dandelion, rosemary, sage, ginger and stevia. Store in a cool, dark, dry place.

2. *To make tea:* Crush a small amount of blend to a fine powder and measure 1 tsp (5 mL) per 1 cup (250 mL) water. Place in a warmed ceramic teapot, add 1 tsp (5 mL) "for the pot" and pour boiling water over herbs. Cover the pot and put a cork in the spout. Steep for about 15 minutes and strain into cups.

Tea blend

Migraine Buster

According to James Duke, "In my own experience, and this is reflected in the medical literature, feverfew works [to prevent and even cure migraines and other headaches] for about two-thirds of those who use it consistently." Take 1 cup (250 mL) daily to avoid migraines.

1 part	feverfew	1 part
1 part	ginkgo	1 part
½ part	lemon balm	½ part
½ part	German chamomile flowers	½ part

1. In an airtight tin or dark-colored jar, combine feverfew, ginkgo, lemon balm and chamomile. Store in a cool, dark, dry place.

2. *To make tea:* Crush a small amount of blend to a fine powder and measure 1 tsp (5 mL) per 1 cup (250 mL) water. Place in a warmed ceramic teapot, add 1 tsp (5 mL) "for the pot" and pour boiling water over herbs. Cover the pot and put a cork in the spout. Steep for about 15 minutes and strain into cups.

Tea blend

Mother's Own

2 parts	red raspberry leaves	2 parts
1 part	rose hips	1 part
1 part	stinging nettle	1 part
1 part	lemon verbena	1 part
1 part	fennel seeds	1 part
½ part	lemon balm	½ part
½ part	alfalfa, aerial parts	½ part

1. In an airtight tin or dark-colored jar, combine raspberry, rose hips, stinging nettle, lemon verbena, fennel, lemon balm and alfalfa. Store in a cool, dark, dry place.

2. *To make tea*: Crush a small amount of blend to a fine powder and measure 1 tsp (5 mL) per 1 cup (250 mL) water. Place in a warmed ceramic teapot, add 1 tsp (5 mL) "for the pot" and pour boiling water over herbs. Cover the pot and put a cork in the spout. Steep for about 15 minutes and strain into cups.

Tea blend

Nettle Tea

2 parts	stinging nettle	2 parts
1 part	dandelion leaves	1 part
1 part	yarrow aerial parts	1 part

1. In an airtight tin or dark-colored jar, combine stinging nettle, dandelion and yarrow. Store in a cool, dark, dry place.

2. *To make tea*: Crush a small amount of blend to a fine powder and measure 1 tsp (5 mL) per 1 cup (250 mL) water. Place in a warmed ceramic teapot, add 1 tsp (5 mL) "for the pot" and pour boiling water over herbs. Cover the pot and put a cork in the spout. Steep for about 15 minutes and strain into cups.

Raspberry Ginger

Tip

Slippery elm bark is, well, slippery. It tends to clump and float on the top of liquids. For this reason, whisk herbs with a wire whisk or fork while slowly pouring in hot water.

1 tbsp	raspberry leaves	15 mL
1 tsp	grated gingerroot or ½ tsp (2 mL) ground)	5 mL
1 tsp	powdered slippery elm bark	5 mL
1½ cups	boiling water	375 mL

1. In a non-reactive teapot, combine raspberry, ginger and elm bark. Whisk while slowly adding boiling water; steep for 15 minutes. Strain into cups and drink warm.

Saw Palmetto

Tea blend

1 part	ground saw palmetto berries	1 part
1 part	green tea	1 part
1 part	chopped fresh nettle root, if available	1 part
½ part	ground gingerroot	½ part

1. In an airtight tin or dark-colored jar, combine palmetto berries, green tea, nettle root and ginger. Store in a cool, dark, dry place.

2. *To make tea:* Crush a small amount of blend to a fine powder and measure 1 tsp (5 mL) per 1 cup (250 mL) water. Place in a warmed ceramic teapot, add 1 tsp (5 mL) "for the pot" and pour boiling water over herbs. Cover the pot and put a cork in the spout. Steep for about 15 minutes and strain into cups.

Tea blend

Spicy Green and Fruit Tea

2 parts	loose dried green tea leaves	2 parts
1 part	chopped dried mango	1 part
1 part	chopped dried papaya	1 part
½ part	chopped dried pineapple	½ part
½ part	anise seeds	½ part
¼ part	crushed cinnamon (or ⅛ part ground cinnamon)	¼ part
⅛ part	ground ginger	⅛ part

1. In an airtight tin or dark-colored jar, blend together green tea, mango, papaya, pineapple, anise, cinnamon and ginger. Store in a cool, dark, dry place.

2. *To make tea:* Crush a small amount of blend to a fine powder and measure 1 tsp (5 mL) per 1 cup (250 mL) water. Place in a warmed ceramic teapot, add 1 tsp (5 mL) "for the pot" and pour boiling water over herbs. Cover the pot and put a cork in the spout. Steep for about 15 minutes, then strain into cups.

Throat Saver Tea Blend

All elements in this soothing tea will help ease a sore throat.

1 part	thyme	1 part
1 part	peppermint	1 part
1 part	sage	1 part
⅛ part	ground gingerroot	⅛ part
	Honey	

1. In an airtight tin or dark-colored jar, combine thyme, peppermint, sage and ginger. Store in a cool, dark, dry place.

2. *To make tea:* Crush a small amount of blend to a fine powder and measure 1 tsp (5 mL) per 1 cup (250 mL) water. Place in a warmed ceramic teapot, add 1 tsp (5 mL) "for the pot" and pour boiling water over herbs. Cover the pot and put a cork in the spout. Steep for about 15 minutes, strain into cups and add honey to taste.

Varicosi Tea

This tea nourishes and tones the veins.

1 part	dandelion leaves	1 part
1 part	yarrow, aerial parts	1 part
1 part	hawthorn, aerial parts	1 part
1 part	linden flower	1 part
½ part	chopped gingerroot or ¼ part ground	½ part

1. In an airtight tin or dark-colored jar, combine dandelion, yarrow, hawthorn, linden flower and ginger. Store in a cool, dark, dry place.

2. *To make tea:* Crush a small amount of blend to a fine powder and measure 1 tsp (5 mL) per 1 cup (250 mL) water. Place in a warmed ceramic teapot, add 1 tsp (5 mL) "for the pot" and pour boiling water over herbs. Cover the pot and put a cork in the spout. Steep for about 15 minutes and strain into cups.

Woman's Own

This nourishing tea increases breast milk in nursing mothers.

Caution: Do not use licorice if you have high blood pressure.

2 parts	motherwort aerial parts	2 parts
1 part	chaste berries	1 part
1 part	red clover flowers	1 part
1 part	powdered licorice (see Caution, left)	1 part
½ part	fennel seeds	½ part
½ part	chopped ginseng or ¼ part powdered	½ part

1. In an airtight tin or dark-colored jar, combine motherwort, chaste berries, red clover, licorice, fennel and ginseng. Store in a cool, dark, dry place.

2. *To make tea:* Crush a small amount of blend to a fine powder and measure 1 tsp (5 mL) per 1 cup (250 mL) water. Place in a warmed ceramic teapot, add 1 tsp (5 mL) "for the pot" and pour boiling water over herbs. Cover the pot and put a cork in the spout. Steep for about 15 minutes and strain into cups.

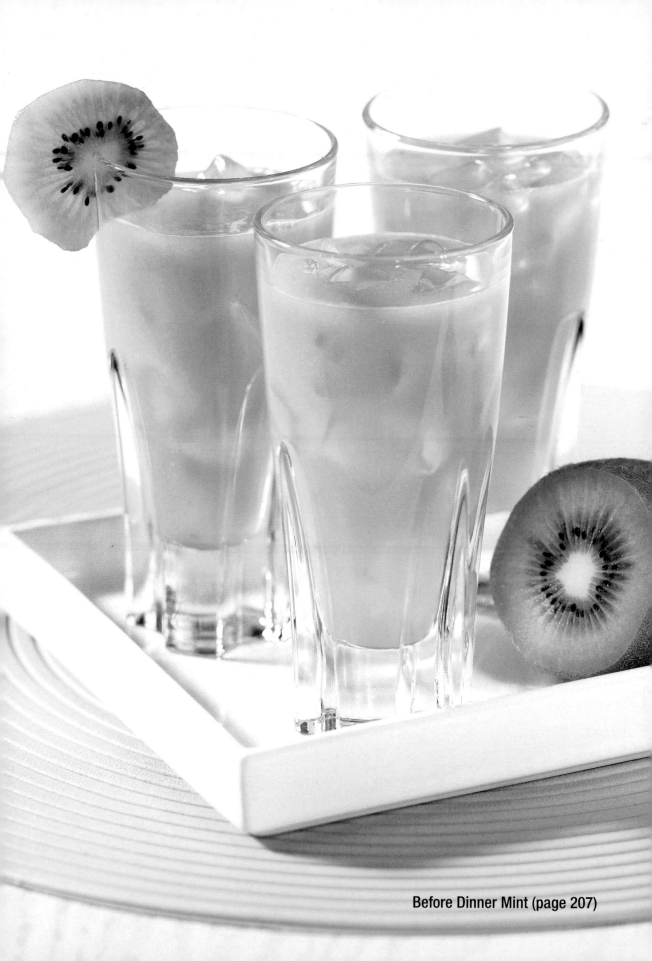

Before Dinner Mint (page 207)

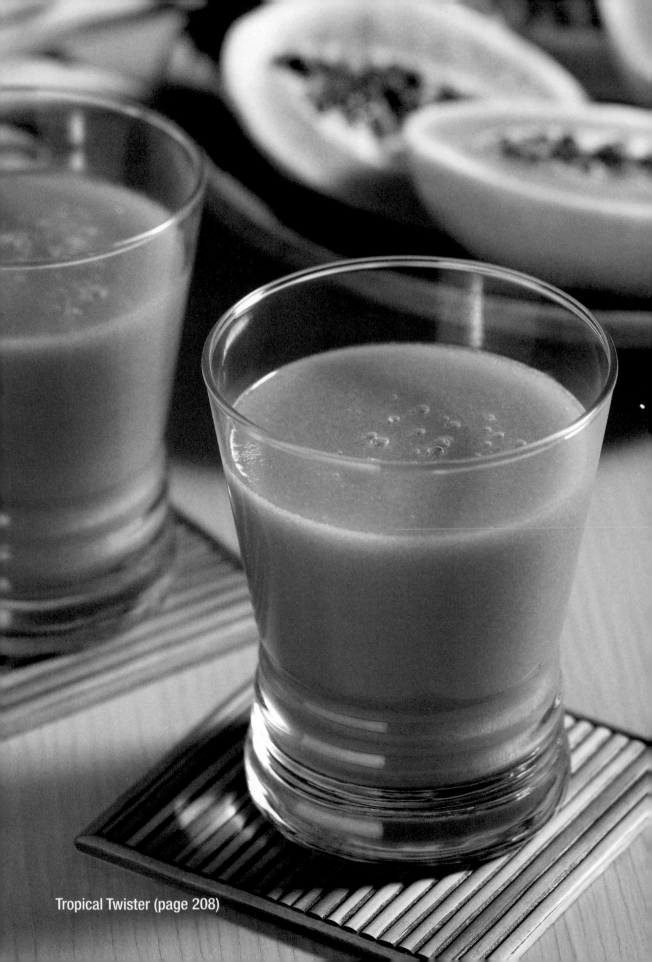

Tropical Twister (page 208)

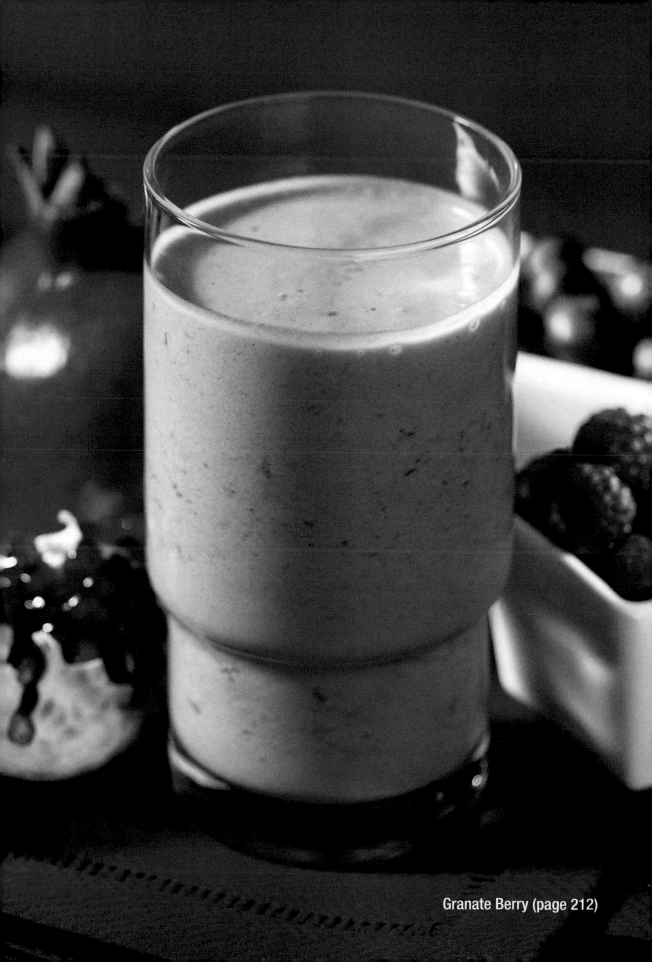

Granate Berry (page 212)

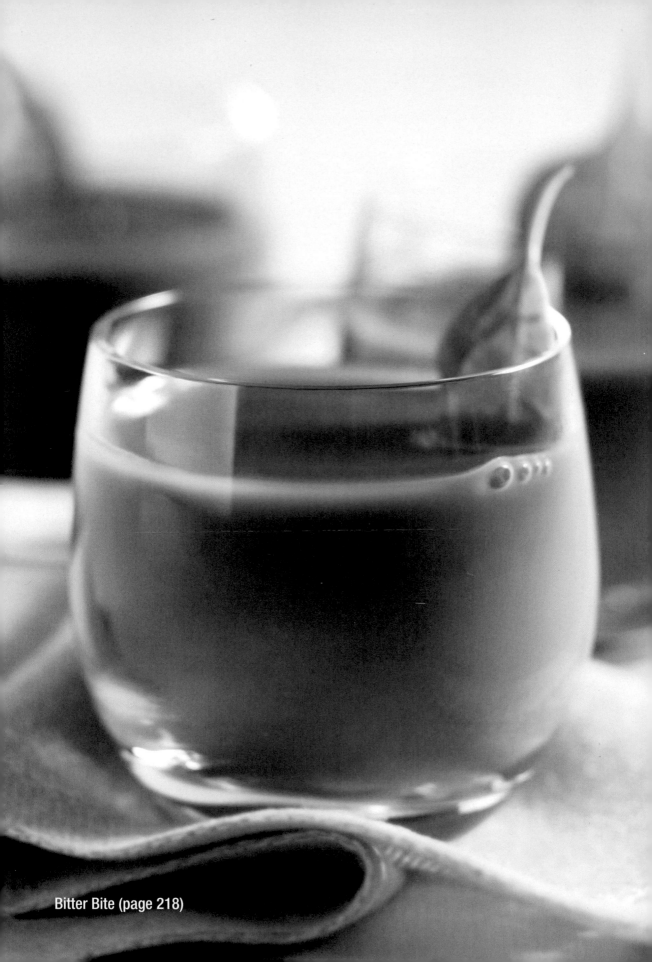

Bitter Bite (page 218)

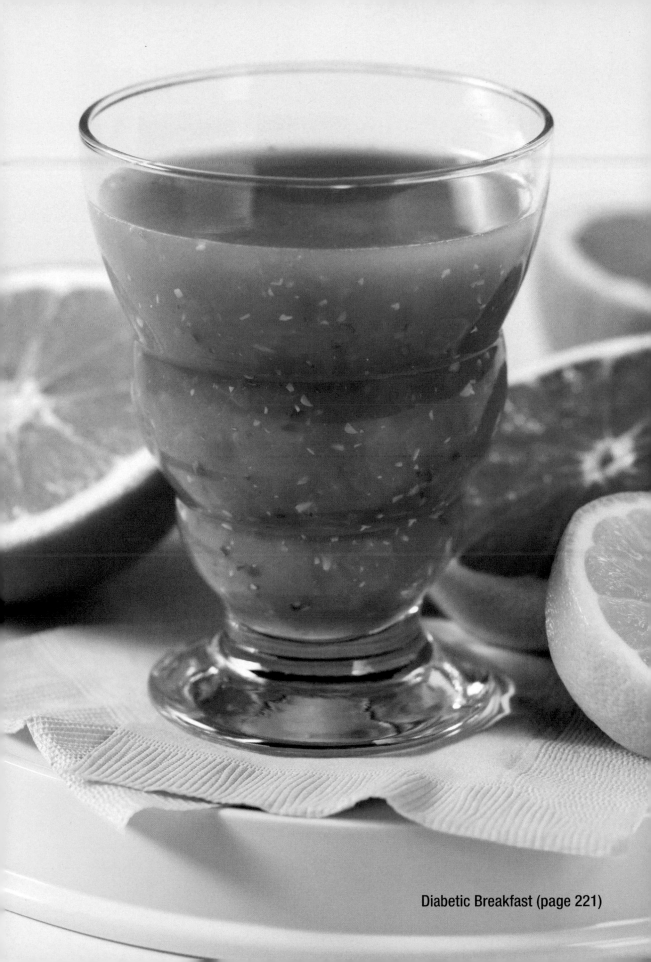

Diabetic Breakfast (page 221)

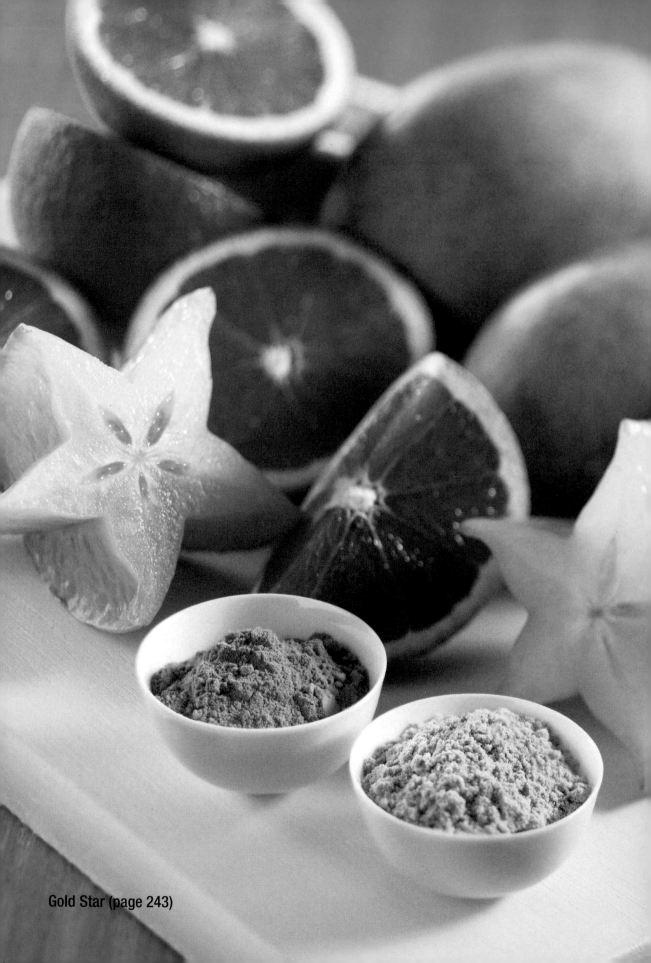

Gold Star (page 243)

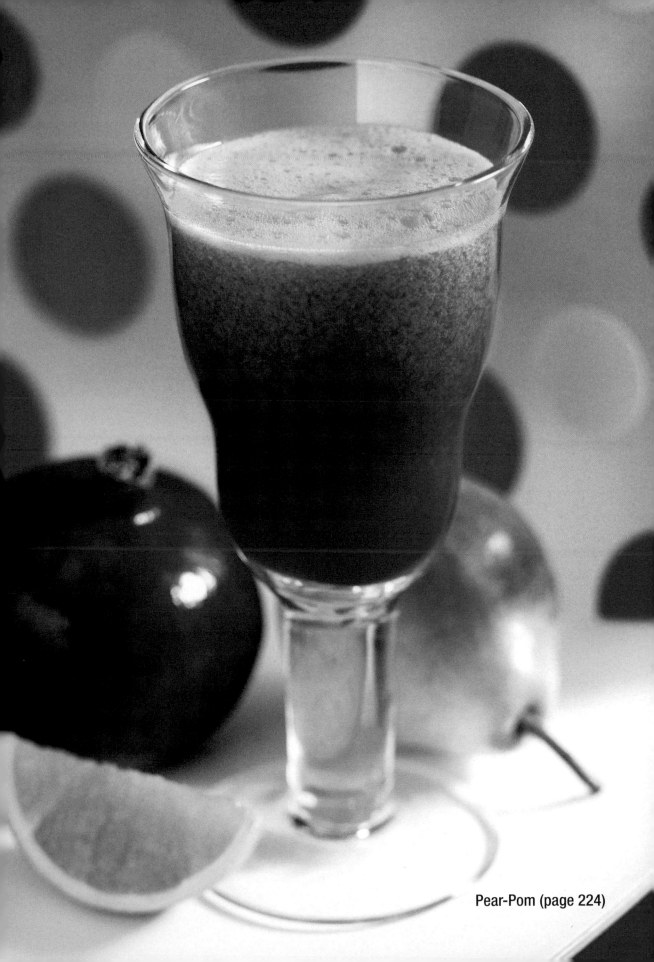

Pear-Pom (page 224)

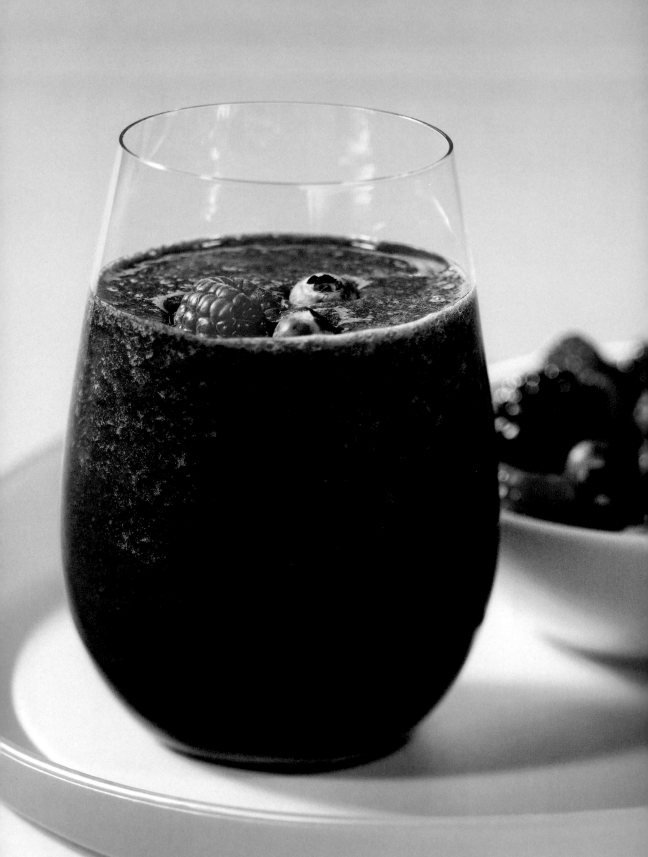

Berry Young (page 229)

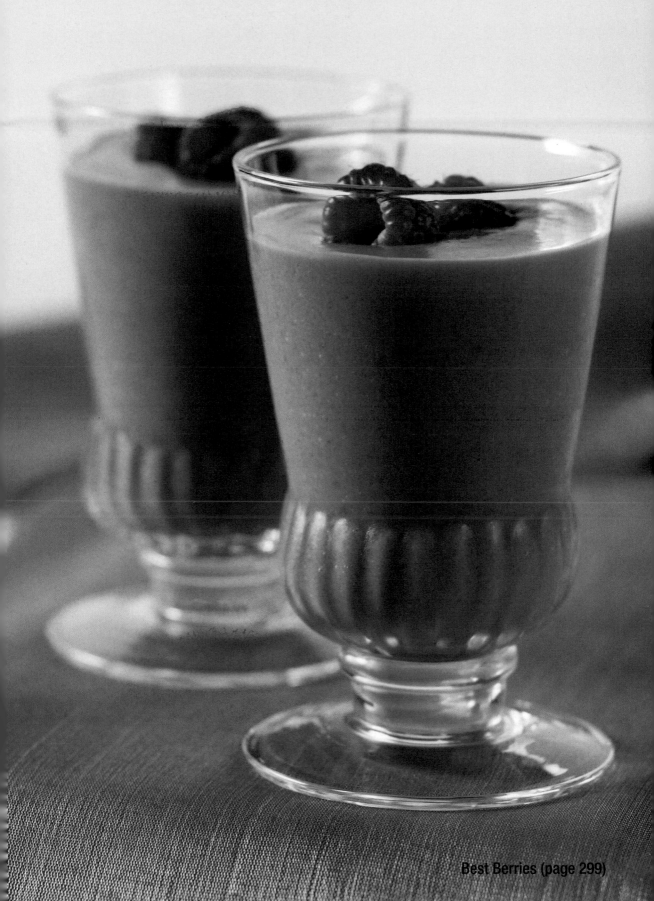

Best Berries (page 299)

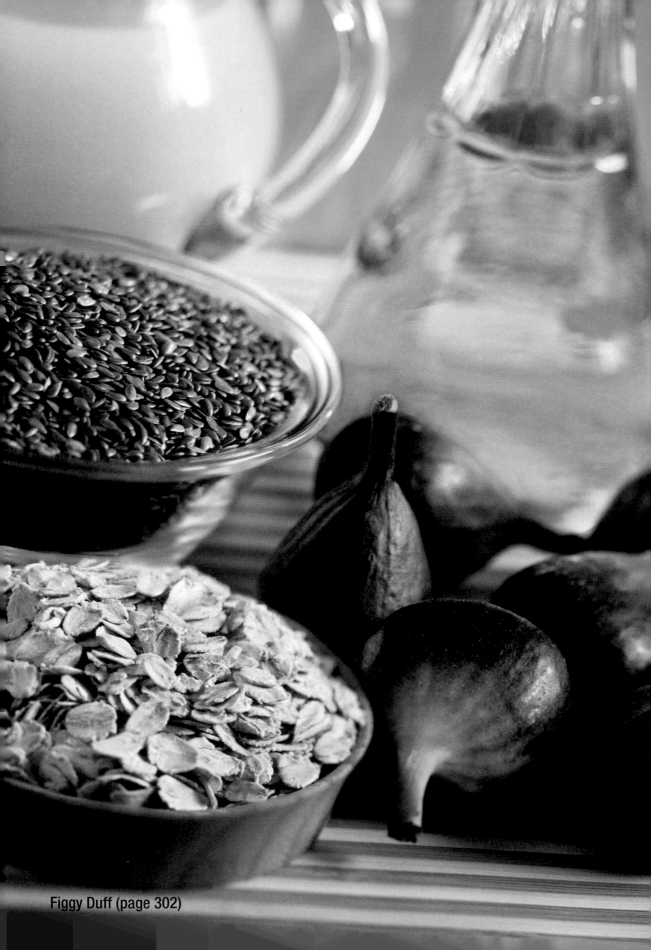

Figgy Duff (page 302)

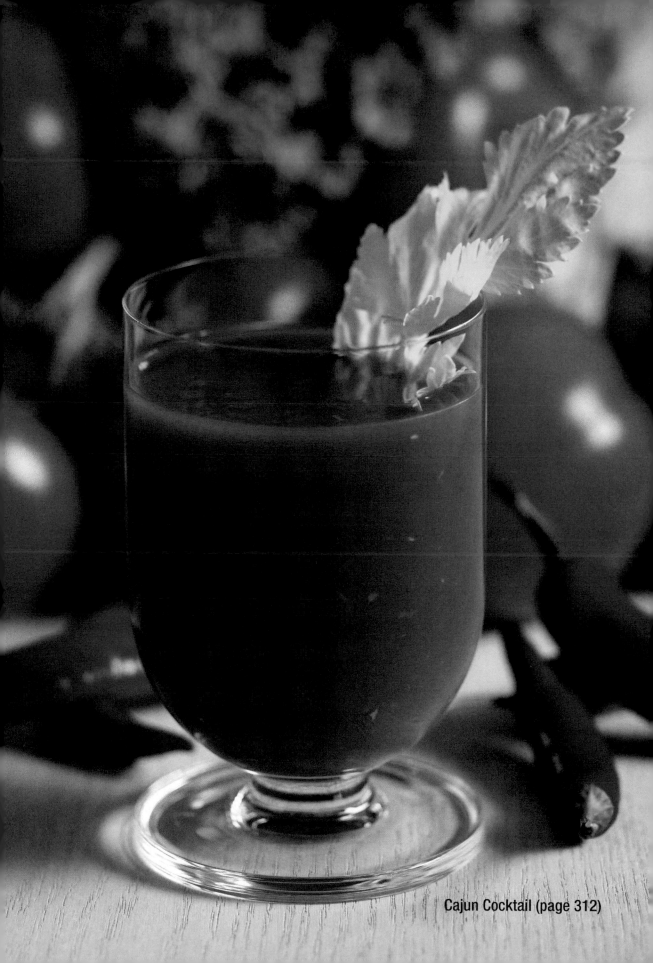

Cajun Cocktail (page 312)

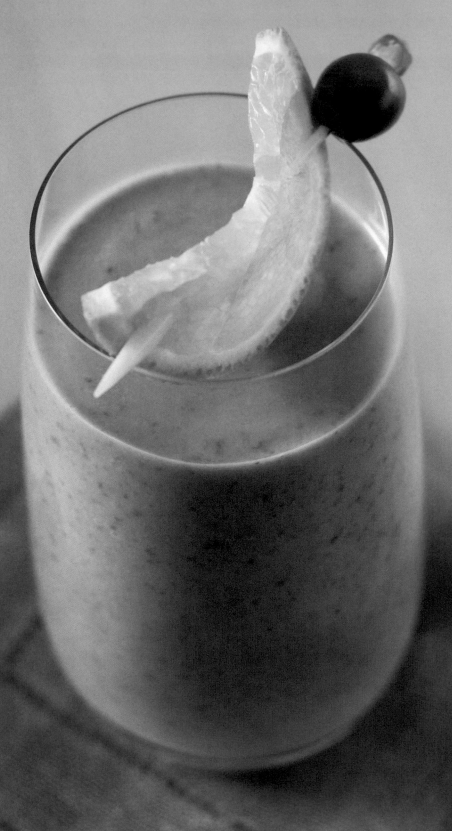

Cran-Orange (page 302)

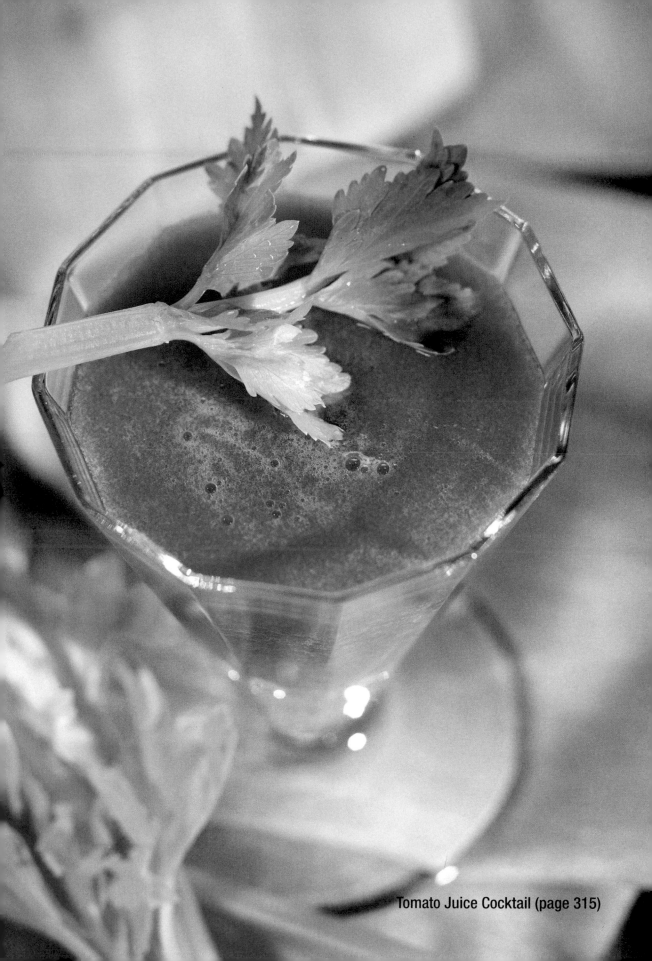

Tomato Juice Cocktail (page 315)

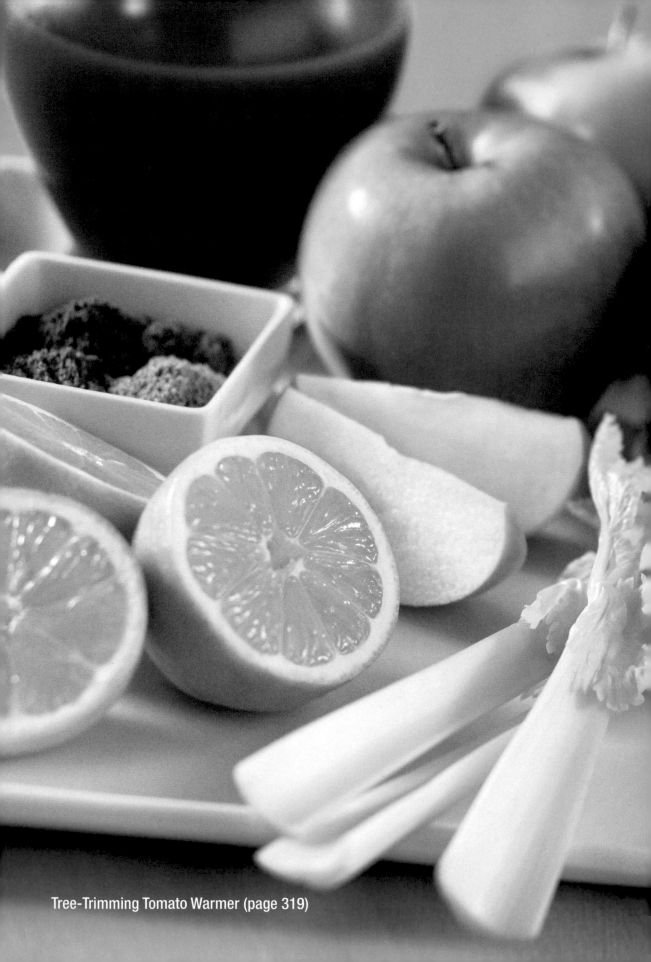

Tree-Trimming Tomato Warmer (page 319)

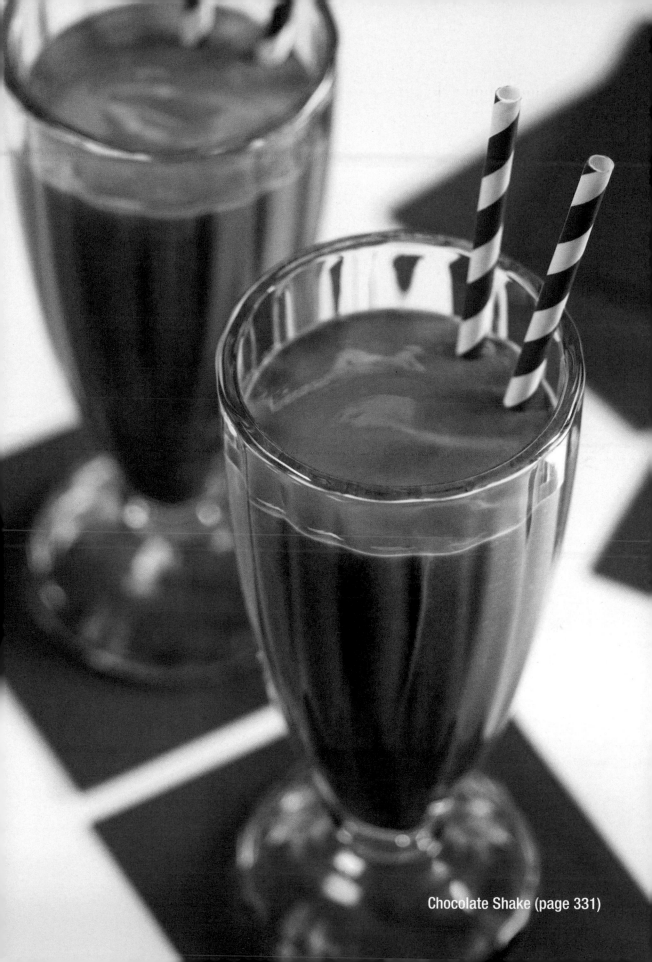

Chocolate Shake (page 331)

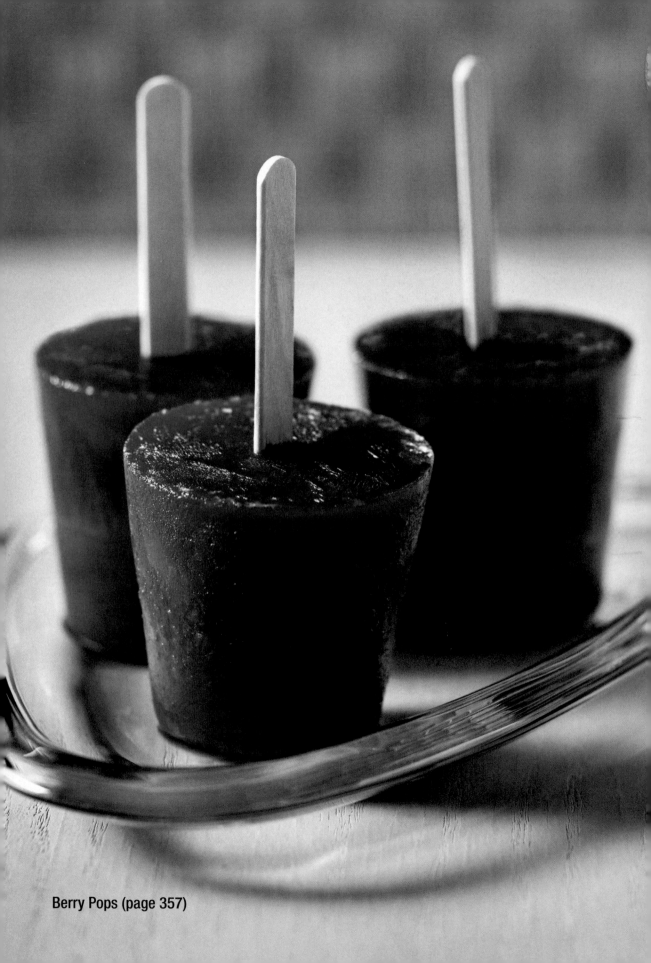

Berry Pops (page 357)

Roughies and Smoothies

Roughies

Our definition of "roughies" is any food that has been made with the pulp from juicing. When fruits, vegetables or herbs are processed in a juice machine, two products are the result — pure raw juice and pulp. While juices contain a concentrated amount of nutrients, the pulp retains the fiber and a substantial amount of nutrients as well. Plan to use pulp from juicing in as many favorite recipes as possible — soup stocks, stews, dips, baked products, sauces and any recipe that calls for a purée of fruit or vegetable.

Versatile fruits or vegetables such as apples, carrots and tomatoes can be juiced first, the pulp collected and kept separate from other juice ingredients to keep their flavors pure for apple sauce, muffins, cakes or tomato sauces and salsas. See the Frozen Treats chapter (pages 341 to 358) for cooling recipes that use pulp.

To use pulp in recipes: Cut out the core and seeds and peel the fruit or vegetable before juicing. For best results, blend pulp using blender or food processor before using or freezing. Measure 2 cups (500 mL) of the blended pulp and transfer to a freezer bag or covered container. Store in the refrigerator if the pulp will be used within a day, or label and freeze until needed.

Apple Rice Pudding

Low in fat, this alternative dessert is delicious.

Tips

Substitute nut or fruit milk (see pages 327 and 328) for soymilk.

Strain the yogurt through a cheesecloth-lined sieve.

2 cups	soymilk	500 mL
¾ cup	rice	175 mL
1 cup	apple pulp	250 mL
½ cup	apple juice	125 mL
3 tbsp	honey	45 mL
½ cup	strained yogurt	125 mL
1 tbsp	finely chopped candied gingerroot	15 mL
½ tsp	ground cinnamon	2 mL
¼ tsp	ground nutmeg	1 mL

1. In a saucepan, combine soymilk and rice. Bring to a light boil over medium-high heat. Cover, reduce heat and simmer gently for 20 minutes or until rice is cooked but still firm.

2. Increase heat slightly and stir in apple pulp, apple juice and honey. Simmer gently for 10 minutes or until liquid is slightly reduced, rice is tender and mixture is thick. Remove from heat and stir in yogurt, ginger, cinnamon and nutmeg.

Applesauce

Makes 4 cups (1 L)

Tips

Add ½ tsp (2 mL) powdered licorice to treat constipation or ½ tsp (2 mL) cayenne pepper or other herbs recommended for specific conditions.

Try carrot and beet juices and more or less water to vary the thickness of the sauce.

2 cups	apple pulp	500 mL
2 cups	filtered water	500 mL
2 cups	apple juice	500 mL
3 tbsp	honey	45 mL
½ tsp	ground cinnamon	2 mL
¼ tsp	ground nutmeg	1 mL

1. In a non-reactive saucepan, combine pulp, water and juice. Bring to a boil over medium-high heat. Reduce heat and simmer for 20 to 30 minutes or until sauce is thick. Stir in honey, cinnamon and nutmeg. Serve warm or at room temperature. Store in covered container in refrigerator.

Avocado Gazpacho

Use any vegetable pulp for this great summer soup.

Caution: Parsley should be avoided during pregnancy and in cases of kidney inflammation.

2 cups	vegetable or chicken stock	500 mL
1	lemon, juiced	1
1 tbsp	white wine vinegar	15 mL
2 cups	vegetable pulp	500 mL
2	celery stalks, cut into chunks	2
½	cucumber, seeded and cut into chunks	½
2	cloves garlic	2
4	sprigs fresh basil	4
1	ripe avocado, cut into chunks	1
1 tbsp	chopped dulse	15 mL
4	sprigs fresh basil or parsley (see Caution, left)	4

1. In a Vita-Mix, food processor or blender, combine stock, lemon juice, vinegar, pulp, celery, cucumber, garlic, basil and avocado. Process on high until smooth (if necessary, process in two batches). Chill and serve garnished with dulse and fresh basil.

Cabbage Salad

Serves 4 to 6

2 cups	cabbage pulp	500 mL
1 cup	carrot-apple pulp	250 mL
3 tbsp	sunflower seeds	45 mL
2 tbsp	raisins	25 mL
2 tbsp	flax seeds	25 mL
1 tbsp	chopped dried apricot	15 mL
¼ cup	hemp oil or olive oil	50 mL
2 tbsp	freshly squeezed lemon juice	25 mL
2 tbsp	soy sauce	25 mL
2	cloves garlic, minced	2
¼ cup	crumbled feta cheese, optional	50 mL

1. In a large salad bowl, combine cabbage pulp, carrot-apple pulp, sunflower seeds, raisins, flax seeds and apricots. Toss to combine.

2. In a small jar with a tight-fitting lid or in a bowl, combine oil, lemon juice, soy sauce and garlic. Shake or whisk to mix thoroughly. Drizzle dressing over salad and toss to coat well. Sprinkle with feta cheese, if using.

Cajun Salsa

Makes 1 cup (250 mL)

Use as a dip for nachos, a spread with bread, or a hot relish for chicken or fish.

Tip

If you like your salsa hot, add a few drops of hot sauce or freshly chopped hot pepper to taste.

1 cup	Cajun Cocktail pulp (see recipe, page 312)	250 mL
2	tomatoes, seeded and coarsely chopped	2
1	clove garlic, finely chopped	1
3 tbsp	olive oil	45 mL

1. In a medium bowl, combine pulp, tomatoes, garlic and olive oil. Toss to combine.

Curry Sauce

Makes 2½ cups (625 mL)

Try using the pulp from Breakfast Cocktail (see recipe, page 311). Serve with cooked rice and steamed or stir-fried vegetables.

2 tbsp	butter	25 mL
1 tbsp	curry powder	15 mL
1 tbsp	garam masala	15 mL
2 cups	nut milk (see pages 327–28) or soymilk	500 mL
1 cup	onion-celery-apple pulp (see left)	250 mL
	Salt and black pepper	

1. In a small non-reactive saucepan, melt butter over medium heat. Stir in curry and garam masala. Cook, stirring, for 1 minute.

2. Whisk in milk and stir in pulp, adjusting heat to keep the mixture at a slight boil. Cook, stirring constantly, for 5 minutes or until sauce is thick. Season to taste with salt and pepper.

Lemon Sauce

Makes 1 cup (250 mL)

Lemon Rice Pudding: In a bowl combine Lemon Sauce with 2 cups (500 mL) cooked rice, 1 cup (250 mL) almond milk and ½ tsp (2 mL) ground cinnamon.

1 cup	pulp from Lemon Aid juice (see recipe, page 171)	250 mL
⅓ cup	freshly squeezed lemon juice	75 mL
3 tbsp	honey	45 mL

1. In a small non-reactive saucepan, combine pulp, lemon juice and honey. Bring to a boil over medium heat. Reduce heat slightly and boil gently, stirring, for 5 minutes or until sauce is thick. Serve warm or at room temperature. Store in covered container in refrigerator.

Papaya Marinade

Makes 1¼ cups (300 mL)

This marinade is delicious with fish and poultry.

Tip
Use kiwi, orange or pineapple pulp if papaya is not available.

1 cup	papaya pulp (see Tip, left)	250 mL
⅔ cup	freshly squeezed orange juice	150 mL
⅓ cup	soy sauce	75 mL
1	clove garlic, minced	1

1. In a shallow baking dish, combine pulp, orange juice, soy sauce and garlic. Arrange items to be marinated in dish, spooning marinade over top to coat both sides. Stand, covered, in refrigerator for 1 hour, turning once or twice.

Thyme Pumpkin Bread

Makes 1 loaf

- Preheat oven to 350°F (180°C)
- 8- by 4-inch (1.5 L) loaf pan, greased

2	eggs	2
2 tbsp	granulated sugar	25 mL
2 tbsp	liquid honey	25 mL
½ cup	olive oil	125 mL
1 cup	pumpkin pulp or squash pulp	250 mL
½ cup	apple pulp	125 mL
½	onion, chopped	½
1 tbsp	Dijon mustard	15 mL
1 cup	all-purpose flour	250 mL
½ cup	whole wheat flour	125 mL
¾ tsp	baking powder	4 mL
½ tsp	baking soda	2 mL
1 tbsp	fresh thyme leaves or 1 tsp (5 mL) dried	15 mL
1 tbsp	chopped fresh oregano or 1 tsp (5 mL) dried	15 mL

1. In a large bowl, beat eggs. Beat in sugar, honey and oil. Stir in squash and apple pulp, onion and mustard.

2. In a medium bowl, stir together all-purpose flour, whole wheat flour, baking powder, baking soda, thyme and oregano.

3. Stir flour mixture into pumpkin mixture. Pour into prepared loaf pan. Bake in preheated oven for 50 to 60 minutes or until a tester comes out clean.

Tomato Sauce

Makes 4 cups (1 L)

Pulp from most tomato juices (such as Cajun Cocktail, page 312, Peppery Tomato Cocktail, page 314, or Tomato Juice Cocktail, page 315) will work in this recipe.

2 tbsp	olive oil	25 mL
3	cloves garlic, minced	3
1	large onion, chopped	1
2 cups	tomato pulp (see left)	500 mL
1 cup	filtered water	250 mL
3 tbsp	soy sauce	45 mL
1 tbsp	balsamic vinegar	15 mL
3 tbsp	chopped fresh basil or 1 tbsp (15 mL) dried	45 mL
2 tbsp	chopped fresh oregano or 1 tbsp (15 mL) dried	25 mL
2 tbsp	fresh thyme leaves or 1 tbsp (15 mL) dried	25 mL
	Salt and black pepper	

1. In a non-reactive saucepan, heat oil over medium heat. Add garlic and onion and sauté for 5 minutes or until soft. Add tomato pulp, water, soy sauce, vinegar, basil, oregano and thyme. Increase heat and bring to a boil. Reduce heat and simmer, stirring occasionally, for 45 minutes to 1 hour or until reduced slightly. Season to taste with salt and pepper.

Smoothies

Smoothies are thick, creamy fruit dishes that are delicious anytime. They are simple combinations of $1/2$ to 1 cup (125 to 250 mL) fresh fruit juice and 1 cup (250 mL) fresh fruit. Bananas are usually included because they thicken the drink. Small amounts of other ingredients such as nuts, seeds, spices and herbs are optional. Nut milks may be used in place of soymilk or some fruit juices. Fruit milks, especially apricot milk, can be substituted for any of the fruit juices in smoothies. See pages 327–28 for information on how to make nut and fruit milks.

To make smoothies: Using a blender or Vita-Mix, place juice or liquid in container and add other ingredients in the order given. Blend for 30 seconds to 1 minute or until smooth. Garnish if desired.

The thick, creamy texture of smoothies makes them as satisfying as a traditional milkshake, but without the use of dairy products (milk, cream or ice cream) or any sweetener. While banana is the most popular thickener in smoothies, other ingredients can be used to produce a similar texture. Nut milks (see pages 327–28), oatmeal or spelt flakes, flax or sesame seeds and nuts serve this purpose as well. Check the texture of the drink while it is still in the container. If too thin, add 1 tbsp (15 mL) oatmeal, nuts or seeds and process again. If too thick, add any fruit juice in increments of $1/4$ cup (50 mL) until the right texture is attained.

Almond-Banana Milk

Serves 1

Almonds work best, but any nut milk is good in this creamy drink.

Tip
See page 329 for directions on freezing bananas.

1 cup	almond milk or soymilk	250 mL
2	bananas, fresh or frozen	2
Pinch	ground nutmeg	Pinch

1. Using a blender, process milk and bananas until smooth. Pour into a glass and sprinkle with nutmeg.

Avocado Pineapple

1 cup	pineapple chunks, fresh or frozen	250 mL
¾ cup	raspberry juice	175 mL
1	avocado, pitted	1

1. Using a blender, process pineapple, raspberry juice, and avocado until smooth. Pour into a glass.

Best Berries

Use any berry — raspberry, strawberry, blueberry or blackberry — for this sweet summer drink.

1 cup	fresh or frozen berries	250 mL
¾ cup	pineapple juice	175 mL
3 tbsp	natural yogurt	45 mL
1	banana	1

1. Using a blender, process berries, pineapple juice, yogurt and banana until smooth. Pour into a glass.

Beta Boost

Tip
When available, substitute 2 fresh, pitted apricots for dried.

½ cup	freshly squeezed orange juice	125 mL
¼ cup	carrot juice	50 mL
½	cantaloupe, seeds intact	½
¼ cup	chopped dried apricots	50 mL
¼ cup	soft tofu	50 mL

1. Using a blender, process orange juice, carrot juice, cantaloupe, apricots and tofu until smooth. Pour into a glass.

Blue Cherry

½ cup	soymilk or nut milk	125 mL
½ cup	fresh or frozen blueberries	125 mL
½ cup	fresh or frozen pitted cherries	125 mL
¼ cup	cranberry juice	50 mL
1	banana	1

1. Using a blender, process soymilk, blueberries, cherries, cranberry juice and banana until smooth. Pour into a glass.

B-Vitamin

Wheat germ is rich in B vitamins. Fish oil, evening primrose oil, flax seed oil, and hemp oil are all rich in the essential fatty acids important to health. Use any of them in this recipe.

1 cup	pineapple chunks, fresh or frozen	250 mL
½ cup	pineapple juice	125 mL
¼ cup	almond milk or soymilk	50 mL
1	banana	1
1 tbsp	wheat germ	15 mL
2 tsp	flax seeds	10 mL
1 tsp	hemp oil	5 mL

1. Using a blender, process pineapple chunks, pineapple juice, milk, banana, wheat germ, flax seeds and oil until smooth. Pour into a glass.

Serves 1

Calming Chamomile Smoothie

Tip
Add 1 tbsp (15 mL) sesame seeds to thicken this drink.

½ cup	soymilk or nut milk	125 mL
1	apple, peeled, cored and cut into pieces	1
¼	cantaloupe, cut into chunks	¼
2 tbsp	natural yogurt	25 mL
1 tbsp	fresh German chamomile flowers or 1 tsp (5 mL) dried	15 mL

1. Using a blender, process soymilk, apple, cantaloupe, yogurt and chamomile until smooth. Pour into a glass.

Serves 1

Cherries Jubilee

2 cups	pitted cherries	500 mL
½ cup	soymilk	125 mL
2	pineapple wedges	2
1	banana	1
1 tbsp	flax seeds	15 mL
⅛ tsp	almond extract, optional	0.5 mL

1. Using a blender, process cherries, soymilk, pineapple, banana, flax seeds and almond extract if using until smooth. Pour into a glass.

Cran-Orange

Tip
Dried cranberries are sweetened. If using fresh cranberries, you may wish to add some honey.

½ cup	dried cranberries	125 mL
¼ cup	freshly squeezed orange juice	50 mL
¼ cup	soft tofu	50 mL
1	orange, seeded	1
1 tbsp	grated gingerroot	15 mL
1 tbsp	liquid honey	15 mL

1. Using a blender, process cranberries, orange juice, tofu, orange, gingerroot and honey until smooth. Pour into a glass.

Figgy Duff

Tip
If fig milk is available, use it instead of pineapple juice and use 2 pineapple wedges in place of the figs and omit the flax seeds.

½ cup	pineapple juice	125 mL
5	figs, fresh or dried	5
2 tbsp	flax seeds	25 mL
2 tsp	oatmeal	10 mL
1 tsp	extra-virgin olive oil or hemp oil	5 mL

1. Using a blender, process pineapple juice, figs, flax seeds, oatmeal and oil until smooth. Pour into a glass.

Frozen Fruit Slurry

Tips

Freeze whole fresh berries when in season and freeze fruit pulp from the juicing process in 2-oz (60 g) paper cups and pop into the Vita-Mix to use in this easy slushy drink you eat with a spoon. See page 329 for how to freeze bananas.

If using a blender, allow fruit and juice to thaw until soft enough to process.

½ cup	freshly squeezed orange juice	125 mL
4	frozen banana chunks	1
4	frozen strawberries	4
¼ cup	frozen fruit juice concentrate	50 mL
1 cup	ice cubes	250 mL

1. In a Vita-Mix or blender, combine orange juice, banana, strawberries, frozen juice concentrate and ice cubes. Secure lid. Process starting at variable speed #1, increasing speed to #10 (or Medium) and to High. Process for 30 to 60 seconds or until ice is chopped (but no longer). Use the tamper while machine is processing. Serve immediately.

Green Energy

A "green" taste, not unpleasant but a definite departure from the traditional smoothie flavors.

Tip

Reduce amount of soymilk to ¼ cup (50 mL) if using frozen spinach.

2 cups	spinach, fresh or frozen	500 mL
½ cup	soymilk	125 mL
¼ cup	apricot milk or soymilk	50 mL
3 tbsp	chopped wheat or barley grass	45 mL
1 tbsp	pumpkin seeds	15 mL
1 tsp	ginkgo, optional	5 mL

1. Using a blender, process spinach, soymilk, apricot milk, grass, pumpkin seeds and ginkgo, if using, until smooth. Pour into a glass.

Liquid Gold

Serves 2 or 3

Tip

For a change, use half freshly squeezed orange juice and half apricot milk (see page 328) and eliminate the dried apricots.

1 cup	freshly squeezed orange juice	250 mL
3 tbsp	freshly squeezed lemon juice	45 mL
2	peaches, peeled and pitted	2
1	mango, pitted	1
4	dried apricots	4
1	banana	1
1	pineapple wedge	1

1. Using a blender, process orange juice, lemon juice, peaches, mango, apricots, banana and pineapple until smooth. Pour into glasses.

Mango Madness

Serves 1

Tip

If using a blender, omit the grapes because the skins are difficult to blend.

1 cup	red or green seedless grapes	250 mL
½ cup	freshly squeezed orange juice	125 mL
1	mango, pitted	1
1	banana	1
1	¼-inch (0.5 cm) piece gingerroot	1
½ tsp	ground cinnamon, optional	2 mL

1. Using a Vita-Mix, process grapes, orange juice, mango, banana, gingerroot and cinnamon if using until smooth. Pour into a glass.

Serves 1

Pineapple-C

1 cup	pineapple chunks	250 mL
½ cup	freshly squeezed orange juice	125 mL
1	lime, juiced	1
¼ cup	hulled strawberries, fresh or frozen	50 mL
2 tbsp	freshly squeezed lemon juice	25 mL

1. Using a blender, process pineapple, orange juice, lime juice, strawberries and lemon juice, until smooth. Pour into a glass.

Serves 1

Plum Lico

Tip

Over-consumption of licorice (more than 1 tsp/5 mL per 1 cup/250 mL) leads to low potassium levels and water retention. If potassium is a concern, add a banana to this or any smoothie recipe.

Caution: Do not use licorice if you have high blood pressure.

1 cup	pitted cherries	250 mL
¼ cup	pineapple juice	50 mL
¼ cup	natural yogurt	50 mL
2	plums, pitted	2
1	grapefruit, seeded and quartered	1
1 tsp	powdered licorice, optional (see Caution, left)	5 mL

1. Using a blender, process cherries, pineapple juice, yogurt, plums, grapefruit and licorice, if using, until smooth. Pour into a glass.

Serves 1 or 2

Prune Smoothie

A good morning starter.

1 cup	soymilk	250 mL
¼ cup	pitted prunes	50 mL
1	banana	1

1. Using a blender, process soymilk, prunes and banana until smooth. Pour into a glass.

The Regular

Orange juice, strawberries and banana is the usual combination for a smoothie.

Tip

For extra punch, add 1 tsp (5 mL) or the contents of 1 gel capsule evening primrose oil or ginkgo to this smoothie.

½ cup	freshly squeezed orange juice	125 mL
4	hulled strawberries, fresh or frozen	4
1	banana	1
2 tbsp	wheat germ	25 mL
1 tbsp	chopped almonds	15 mL

1. Using a blender, process orange juice, strawberries, banana, wheat germ and almonds until smooth. Pour into a glass.

Sea-Straw Smoothie

Use kelp or any other sea herb in this high-calcium drink.

½ cup	freshly squeezed grapefruit juice	125 mL
6	hulled fresh strawberries, fresh or frozen	6
3 tbsp	chopped dates	45 mL
1 tsp	crushed dulse	5 mL

1. Using a blender, process grapefruit juice, strawberries, dates and kelp until smooth. Pour into a glass.

Smart Smoothie

½ cup	freshly squeezed orange juice	125 mL
¼ cup	blueberries, fresh or frozen	50 mL
¼ cup	seedless grapes	50 mL
1 cup	spinach, fresh or frozen	250 mL
1 tbsp	flax seeds	15 mL
1 tsp	ginkgo, optional	5 mL
1 tsp	skullcap	5 mL
1 tsp	lecithin	5 mL

1. Using a blender, process orange juice, blueberries, grapes, spinach, flax seeds, ginkgo, if using, skullcap and lecithin until smooth. Pour into glasses.

Serves 1	**Spa Special**	
¼ cup	freshly squeezed grapefruit juice	50 mL
¼ cup	soft tofu	50 mL
¼ cup	blueberries, fresh or frozen	50 mL
3	strawberries, fresh or frozen	3
1 tsp	milk thistle	5 mL

1. Using a blender, process grapefruit juice, tofu, blueberries, strawberries and milk thistle until smooth. Pour into a glass.

Serves 1	**Taste of the Tropics**	
½ cup	freshly squeezed orange juice	125 mL
1	lime, juiced	1
2	papayas, seeded	2
2	pineapple wedges	2
1	banana	1
1	sprig fresh mint, optional	1

1. Using a blender, process orange juice, lime juice, papayas, pineapple, banana and mint if using until smooth. Pour into a glass.

Serves 2	**Tropi-Cocktail**	
½ cup	natural yogurt	125 mL
¼ cup	apricot milk or soymilk	50 mL
1	papaya, seeded	1
1	banana	1
1	mango, pitted	1
¼	cantaloupe, cut into chunks	¼

1. Using a blender, process yogurt, apricot milk, papaya, banana, mango and cantaloupe until smooth. Pour into glasses.

Tropics

Tip
For extra relief from heartburn, add 1 tbsp (15 mL) slippery elm powder.

½ cup	coconut milk	125 mL
1	papaya, seeded	1
1	banana	1
1	kiwifruit, cut in half	1
½ cup	pineapple chunks	125 mL

1. Using a blender, process coconut milk, papaya, banana, kiwifruit and pineapple until smooth. Pour into glasses.

Watermelon Smoothie

1 cup	watermelon chunks	250 mL
1 cup	blueberries, fresh or frozen	250 mL
⅓ cup	natural yogurt	75 mL
2 tbsp	pumpkin seeds, optional	25 mL

1. Using a blender, process watermelon, blueberries, yogurt and pumpkin seeds, if using, until smooth. Pour into glass.

Specialty Drinks

Cocktail Juices

Cocktails are relatively new inventions, arising early in the 18th century as brandy-sugar-champagne mixtures. Today, any short, cold drink based on alcohol or liqueur, stirred or shaken, served neat, on the rocks or blended with ice, is called a cocktail.

The following drinks have all the pizzazz of traditional cocktails with one exception: the fruit and vegetables *are* the drink, not just the decoration. They are the new-age cocktails, still using the 'cocktail' moniker because of their complex blend of ingredients, spices and herbs. With these drinks, cocktail hour starts at breakfast and continues all day!

Apple Spice Cocktail

Serves 2

4	apples	4
1	carrot	1
1	stalk celery	1
1	1-inch (2.5 cm) piece gingerroot	1
¼ tsp	ground cardamom	1 mL
¼ tsp	ground nutmeg	1 mL

1. Using a juicer, process apples, carrot, celery and gingerroot. Pour into a carafe or pitcher and whisk in cardamom and nutmeg. Pour into glasses.

Berry Fine Cocktail

Serves 2

2 cups	raspberries	500 mL
2	oranges	2
½ cup	whole cranberries, fresh or frozen	125 mL
½ cup	hulled fresh strawberries	125 mL

1. Using a juicer, process raspberries, oranges, cranberries and strawberries. Whisk and pour into glasses.

Breakfast Cocktail

A sweet blend of goodness
— even the pastel orange
color lends a cheerful note.

Tip

Save pulp for use in Curry
Sauce (see recipe,
page 294). Peel, core and
seed squash and apples if
planning to use pulp later.

¼	acorn or butternut squash, cut to fit tube	¼
2	apples	2
1	carrot	1
1	1-inch (2.5 cm) piece gingerroot	1
¼ cup	natural yogurt	50 mL

1. Using a juicer, process squash, apples, carrot and gingerroot. Whisk in yogurt. Pour into a carafe or large glasses.

Cabbage Cocktail

Serves 2 or 3

Tip

Caution: Parsley should be
avoided during pregnancy
and in cases of kidney
inflammation.

¼	head cabbage, cut to fit tube	¼
2	carrots	2
2	stalks celery	2
1	clove garlic	1
3	sprigs fresh parsley (see Caution, left)	3
2	parsnips	2
2	sprigs fresh dill	2
1	beet	1
1	apple	1
½ tsp	fennel seeds, optional	2 mL

1. Using a juicer, process cabbage, carrots, celery, garlic, parsley, parsnips, dill, beet and apple. Whisk and pour into a carafe or large glasses. Whisk in fennel seeds, if using.

Cajun Cocktail

Tip

If fresh chile pepper is not available, substitute 1 or 2 drops hot sauce or Jamaican jerk sauce. See page 189 for directions on juicing chile peppers. Plan to use pulp for Cajun Salsa (see recipe, page 294).

Caution: Parsley should be avoided during pregnancy and in cases of kidney inflammation.

3	tomatoes	3
3	sprigs fresh parsley (see Caution, left)	3
2	stalks celery, leaves intact	2
1	clove garlic	1
½	cucumber	½
½	lime	½
½ tsp	prepared horseradish	2 mL
Dash	Worcestershire sauce	Dash
1	fresh chile pepper	1

1. Using a juicer, process tomatoes, parsley, celery, garlic, cucumber and lime. Pour into a carafe or pitcher. Whisk in horseradish and Worcestershire sauce.

2. In a separate container, juice chile pepper (see note, left). Whisk chile juice into cocktail ½ tsp (2 mL) at a time, tasting before adding more. Pour into glasses.

Cauliflower Cocktail

Tip

Use any sea herb in place of the kelp.

½	head cauliflower, cut to fit tube	½
1	spear broccoli	1
3	tomatoes	3
2	carrots	2
2	stalks celery	2
1	apple	1
1 tsp	crumbled kelp	5 mL

1. Using a juicer, process cauliflower, broccoli, tomatoes, carrots, celery and apple. Whisk and pour into glasses. Sprinkle with kelp.

Citrus Cocktail

Tip
Use any melon for this recipe.

½	melon, cut to fit tube	½
1 cup	hulled fresh strawberries	250 mL
1	1-inch (2.5 cm) piece gingerroot	1
1	orange	1
1	grapefruit, cut to fit tube	1
¼ cup	natural yogurt	50 mL
1 tbsp	wheat germ or finely ground almonds	15 mL

1. Using a juicer, process melon, strawberries, gingerroot, orange and grapefruit. Pour into a carafe. Whisk in yogurt and wheat germ. Pour into glasses.

Melon Cocktail

½	melon, cut to fit tube	½
4	oranges	4
1	carrot	1
1	2-inch (5 cm) slice watermelon, cut to fit tube	1

1. Using a juicer, process melon, oranges, carrot and watermelon. Whisk and pour into glasses.

Melon Morning Cocktail

1	2-inch (5 cm) slice watermelon, cut to fit tube	1
¼	cantaloupe	¼
2	oranges	2
2	pineapple wedges	2

1. Using a juicer, process watermelon, cantaloupe, oranges and pineapple. Whisk and pour into glasses.

Orange Cream Cocktail

Tip

You can replace the orange sherbet with lemon or lime sherbet.

Add 1 oz (30 mL) orange liqueur for a dessert cocktail.

3	oranges	3
2	pineapple wedges	2
1	lime	1
1	lemon	1
½ cup	orange sherbet	125 mL
2	sprigs fresh mint	2

1. Using a juicer, process oranges, pineapple, lime and lemon. Whisk and pour into glasses. Divide sherbet in half and scoop into each glass. Garnish with mint sprig.

Peppery Tomato Cocktail

Caution: Parsley should be avoided during pregnancy and in cases of kidney inflammation.

3	tomatoes	3
1	handful watercress	1
1	green bell pepper, trimmed	1
1	clove garlic	1
3	sprigs fresh parsley (see Caution, left)	3
2	carrots	2
¼	fresh fennel bulb	¼
½ tsp	cayenne pepper	2 mL

1. Using a juicer, process tomatoes, watercress, green pepper, garlic, parsley, carrots and fennel. Whisk together with cayenne and pour into glasses.

Pineapple-Kiwi Cocktail

Serves 4

Tip

This is a very sweet drink, so you may wish to balance it by adding a lemon and up to 2 cups (500 mL) mineral water.

½	pineapple, cut into wedges	½
3	kiwifruits	3
2	oranges	2

1. Using a juicer, process pineapple, kiwifruits and oranges. Whisk and pour into glasses.

Tomato Juice Cocktail

Serves 4

The sodium in the celery lends its natural salt to this refreshing late-summer cooler.

Caution: Parsley should be avoided during pregnancy and in cases of kidney inflammation.

3	tomatoes	3
1	handful fresh basil	1
1	small zucchini	1
1	clove garlic	1
3	sprigs fresh parsley (see Caution, left)	3
1	stalk celery	1
1	beet	1
⅛ tsp	cayenne pepper, optional	0.5 mL

1. Using a juicer, process tomatoes, basil, zucchini, garlic, parsley, celery and beet. Whisk together with cayenne and pour into glasses.

Mulled Juices

Heating juices gives them a warming quality that's ideal when you are suffering from a cold or when it's cold outside. Keep in mind that heat-sensitive nutrients are lost when juices are heated. Our use of the term "mulled" takes liberty with the term, since it usually applies only to red wine or cider.

Use preheated mugs or glasses to keep the mulled juices warm once served. To preheat mugs, pour boiling water into them and let stand. Drain and fill with hot mulled juice.

Blazing Bullshot

Serves 4

Tip
Use any combination of vegetables for the vegetable juice.

3 cups	beef bouillon or vegetable stock	750 mL
1	fresh chile pepper	1
1 cup	tomato or mixed vegetable juice	250 mL
¼ cup	freshly squeezed lemon juice	50 mL
Splash	Worcestershire sauce	Splash
1 tsp	garam masala, optional	5 mL
4	stalks celery, leaves intact, optional	4

1. In a saucepan over medium heat, combine bouillon and chile pepper. Heat until just simmering. Cover, reduce heat and simmer for 10 minutes.

2. Remove from heat and whisk in tomato juice, lemon juice, Worcestershire sauce and garam masala, if using. Remove chile pepper and pour hot mixture into glasses. Cut pepper lengthwise into quarters and use as garnish with celery stalks, if desired.

Hot Spiced Apples

Serves 2

2 cups	apple juice or water	500 mL
3	apples, peeled, cored and sliced	3
2	plums, pitted and coarsely chopped	2
¼ cup	chopped raisins or dates	50 mL
¼ cup	rolled oats	50 mL
1 tbsp	finely chopped candied ginger	15 mL
¼ tsp	ground cinnamon	1 mL
¼ tsp	ground nutmeg	1 mL

1. In a saucepan over high heat, bring apple juice to a boil. Stir in apples, plums, raisins, oats and ginger. Reduce heat to medium and simmer for 10 minutes or until fruit is soft.

2. Remove from heat, stir in cinnamon and nutmeg and let cool slightly. Pour into a blender and blend at low speed until smooth. Pour into mugs and thin with boiling water if too thick.

Hot Spiced Pear Nectar

Serves 2 or 3

Tip
Use poblano or New Mexican chiles if available, or use a cayenne pepper and discard after heating the drink.

6	pears	6
2	apples	2
1	lemon	1
½	fresh chile pepper	½
2 tbsp	maple syrup or molasses	25 mL
3	allspice berries	3
1	2-inch (5 cm) cinnamon stick	1

1. Using a juicer, process pears, apples, lemon and chile. Transfer juice to a saucepan. Over medium heat, stir in maple syrup, allspice berries and cinnamon. Bring to just under a boil. Cover, reduce heat and simmer for 5 minutes. Strain into heated mugs.

Serves 4	**Mulled Cranberry**	

2 cups	fresh cranberry juice	500 mL
1 cup	apple juice	250 mL
1 cup	beet juice	250 mL
½ cup	filtered water	125 mL
1 tbsp	fresh stevia leaves or 1 tsp (5 mL) powdered stevia	15 mL
3	whole cloves	3
3	allspice berries	3
1	2-inch (5 cm) cinnamon stick	1

1. In a saucepan over medium heat, combine cranberry juice, apple juice, beet juice, water, stevia, cloves, allspice berries and cinnamon. Over high heat, bring to just under a boil. Cover, reduce heat and simmer for 5 minutes. Strain into hot mugs.

Serves 4	**Pineapple Cranberry Sizzler**	

Tip

For a deeper pineapple taste, add 2 or 3 bruised pineapple sage leaves (*Salvia elegans*), if available, to the pot while it is simmering.

Caution: Do not use licorice if you have high blood pressure.

2 cups	pineapple juice	500 mL
1 cup	fresh cranberry juice	250 mL
½ cup	apple cider or apple juice	125 mL
1	2-inch (5 cm) piece licorice (see Caution, left)	1
5	whole coriander seeds	5
2 tbsp	liquid honey	25 mL
1 tsp	fenugreek seeds	5 mL

1. In a saucepan over medium heat, combine pineapple juice, cranberry juice, apple cider, licorice, coriander, honey and fenugreek. Bring to just under a boil. Cover, reduce heat and simmer for 5 minutes. Strain into hot mugs.

Tree-Trimming Tomato Warmer

4	apples	4
1	lemon	1
1 tbsp	curry powder	15 mL
1 tsp	ground cinnamon	5 mL
1 tsp	ground cumin	5 mL
4 cups	tomato juice	1 L
4	stalks celery	4

1. Using a juicer, process apples and lemon.

2. In a saucepan combine curry, cinnamon and cumin. Toast spices over low heat, stirring constantly, for 2 minutes or until spices are aromatic. Be careful not to let the spices burn. Add apple-lemon juice and tomato juice. Increase heat and bring to a light boil, stirring.

3. Remove from heat, pour into heated mugs and garnish with celery stalks.

Juice Punches

The *Dictionary of Gastronomy* suggests that the word "punch" comes from the Hindi word panch, meaning five, because five ingredients — arrack, lime, sugar, spices and water — were used. In its "Glossary of Culinary Terms," *Mrs. Beeton's Household Management* gives the following definition: "Punch á la Romaine (Fr). A kind of soft white ice, made from lemon-juice, white of egg, sugar, and rum. It is served in goblets and acts as a digestive." And *The New Larousse Gastronomique* explains it thus: "Punch: A drink said to have originated among English sailors, and which, about 1552, consisted of a simple mixture of cane spirit and sugar, heated."

Whatever its origins, punch has come to be known as a mixture of fruit juices served over ice with or without alcohol. Some punches require a simple syrup (a mixture of sugar and water, boiled to thicken it) especially if lemons are a major ingredient. Most of the recipes here rely on the natural sugars in the fruit as sweeteners.

Apple-Orange Punch

Serves 6

Make this punch in the fall, when apple cider is fresh and widely available. Use some of the orange and lime peel as garnish.

Tip

You can use frozen orange, lemon or lime sherbet in place of the homemade Orange-Melon Sherbet.

4	beets	4
6	apples	6
3	oranges	3
1	lime	1
1	1-inch (2.5 cm) piece gingerroot	1
4 cups	fresh apple cider	1 L
6	scoops frozen Orange-Melon Sherbet (see recipe, page 354)	6

1. Using a juicer, process beets, apples, oranges, lime and gingerroot. Whisk together with cider and chill. *To serve:* Pour into a punch bowl and float sherbet on top.

Berry Combo

Serves 6

Perfect for spring gatherings, this punch has a vibrant pink color that brightens the buffet table. If available, float sweet cicely flowers or rose petals on top.

Native Cranberries

Chief Pakimintzen of the Delaware Indians offered cranberries as a gesture of peace. Over time, "pakimintzen" came to be the Delawares' word for "cranberry eater."

The Pequot Indians of Cape Cod and the Leni-Lenape tribes of New Jersey called the cranberry *ibimi*, meaning "bitter berry."

4 cups	water	1 L
2 cups	blackberries or raspberries, fresh or frozen	500 mL
1½ cups	coarsely chopped rhubarb	375 mL
1 cup	cranberries, chopped	250 mL
2 tbsp	granulated sugar (or to taste)	25 mL
1 tsp	powdered stevia	5 mL
½	pineapple, cut into wedges	½
4	beets	4
1	lemon	1
¼ cup	chopped fresh sweet cicely	50 mL
2 tbsp	finely grated gingerroot	25 mL
	Ice, optional	

1. In a saucepan over medium-high heat, bring water, blackberries, rhubarb, cranberries, sugar and stevia to a boil. Reduce heat and simmer, stirring occasionally, for 15 minutes. Strain through a sieve, pressing on solids to extract all liquid. Discard solids. Chill.

2. *To serve:* Using a juicer, process pineapple, beets and lemon. Whisk and add to punch bowl, with chilled rhubarb-berry juice. Whisk in sweet cicely and gingerroot and serve over ice, if desired.

Serves 6	# Fruit Punch	
4	oranges	4
1	pineapple, cut into wedges	1
1	lemon	1
1 cup	soft tofu	250 mL
3	bananas	3
2 cups	hulled fresh strawberries	500 mL
1 cup	raspberries	250 mL
3 cups	mineral water	750 mL
2 cups	ice cubes	500 mL

1. Using a juicer, process oranges, pineapple and lemon. Whisk and pour into a large glass jar with a lid. Chill until ready to serve.

2. Just before serving, divide each of tofu, bananas, strawberries and raspberries into 2 equal portions. Measure 2 cups (500 mL) of chilled orange-pineapple juice and set aside. Pour remaining juice into punch bowl.

3. Using a blender, process 1 cup (250 mL) of reserved orange-pineapple juice with one portion of tofu, bananas, strawberries and raspberries. Add to punch bowl. Process remaining 1 cup (250 mL) of juice, tofu and fruit. Add to punch bowl. Whisk until combined. Stir in mineral water, add ice and serve immediately.

Serves 4	**Gardener's Lemonade**	
1 cup	water	250 mL
⅓ cup	granulated sugar	75 mL
6	lemons	6
3 cups	hot water	750 mL
1 tbsp	chopped fresh lemon balm	15 mL
1 tbsp	chopped fresh mint	15 mL
1 tbsp	chopped fresh bergamot, optional	15 mL
3	fresh linden flowers, optional	3
	Extra tea herbs (see page 324), optional	

1. In a small saucepan over medium heat, combine 1 cup (250 mL) water and sugar. Heat, stirring constantly, until sugar has completely dissolved. Bring to a boil and cook, without stirring, for 1 minute or until the syrup is clear. Set aside to cool.

2. Peel the rind of 2 lemons in one continuous strip. Set strips aside. Cut all 6 lemons in half.

3. Using a citrus press or cone hand juicer, juice lemons and strain into a large pitcher. Stir in cooled syrup, hot water, lemon balm, mint, bergamot, if using, linden flowers, if using, and reserved lemon rind strips. Set in sun or leave on kitchen counter to steep for 1 hour or more. Remove herbs and lemon peel and chill or serve over ice. Garnish with fresh leaves of lemon balm, bergamot or linden flowers and mint sprigs, if desired.

Tea Herbs

The following herbs make excellent herbal teas. Use them alone or in combination.

Anise hyssop (*Agastache foeniclum*, see Hyssop, page 137). Scented of anise and mint. Best if blended with other tea herbs.

Bergamot (*Mondara*). The whole plant smells pleasantly of orange and the taste is slightly citrus.

German chamomile (*Matricaria*, see page 133). Lends a flowery, apple-like taste.

Lavender (*Lavendula*, see page 137). A flowery, distinct flavor. Best blended with other tea herbs.

Lemon balm (*Melissa officianalis*, see page 138). The sweet, strong lemon smell and taste makes it a popular tea herb, alone or in blends.

Lemon verbena (*Aloysia triphylla*, see page 138). Rich lemon taste.

Linden flower (*Tilia cordata*, see page 139). A mild-flavored, gently calming herb.

Mint (*Mentha*, see pages 143 and 147). Many varieties available including ginger, lime and apple.

Roses (*Rosa*, see page 145). Use petals and hip. Do not use flower shop roses.

Scented geraniums (*Pelagonium*). Use the highly aromatic leaves from more than 150 different *Pelagoniums*.

Sweet cicely (*Myrrhis odoratat*). A very sweet, anise-flavored leaf that is commonly used in tea blends.

Thyme (*Thymus*, see page 149). Many different flavors including nutmeg, orange and lemon.

Serves 6

Lavender Punch

Serves 6

Roman Punch No. 1

"Grate the yellow rind of four lemons and two oranges upon two pounds of sugar. Squeeze the juice of the lemons and oranges; cover it and let it stand until next day. Strain it through a sieve, mix with the sugar; add a bottle of champagne and the whites of eight eggs beaten to a stiff froth. It may be frozen or not, as desired. For winter use snow instead of ice." *Serves 8*

From the *White House Cookbook* by Hugo Zieman and Mrs. F.L. Gilette, Toronto: The Copp Clark Co. Limited, 1887.

2 cups	water	500 ml
1	2-inch (5 cm) stick cinnamon	1
2	star anise pods and seeds	2
3	allspice berries	3
2	whole cloves	2
1	stick astragalus root, optional	1
3 tbsp	fresh lavender flower buds or 1 tbsp (15 mL) dried	45 mL
4	oranges	4
3	lemons	3
3 cups	red grapes	750 mL
3 cups	mineral water	750 mL
	Honey, to taste, optional	

1. In a medium saucepan over medium heat, combine water, cinnamon, star anise, allspice, cloves and astragalus, if using. Bring to a light boil over high heat. Cover, reduce heat and simmer gently for 5 minutes. Remove from heat and stir in lavender flowers. Cover and let stand for 10 minutes. Strain into a covered jar or container, discard solids. Chill until ready to serve.

2. *To serve:* Using a juicer, process oranges, lemons and grapes. Whisk and add to a punch bowl. Stir in chilled lavender water and mineral water. Serve over ice, and sweeten to taste with honey, if desired.

Summer Flower Nectar

Serves 6

¼ cup	fresh calendula petals	50 mL
¼ cup	chopped fresh lemon balm	50 mL
3 tbsp	fresh rose petals	45 mL
1 tbsp	fresh lavender flowers	15 mL
1 tbsp	grated orange zest	15 mL
1 tsp	chopped gingerroot	5 mL
4 cups	boiling water	1 L
5 tbsp	liquid honey	75 mL
3	peaches, pitted	3
3	apricots, pitted	3
3	nectarines, pitted	3
2	oranges	2
2	2-inch (5 cm) slices watermelon, cut to fit tube	2
3 cups	mineral water	750 mL
3	whole roses, optional	3
3	whole calendula flowers, optional	3

1. Place calendula, lemon balm, rose petals, lavender, orange zest and gingerroot in a teapot. Pour in boiling water and steep for 5 minutes. Strain tea into a pitcher or container, discard solids. Add honey and stir until dissolved. Chill until ready to serve.

2. *To serve:* Using a juicer, process peaches, apricots, nectarines, oranges and watermelon. Whisk and pour into a punch bowl. Stir in mineral water and chilled tea. Garnish with whole flowers, if desired, and serve over ice.

Milk Substitutes

Milk allergies, or a separate condition called lactose intolerance (see page 364), cause a significant number of people to experience painful symptoms that make it necessary to eliminate milk and dairy products from their diet. In addition to milk, cream and butter, problematic foods can include processed products like cereals, baking mixes and baked goods that contain milk, milk solids, cheese (or cheese flavoring), whey, curds, and even margarine.

Fermented dairy foods, such as natural yogurt, contain live bacteria that help digest lactose and may not irritate allergies. Soymilk and nut milks are the best substitutes for dairy milk.

Soymilk

Soymilk (and tofu) is widely available in supermarkets and alternative/health stores, but can easily be made at home (see *Rodale's* reference, Bibliography, page 367). Soymilk and tofu should be used with some caution, however, since there is growing concern over the use of genetically modified and chemically sprayed soybeans for most commercial soy products.

Nut milk

Nuts make a pleasant, thick liquid that can be used in some sauces and desserts. Use unsalted, organic almonds, pecans, cashews or walnuts (any nut or seed will work) with the skins still on. Nuts contribute protein, vitamin E and fiber to the diet, but should be taken in small amounts since they have a high fat content (although mostly unsaturated and with essential fatty acids). Nut milks make a thicker shake or smoothie than soymilk.

As you might expect, anyone with an allergy to nuts cannot use nut milks. However, for healthy teens with high-energy demands, nut milks can be used regularly in any of the milk shake recipes in this section.

To make nut milk: Combine the nuts with other ingredients as listed below in a clean jar with a lid. Note that boiled water should not be boiling when added. Shake well, cool, blend using a blender or food processor, and use immediately. Or return to the jar and place in refrigerator for up to 2 or 3 days.

Almond: 1 cup (250 mL) finely chopped almonds, 1 tbsp (15 mL) finely chopped dates, 1 tbsp (15 mL) flax seeds, 1-inch (2.5 cm) piece vanilla bean, 2 cups (500 mL) just-boiled water

Cashew: 1 cup (250 mL) finely chopped cashews, 1 tbsp (15 mL) finely chopped dried dulse, 1 tbsp (15 mL) finely chopped raisins, 1-inch (2.5 cm) piece vanilla bean, 2 cups (500 mL) just-boiled water

Pecan: 1 cup (250 mL) finely chopped pecans, 1 tbsp (15 mL) finely chopped raisins, 1 tbsp (15 mL) flax seeds, 1-inch (2.5 cm) piece vanilla bean, 2 cups (500 mL) just-boiled water

Walnut: 1 cup (250 mL) finely chopped walnuts, 1 tbsp (15 mL) finely chopped dates, 1 tbsp (15 mL) flax seeds, 1-inch (2.5 cm) piece vanilla bean, 2 cups (500 mL) just-boiled water

Fruit milk

Coconut/carob milk. Use fresh coconut and shred it, freezing the remainder if necessary. If fresh coconut is unavailable, use the unsweetened dried type available at some alternative/health stores. Coconut is naturally sweet and when blended with carob, it is even sweeter. Use coconut milk to replace dairy and sugar in shakes, puddings and other desserts.

To make coconut milk: In a blender or food processor, combine ½ cup (125 mL) shredded fresh coconut (or ⅓ cup/75 mL shredded dried), 3 tbsp (45 mL) powdered carob (optional), 1-inch (2.5 cm) piece vanilla bean and ½ cup (125 mL) just-boiled water. Cool and process until smooth. Add more water if a thinner product is desired. Use immediately or store in refrigerator up to 1 week.

Date milk. Date sugar is commonly used in commercial products as a sweetener. Using date milk is like using sugar (although it provides some fiber and a few nutrients), so use it sparingly. Make the milk with pitted dates.

To make date milk: In a blender or food processor, combine ¼ cup (50 mL) chopped dates, 1-inch (2.5 cm) piece vanilla bean and ½ cup (125 mL) just-boiled water. Cool and process until smooth. Use immediately or store in refrigerator for up to 1 week.

Fig milk. Figs have antibacterial, cancer-fighting properties and make a sweet milk that can be used with yogurt or tofu in shakes and other recipes. Use fresh figs if available. Dried figs are tough and should be coarsely chopped by hand before processing in the blender or food processor.

To make fig milk: In a blender or food processor, combine ¼ cup (50 mL) chopped figs, 1-inch (2.5 cm) piece vanilla bean and ½ cup (125 mL) just-boiled water. Cool and process until smooth. Use immediately or store in refrigerator for up to 1 week.

Apricot milk. Sweet, yet slightly tart, this fruit milk has a unique taste. Use it in any of the fruit shakes or smoothies in this book. Look for organic apricots without sulphur added in the drying process.

To make apricot milk: In a blender or food processor, combine ¼ cup (50 mL) chopped dried apricots, 1-inch (2.5 cm) piece vanilla bean and ½ cup (125 mL) just-boiled water. Cool and process until smooth. Use immediately or store in refrigerator for up to 1 week.

Serves 1		

Apple Pie

1 cup	soymilk or apricot milk	250 mL
2	apples, peeled, cored and quartered	2
2 tbsp	spelt flakes	25 mL
¼ tsp	ground cinnamon	1 mL
⅛ tsp	ground nutmeg	0.5 mL

1. In a blender, process soymilk, apples, spelt, cinnamon and nutmeg until smooth. Pour into a glass.

Serves 1		

Avocado Shake

1 cup	soymilk or nut milk	250 mL
1	avocado, pitted	1
1	grapefruit, quartered	1
½	lemon, juiced	½
1 tbsp	molasses	15 mL

1. In a blender, process soymilk, avocado, grapefruit, lemon juice and molasses until smooth. Pour into a glass.

Serves 1		

Banana Frappé

Tip

To freeze bananas: Choose fully yellow bananas with no bruises or brown spots. Peel and cut each into four chunks and arrange on a baking sheet. Freeze in the coldest part of the freezer for 30 minutes. Place the chunks in one large or several individual freezer bags. Seal and store the chunks in the freezer for four to six months. Four frozen chunks equal one whole fresh banana.

1 cup	almond milk or soymilk	250 mL
½ cup	soft tofu	125 mL
4	frozen banana chunks	4
1 tbsp	powdered carob	15 mL
¼ tsp	almond extract, optional	1 mL
Pinch	ground nutmeg	Pinch

1. In a blender, process almond milk, tofu, banana, carob and almond extract if using, until smooth. Pour into a glass and garnish with nutmeg.

Berry Frappé

Serves 1 or 2

Tip

Any berries — blueberries, raspberries, gooseberries, strawberries, blackberries or even currants — work well in this shake.

1 cup	soymilk or nut milk	250 mL
½ cup	soft tofu	125 mL
½ cup	berries, fresh or frozen	125 mL
½	lemon, juiced	½

1. In a blender, process soymilk, tofu, berries and lemon juice until smooth. Pour into 1 large or 2 smaller glasses.

Beta Whiz

Serves 1 or 2

This drink is thick with the distinctive taste of cantaloupe. For a thinner consistency, increase either the orange or carrot juice by ¼ cup (50 mL) or to taste.

½ cup	apricot milk or soymilk	125 mL
¼ cup	carrot juice	50 mL
¼	cantaloupe, cut into chunks	¼
1 tbsp	chopped almonds	15 mL
1 tbsp	buckwheat flakes	15 mL

1. In a blender, process apricot milk, carrot juice, cantaloupe, almonds and buckwheat until smooth. Pour into 1 large or 2 smaller glasses.

Carob-Orange Shake

Serves 1

1 cup	freshly squeezed orange juice	250 mL
½ cup	yogurt	125 mL
2 tbsp	powdered carob	25 mL
1 tsp	grated orange peel, optional	5 mL

1. In a blender, process orange juice, yogurt, carob and orange peel if using until smooth. Pour into a glass.

Chocolate Shake

1 cup	pecan milk or soymilk	250 mL
½ cup	soft tofu	125 mL
4	frozen banana chunks	4
2 tbsp	powdered carob	25 mL

1. In a blender, process pecan milk, tofu, banana and carob until smooth. Pour into 1 large or 2 smaller glasses.

Date and Nut Shake

Tip

If not using date milk, add 1 tbsp (15 mL) chopped dates. Thicken with oats or banana if desired.

1 cup	date milk or soymilk	250 mL
½ cup	soft tofu	125 mL
2	pears, peeled and cored	2
1 tbsp	chopped almonds	15 mL

1. In a blender, process date milk, tofu, pears and almonds until smooth. Pour into 1 large or 2 smaller glasses.

Hot Carob

This makes a great nightcap.

2 cups	date or fig milk or soymilk	500 mL
3 tbsp	powdered carob	45 mL
½ tsp	ground cinnamon	5 mL

1. In a saucepan over medium-low heat, scald milk (heat until little bubbles form around the edge of the pan). Whisk in carob and cinnamon and simmer gently until blended. Serve immediately in warmed mugs.

Hot Nut Chai

Use any nut milk for this recipe.

Tip
Add 1 tbsp (15 mL) powdered carob if desired.

2 cups	nut milk	500 mL
2 tsp	Indian Chai Blend (see recipe, page 336)	10 mL

1. In a saucepan over medium-low heat, scald milk (heat until little bubbles form around the edge of the pan). Whisk in Indian Chai Blend and simmer gently for about 10 minutes. Strain into hot mugs and serve immediately.

Strawberry Shake

1½ cups	hulled strawberries, fresh or frozen	375 mL
½ cup	orange or pomegranate juice	125 mL
½ cup	soft tofu	125 mL
½ tsp	vanilla extract	2 mL

1. In a blender, process strawberries, orange juice, tofu and vanilla until smooth. Pour into a glass.

Tropical Shake

1 cup	coconut or fruit milk or soymilk	250 mL
1 cup	chopped pineapple	250 mL
½ cup	soft tofu	125 mL
1	mango, pitted	1
1	star fruit	
¼ tsp	powdered star anise	1 mL

1. In a blender, process coconut milk, pineapple, tofu, mango, star fruit and star anise until smooth. Pour into glasses.

Coffee Substitutes

There is no herb that imitates the taste of coffee or that has the caffeine found in coffee. The recipes that follow have a fragrant taste quite unique and delicious on their own, and no milk is needed, although you might try a drop or two of nut milk (see pages 327–28) in them. When taken on a regular basis in place of coffee, they will act as tonics and provide significant healing benefits.

To harvest roots you have grown or those gathered from the wild, wait until after the tops of the plants have died back in the fall (be sure to note the location of the plants first), but before the ground is frozen, to dig up the roots.

To roast fresh roots: Preheat oven to 300°F (150°C). Scrub roots well and chop to a uniform medium size (about the size of dried peas). Spread on an ungreased baking sheet and bake in preheated oven, stirring after 20 minutes, for 45 minutes or until golden. Reduce oven temperature to 200°F (100°C); bake for 1 hour or until thoroughly dry, stirring every 20 minutes. Cool before blending or storing.

To roast dried roots: Most alternative/health stores sell the herb roots listed below in chopped, dried form. Roasting gives a richer taste to the blend but is strictly optional. Spread dried roots on an ungreased baking sheet and roast at 300°F (150°C), stirring once, for 20 minutes or until lightly browned.

To brew root coffee: Just before using, grind small amounts at a time with a mortar and pestle, coffee grinder or mini food processor. Use 1 tbsp (15 mL) ground roots for every 1 cup (250 mL) of water. Brew in a coffee maker as you would regular coffee. Use stevia or honey to sweeten if desired.

Use any or all of the roots listed below to blend your own rich-tasting coffee substitute. All of the roots are available in dried form in alternative/health stores and most may be wildcrafted.

Astragalus root (*Astragalus membranacus,* see page 124). Either whole root or cut or powdered, astragalus can be used in coffee substitute blends.
Burdock root (*Arctium lappa,* see page 126). A healing root which lends a nutty taste to roasted herb root blends.
Chicory root (*Cichorium intybus*). The most common coffee substitute and closest in taste. However, unlike coffee, chicory does not have caffeine and is mildly liver-supportive. The large roots can be used alone but are best blended with other roasted herb roots, nuts, grains, seeds or spices.
Dandelion root (*Taraxacum officinalis,* see page 130). A common root, fairly mild in taste, and best blended with other roasted herb roots or spices.
Echinacea root (*Echinacea angustifolia* or *E. purpurea,* see page 131). Available in dried, whole or cut form (or fresh from growers in the fall). It is a good root to add to winter coffee blends, and helps stimulate the immune system.
Ginseng root (*Panax quinquefolius,* see page 134). An excellent coffee substitute that restores both physical and mental functions. If taken regularly, it improves resistance to disease and stress. And, unlike coffee, it is not addictive.

Licorice (*Glycyrrhiza glabra*, see page 139). Adds a sweet, slightly anise taste to all root blends, and helps to activate healing properties in other herbs. Do not use in cases of high blood pressure.

Marshmallow root (*Althaea officinalis*, see page 139). A mild-tasting root that offers medicinal benefits.

Yellow dock root (*Rumex crispus*, see page 151). A cleansing herb with strong laxative properties, it can be blended with other roots and used for specific remedies, but is not a general coffee substitute.

Coffee

When coffee (*Coffea arabica*) was introduced to Europeans in the 1600s, it was dispensed by physicians as a drug. But the stimulating beverage soon became popular and, in 1652, the first coffee shop had opened in London.

Now known to boost mental proficiency, act as a mild antidepressant, stimulate physical ability and stamina, mitigate asthma attacks, protect teeth from cavities and perhaps help deflect cancer, coffee taken in moderate amounts (no more than 2 cups/500 mL per day) may actually be useful in specific circumstances.

But caffeine has many less desirable side effects: it directly stimulates the heart and raises blood pressure; it appears to promote heart disease in people at risk, as well as those who consume 5 cups (1.25 L) or more per day. Coffee may be a factor in fibrocystic breast disease. It depletes the body of B vitamins, magnesium, zinc and calcium. Excess coffee is associated with anxiety and depression. Caffeine increases the effects of stress and aggravates symptoms of anxiety, tension, irritability and hypoglycemia. Coffee interferes with hormonal balance, disturbing the normal menstrual cycle. Coffee can trigger headaches in some people, even if taken moderately, and often when withdrawn. Coffee can seriously impair the ability to get to sleep as well as the quality of sleep. Coffee is contraindicated in people prone to ulcers, chronic diarrhea, kidney stones and gout, anxiety, tension, depression, hypoglycemia, menstrual disturbances, breast lumps, high blood pressure, arthritis, during pregnancy, and those who suffer panic attacks.

All in all, herbalists believe that the benefits do not outweigh the negative effects of coffee consumption. They recommend juices and coffee substitutes as a healthier, more nutritious alternative.

Anxiety Antidote

This is a very mild-tasting blend. For a richer taste, add 1 tsp (5 mL) carob for each cup to be brewed.

Tip

A few drops of valerian tincture can be added to a cup of this soothing drink if taken before bedtime. Note, however, that some people experience adverse effects from valerian.

- Preheat oven to 300°F (150°C)
- Large baking sheet, ungreased

1 cup	chopped chicory root	250 mL
1 cup	chopped marshmallow root	250 mL
½ cup	finely chopped almonds	125 mL
½ cup	rolled oats	125 mL
1 tbsp	ground ginseng	15 mL
1 tsp	ground cloves	5 mL
½ tsp	ground allspice, optional	2 mL
¼ tsp	ground nutmeg	1 mL

1. Spread chicory roots, marshmallow roots, almonds and oat flakes on baking sheet. Roast in preheated oven, stirring once, for 20 minutes or until lightly browned. Set aside to cool.

2. In a bowl combine roasted mixture with ginseng, cloves, allspice, if using, and nutmeg. Transfer to an airtight jar to store.

3. Grind a small amount and use 1 tbsp (15 mL) for every 1 cup (250 mL) water.

Easy Root Coffee

Using the powdered form of roots makes them easy to blend — an "instant" coffee substitute. To make 1 cup (250 mL) Easy Root Coffee, measure 1 tbsp (15 mL) root blend into a mug and pour boiling water over. Stir and allow solids to settle on the bottom (or strain) before drinking.

½ cup	powdered chicory root	125 mL
¼ cup	powdered dandelion root	50 mL
¼ cup	powdered burdock root	50 mL
¼ cup	powdered carob	50 mL
1 tbsp	ground ginseng	15 mL

1. In a mixing bowl, combine chicory, dandelion, burdock, carob and ginseng. Transfer to an airtight jar to store.

**Makes about
⅓ cup (75 mL)
blend**

For a sweet sip of the East, try this spice blend. If you prefer it sweeter than it already is, use any of the fruit milks when making the chai, or add powdered stevia (½ tsp/2 mL to each ⅓ cup/75 mL of the blend).

Indian Chai Blend

2 tbsp	fennel seeds	25 mL
1 tbsp	cardamom seeds	15 mL
1 tbsp	coriander seeds	15 mL
1 tbsp	fenugreek seeds	15 mL
2	whole cloves	2
2	star anise pods with seeds	2
1	2-inch (5 cm) cinnamon stick, crushed or broken into pieces	1

1. In a small saucepan over medium-high heat, combine fennel, cardamom, coriander, fenugreek, cloves, star anise and cinnamon pieces. Toast for 40 seconds or until seeds begin to sizzle and pop. Set aside to cool.

2. Using a mortar and pestle, coffee grinder or small food processor, grind toasted mixture. Transfer to a clean jar with a lid, label and store in a cool dry place. Use 1 tsp (5 mL) blend per 1 cup (250 mL) water.

Indian Chai Tea

Serves 1

A warming drink to take at bedtime, this tea can be prepared with any of the strained nut or fruit milks (see pages 327–28). If using fruit milk, combine with an equal amount of regular or soymilk to make up 1 cup (250 mL). For more sweetness, increase the proportion of fruit milk.

2 tsp	Indian Chai Blend (see recipe, page 336)	10 mL
¼ cup	water	50 mL
1 cup	skim milk or soymilk or almond milk	250 mL
1	bag green tea or 1 tsp (5 mL) loose green tea leaves	1
Pinch	freshly grated nutmeg	Pinch

1. In a small saucepan over medium heat, combine Indian Chai Blend, water and milk. Bring to a boil, reduce heat and gently simmer for 10 minutes. Turn off heat and add green tea bag or stir in leaves. Cover and leave saucepan on burner. Steep for 3 to 5 minutes and strain into a cup. Sprinkle with grated nutmeg and serve immediately.

Indian chai

Indian chai — tea boiled with spices and milk — is starting to bubble up in tony areas of cities and airport kiosks all over North America. Little has been written about this now trendy beverage, although one book describes it as follows:

[In India...] generally the tea is boiled in an open pot together with a few green (unbleached) cardamom seeds, a pinch of fennel, and sugar. Milk is added to the boiling liquid — about one part milk to four parts water. This sweet, fragrant brew is served all over India, in cups and glasses in the cities and towns, and sometimes in crude earthenware "glasses" — which look like miniature flower pots — in remoter villages. Every station of the Indian railway has at least one tea stand, and at any hour of the day or night, as a train lumbers in, the air is filled with cries of the tea vendors — "chay-ya! chay-ya!"

The Book of Coffee and Tea: A Guide to the Appreciation of Fine Coffees, Teas, and Herbal Beverages. Joel, David and Karl Schapira. New York: St. Martin's Press, 1975.

Root Coffee Blend

Makes 2½ cups
(625 mL) root
blend

Tip

See page 333 for tips on
harvesting your own fresh
roots.

Caution: Do not use licorice
if you have high blood
pressure.

- Preheat oven to 300°F (150°C)
- Large rimmed baking sheet, ungreased

6 to 8	chopped fresh dandelion roots	6 to 8
4 to 6	chopped fresh burdock roots	4 to 6
3 to 4	chopped fresh chicory roots	3 to 4
1	2-inch (5 cm) piece cinnamon stick	1
¼ cup	chopped fresh or dried licorice (see Caution, left)	50 mL
1 tbsp	ground ginseng	15 mL

1. Spread dandelion, burdock and chicory roots on baking sheet. Bake in preheated oven, stirring after 20 minutes, for 45 minutes or until golden. Reduce oven temperature to 200°F (100°C) and roast for 45 minutes to 1 hour or until thoroughly dry, stirring every 20 minutes. Set aside to cool.

2. Meanwhile, using a mortar and pestle, food processor or blender, crush cinnamon stick.

3. In a bowl combine roasted roots, crushed cinnamon, licorice and ginseng. Transfer to an airtight jar to store. Roots must be thoroughly dried before storing.

4. Grind a small amount and use 1 tbsp (15 mL) for every 1 cup (250 mL) water.

Coffee blend

Seed Power Coffee

Roasted or unroasted, this blend makes a delicate drink. Chopped fresh roots are best, but you may use dried roots in this recipe.

• Preheat oven to 300°F (150°C)
• Large rimmed baking sheet, ungreased

1 part	pumpkin seeds	1 part
1 part	sunflower seeds	1 part
½ part	sesame seeds	½ part
1 part	chopped chicory root	1 part
½ part	ground ginkgo	½ part
¼ part	powdered carob	¼ part

1. For an unroasted blend, proceed with step 2. Otherwise, spread pumpkin seeds, sunflower seeds, sesame seeds and chicory on baking sheet. Roast in preheated oven, stirring once, for 20 minutes or until lightly browned. Set aside to cool.

2. In a medium bowl, combine seeds, chicory, ginkgo and carob. Stir well to mix. Transfer to a clean jar with lid.

3. Grind a small amount and use 1 tbsp (15 mL) for every 1 cup (250 mL) water.

Coffee blend

Winter Coffee

1 part	chopped chicory root	1 part
1 part	chopped burdock root	1 part
¾ part	powdered carob	¾ part
½ part	chopped echinacea root	½ part
¼ part	chopped astragalus root	¼ part
¼ part	chopped orange peel	¼ part

1. In a medium bowl, combine chicory root, burdock root, carob, echinacea, astragalus and orange peel. Stir well to mix. Transfer to a clean jar with lid.

2. Grind a small amount and use 1 tbsp (15 mL) for every 1 cup (250 mL) water.

Drying citrus peel

Herb tea and root coffee blends can be enriched with the use of dried citrus peel. Use organic fruit only — much of the chemicals from pesticides are concentrated in the peel. To dry, remove peel, coarsely chop and place on a drying rack or in a sieve so that air can circulate freely. Keep in a warm dark place for at least a week. When absolutely dry, transfer to a glass jar and store in a cool, dark, dry place.

Frozen Treats

Frozen Treats

Holistic health practitioners all agree that sugar is a major contributor to diabetes, hypoglycemia and tooth decay — and, for this reason, should be avoided. Similarly, honey and other natural, non-herb sweeteners should be used only in very small amounts or not at all. Stevia (see page 148) is a good substitute in cases where the specific chemistry of sugar is not essential. Unfortunately, sugar (or honey) is necessary in frozen desserts — without it the dessert crystallizes and freezes the liquids into one solid block. To ensure a soft, spoonable texture, frozen desserts must contain enough sugar to lower their freezing point; the more sugar, the softer the consistency.

The recipes in this section represent something of a compromise: They do not contain enough sugar to keep them from freezing completely, but they do have enough to give them a pleasant texture. We have included only as much sugar (or honey) as is absolutely necessary, so don't try to reduce the amounts any further or the recipes won't work.

Still, given that sugar is so undesirable, why provide these recipes at all? We offer them because they enable you to use some of the pulp that is produced from juicing. Because they contain far less sugar and only fresh, natural ingredients that contain no other chemicals or additives, these frozen treats are certainly preferable to commercial ice cream and sherbet. And the ice pops in this section are a better bet for kids than the colored, sugared water they get from the store.

Of course, boiling and freezing juice, no matter how fresh it is, will destroy vitamin C, enzymes and other heat-sensitive phytonutrients. The best alternative is to make "instant" frappé or frozen yogurt using the Vita-Mix (see page 9). This uses the whole fruit with pulp and does not require any sweeteners, except a small amount according to individual taste.

To use pulp from juice recipes: Pulp from any of the fruit juice or fruit juice cocktails may be used to make sherbets, ices or frappés, frozen yogurt or popsicles. Pulp from some of the sweeter vegetable juices such as carrot, beet, parsnip or fennel may also be used if blended with fruit pulp. To use pulp for frozen desserts, cut out the core and seeds and peel the fruit or vegetable before juicing. For best results, blend pulp using blender or food processor before using in frozen treats. Measure 2 cups (500 mL) of the blended pulp and chill if the frozen dessert will be made within a day, or label and freeze until ready to use.

Frappés

The term frappé comes from the French, meaning "chilled" or "iced." Simple mixtures made from water, sugar and chopped fruit, frappés are frozen to a mushy consistency. Frappés are coarser (with a texture resembling that of coarse rock salt) than any of the other iced desserts. To make frappé from chilled or frozen pulp, the pulp need only be thawed enough to blend with other ingredients.

Freezing ices, frappés, sherbets and yogurt: Freezing times given in recipe are approximate. Actual results will depend on the freezer and the pan. Deep-sided metal loaf pans are best because with each stirring, air is incorporated and the mixture tends to expand. The recipes in this section give directions for freezing the mixture in a 9-by 5-inch (2 L) metal loaf pan in a chest freezer. However, if your freezer has a "fast freeze" compartment or if a square, shallow metal pan is used, freezing times will be shorter. All of the frozen treats can be made with an ice cream machine. Follow manufacturer's directions when using this appliance.

To "ripen" frozen ices: Unless timed perfectly, most ices will be too hard to serve directly from the freezer. In order to make them easy to serve and to bring out their best flavor, iced desserts require "ripening" or softening. To ripen, set the iced dessert in the refrigerator for 45 minutes to 2 hours before serving, depending on the pan (wide, shallow pans thaw more quickly) and the degree to which the ice is frozen.

Serves 4 to 6

Frappé

Tips

Be sure to trim off the white pith and remove seeds before juicing the citrus fruits used in this recipe. Save and freeze the pulp from fruit juices for use in homemade frozen ices.

Any fruit juice works well in this recipe.

- 9- by 5-inch (2 L) metal loaf pan

2 cups	chilled or frozen fruit pulp	500 mL
2 cups	freshly squeezed orange juice or apple juice	500 mL
1	lemon, juiced	1
¾ cup	granulated sugar or liquid honey	175 mL

1. In a blender combine pulp, freshly squeezed orange juice, lemon juice and sugar. Blend for 10 seconds on High. Pour into loaf pan. Freeze for 2 hours or until a mushy consistency is reached.

2. Stir mixture and return to freezer for 1 hour or just until firm enough to scoop. If it freezes solid, ripen in the refrigerator (see above) to soften.

Instant Frappé

To make instant frappé you will need a Vita-Mix machine. The benefits of this method are that you can use the peel, core and seeds of most fruit, and sugar is not required. To sweeten, just add ½ tsp (2 mL) powdered or liquid stevia to taste.

2 cups	fruit or fruit-vegetable pulp	500 mL
½ cup	fruit juice	125 mL
1 to 2 tbsp	liquid honey or maple syrup, optional	15 to 25 mL
3 cups	ice cubes	750 mL

1. Combine pulp, juice, honey, if using, and ice cubes in Vita-Mix bowl. Secure lid. Process at variable speed #1, increasing speed to #10 and to High. Process for 30 to 60 seconds or until ice is chopped (but no longer). Serve immediately.

Berry Rosemary Frappé

The rosemary is optional here, but it adds a fragrant bite that complements the sweetness of the berries.

Tip

Berry pulp from any berry juice such as Berry Best, page 163 will work in this delicious iced dessert.

• 9- by 5-inch (2 L) metal loaf pan

2 cups	water	500 mL
2 cups	berry pulp	500 mL
½ cup	liquid honey	125 mL
2 tsp	fresh rosemary, optional	10 mL

1. Using a blender, process water, pulp, honey and rosemary, if using, until blended.

2. Pour mixture into loaf pan. Freeze for 2 hours or until a mushy consistency is reached. Stir with a fork and return to freezer for 1 hour or until firm. If consistency is too hard, ripen in the refrigerator to soften.

Carrot, Fennel & Orange Frappé

● 9- by 5-inch (2 L) metal loaf pan

2 cups	water	500 mL
½ cup	granulated sugar	125 mL
2 cups	pulp from Carrot Fennel Orange juice (see recipe, page 165)	500 mL

1. In a saucepan, combine water and sugar. Bring to a boil over medium-high heat and cook for 3 minutes without stirring. Remove from heat and set aside to cool.

2. In loaf pan, combine sugar syrup and pulp. Freeze for 2 hours or until a mushy consistency is reached. Stir with a fork and return to freezer for 1 hour or until firm. If consistency is too hard, ripen in the refrigerator to soften.

Grapefruit Frappé

● 9- by 5-inch (2 L) metal loaf pan

2 cups	water	500 mL
¾ cup	granulated sugar	175 mL
1 cup	pulp from Grapefruit juice (see recipe, page 169)	250 mL

1. In a saucepan, combine water and sugar. Bring to a boil over medium-high heat and cook for 3 minutes without stirring. Remove from heat and set aside to cool.

2. In loaf pan, combine sugar syrup and grapefruit pulp. Freeze for 2 hours or until a mushy consistency is reached. Stir with a fork and return to freezer for 1 hour or until firm. If consistency is too hard, ripen in the refrigerator to soften.

Lavender Fennel Frappé

Serves 4 to 6

- 9- by 5-inch (2 L) metal loaf pan

2 cups	water	500 mL
¼ cup	liquid honey	50 mL
5 or 6	lavender stems and flowers	5 or 6
½	vanilla bean	½
2 cups	fennel pulp or fennel combination pulp (such as Pear Fennel juice, see recipe, page 173)	500 mL

1. In a saucepan, combine water and honey. Bring to a boil over medium-high heat and cook for 2 to 3 minutes without stirring. Remove from heat and stir in lavender and vanilla bean. Set aside to cool.

2. When cooled, strain lavender mixture into loaf pan, discarding solids. Stir in pulp and freeze for 2 hours or until a mushy consistency is reached. Stir with a fork and return to freezer for 1 hour or until firm. If consistency is too hard, ripen in the refrigerator to soften.

Pineapple Sage Frappé

Serves 4 to 6

Tip
Pineapple sage is a tender perennial with sweet, fragrant pineapple flavor. If you can find this herb, use it in this or any of the fruit juice recipes.

- 9- by 5-inch (2 L) metal loaf pan

2 cups	water	500 mL
2 cups	pulp from Pineapple Citrus juice (see recipe, page 174)	500 mL
½ cup	liquid honey	125 mL
1 tbsp	chopped fresh pineapple sage, optional	15 mL

1. Using a blender, process water, pulp, honey and sage leaves until blended. Pour mixture into loaf pan. Freeze for 2 hours or until a mushy consistency is reached. Stir with a fork and return to freezer for 1 hour or until firm. If consistency is too hard, ripen in the refrigerator to soften.

Honey

Referred to as "the white man's fly" by Native Americans, the honeybee was introduced to North America in the seventeenth century by English colonists. It quickly became important for pollinating food crops and providing a sweet alternative to sugar from cane, beets and molasses.

To produce 1 tsp (5 mL) of honey, worker bees, which collect the nectar and flower pollen, will fly a distance equivalent to once around the world. A colony of workers must visit and extract nectar from about 2 million flowers to produce only 1 lb (500 g). In early human history, when honey was taken from hives, they were often destroyed in the process. Thankfully, in the mid-1800s, a wooden hive structure was invented that permitted the harvesting of honey without harming the bees. Variations on that box are still used by modern beekeepers.

The color and flavor of honey differ from region to region and country to country, depending on the types of flowers from which the nectar is gathered. Some common North American bee plants are listed below.

Alfalfa. An important honey plant in most of western North America, alfalfa honey is white or extra-light amber in color and mild in taste.

Buckwheat. Plants grow in cool, moist climates and produce a dark brown and distinct strongly flavored honey early in the season.

Clover. The most important (and popular) honey plant in North America, clover produces a honey that varies in color from water-white to extra-light amber and has a mild, delicate flavor.

Eucalyptus. With more than 500 distinct species and hybrids of eucalyptus, the honey from this plant varies greatly in color and taste but is generally a bold-flavored honey with a slightly medicinal aftertaste.

Orange blossom. Often derived from a combination of citrus blossom sources, the honey is white to extra-light amber with the distinctive fragrance of oranges. This honey is abundant in the southern United States.

Sage. Found mostly along the California coast and Sierra Nevada mountain range, sage shrubs produce a mild, delicately flavored honey that is usually white in color.

Sunflower. A gold colored honey with a unique but delicate flavor from sunflowers that grow in abundance in Manitoba and the central United States.

For more information about honey and honey production, visit www.honey.com or http://www.honey.com/consumers/honeyinfo/default.asp.

Ices

Made only from water, flavored water, fruit juices and syrup (no pulp is used in true ices), the texture of ices falls between the coarse frappé and the finer sherbet.

Sugar, sugar everywhere

The human predilection (or weakness) for sugar is such that it is now added in significant quantities to many commercially prepared food products, ranging from baby foods and vegetables to sauces, juices — even salt! We can't get away from it. Sugar comes from sugarcane, sorghum, corn syrup, sugar beets, and sugar maple. Its component parts — dextrose (corn sugar), sucrose (cane sugar), fructose (fruit sugar), glucose or lactose (milk sugar) — are what we find in most commercially prepared foods.

And the result of eating all that sugar? Apart from supplying excess calories, sugar depletes the immune system, causes tooth decay and contributes to diabetes and hypoglycemia. Worse for children, high-sugar foods can replace nutritious foods and deprive young bodies of the nutrients necessary for growth and good health.

Green Tea Ice

• 9- by 5-inch (2 L) metal loaf pan

1	bag green tea or 1 tsp (5 mL) loose green tea leaves	1
2 tsp	Digestive Seed Tea (see recipe, page 211) or fennel seeds	10 mL
1	star anise pod, seeds intact	1
½	vanilla bean	½
3 cups	boiling water	750 mL
½ cup	granulated sugar	125 mL
2 tbsp	freshly squeezed lemon juice	25 mL

1. In a large, non-reactive teapot, combine green tea, Digestive Seed Tea, anise and vanilla bean. Pour in boiling water, cover and steep for 5 minutes.

2. In a loaf pan, strain hot tea over sugar, stirring to dissolve. Set aside to cool.

3. When cooled, stir in lemon juice. Freeze for 2 hours or until a mushy consistency is reached. Stir with a fork and return to freezer for 1 hour or until firm. If frozen solid when ready to serve, ripen in the refrigerator to soften.

Lemon Ice

A wonderfully tart, lip-smuckering frozen dessert.

● 9- by 5-inch (2 L) metal loaf pan

4	lemons	4
2 cups	boiling water	500 mL
1/3 cup	liquid honey	75 mL
1/4 cup	chopped fresh lemon balm	50 mL

1. Grate the zest from one lemon and set aside. Using a citrus press or cone hand juicer, juice the lemons.

2. In loaf pan, combine boiling water, lemon juice, lemon zest, honey and lemon balm. Freeze for 2 hours or until a mushy consistency is reached. Stir with a fork and return to freezer for 1 hour or until firm. If consistency is too hard, ripen in the refrigerator to soften.

Minty Ice

● 9- by 5-inch (2 L) metal loaf pan

2 cups	water	500 mL
1/2 cup	granulated sugar	125 mL
1/4 cup	chopped fresh mint	50 mL
1	lime, juiced	1

1. In a saucepan, combine water, sugar and mint. Bring to a boil over medium-high heat and cook for 3 minutes without stirring. Remove from heat and set aside to cool.

2. Stir lime juice into cooled mint mixture and pour into loaf pan. Freeze for 2 hours or until a mushy consistency is reached. Stir with a fork and return to freezer for 1 hour or until firm. If consistency is too hard, ripen in the refrigerator to soften.

Serves 4 to 6

Strawberry-Beet Ice

- 9- by 5-inch (2 L) metal loaf pan

2 cups	strawberry and beet pulp	500 mL
2 cups	water	500 mL
⅓ cup	liquid honey	75 mL

1. In loaf pan combine pulp, water and honey. Freeze for 2 hours or until a mushy consistency is reached. Stir with a fork and return to freezer for 1 hour or until firm. If consistency is too hard, ripen in the refrigerator to soften.

Serves 4 to 6

Tarragon Ice

- 9- by 5-inch (2 L) metal loaf pan

2 cups	water	500 mL
½ cup	granulated sugar	125 mL
3 tbsp	chopped fresh tarragon	45 mL
2	lemons, juiced	2

1. In a saucepan, combine water, sugar and tarragon. Bring to a boil over medium-high heat and cook for 3 minutes without stirring. Remove from heat and set aside to cool.

2. Stir lemon juice into cooled tarragon mixture and pour into loaf pan. Freeze for 2 hours or until a mushy consistency is reached. Stir with a fork and return to freezer for 1 hour or until firm. If consistency is too hard, ripen in the refrigerator to soften.

Sweet Alternatives

Aztec sweet herb (*Phyla scaberrima*, formerly *Lippia dulcis*). A perennial herb used by the Aztecs. The compound hernandulcin, found in the leaves, stems and roots, is about three times as sweet as sucrose but has a somewhat bitter aftertaste.

Date sugar. A coarse, dark mealy substance from ground-up dehydrated dates. High in fiber, vitamins and minerals, it is fine in baked products but does not dissolve in drinks or liquids.

Honey. See page 347.

Katemfe (*Thaumatococcus daniellii*). A perennial herb of the arrowroot family found in the East and West African rain forests. The sweet protein thaumatin, found in fruit of the plant, is up to 1,600 times as sweet as sucrose but loses its sweetness if heated.

Licorice (*Glycyrrhiza glabra*, see page 139). Its wrinkled, thick brown roots contain glycyrrhizin, a compound that is 50 to 150 times as sweet as cane sugar. The elderly or people with high blood pressure or heart, kidney, or liver disease should avoid licorice.

Molasses (see page 152). The stronger tasting, crude blackstrap molasses is preferred nutritionally to the other lighter types. Molasses is a concentrated syrupy by-product of sugar cane refining and is rich in B vitamins, vitamin E, iron, calcium, magnesium, potassium, chromium, manganese and zinc.

Stevia (*Stevia rebaudiana*, see page 148). Known as the "sweet herb" and used in Paraguay and Central America since pre-Columbian times, stevia is 200 to 300 times as sweet as sucrose with none of the side effects or calories. A mild aftertaste is detectable in juices or fruit desserts where stevia is used. Widely available in alternative/health stores, stevia is the easiest of the sweet herbs to find and use even though it is still prevented from being used as a sugar substitute in the United States.

Other fruits and berries offering sweet alternatives to sugar include serendipity berries (*Dioscoreophyllum cumminsii*) and miracle fruit (*Synsepalum dulcificum*).

Sherbets

Also called sorbet, sherbet is a smooth, frozen sugar-fruit-water mixture. Because of their high liquid content, sherbets require stabilizers to keep the texture solid and smooth but without freezing too hard. Dissolved gelatin, softened marshmallows and beaten egg whites are used for this purpose.

Sherbets are usually served in chilled sherbet glasses but individual servings can be molded in the shape of an egg and served on a chilled dessert plate with fruit or herb garnishes. Unlike mousses or cream molded frozen desserts, sherbets are not usually served with sauces.

Basil-Pear Sherbet

Serves 4 to 6

● 9- by 5-inch (2 L) metal loaf pan

2 cups	pulp from Autumn Refresher juice (see recipe, page 163)	500 mL
2 cups	water	500 mL
½ cup	granulated sugar	125 mL
2 tbsp	chopped fresh basil	25 mL
2	egg whites	2

1. In loaf pan combine pulp, water, sugar and basil. Freeze for 1 to 2 hours or until a mushy consistency is reached.

2. Beat egg whites in a bowl until stiff but not dry. Remove sherbet from freezer and beat with a fork for 20 seconds. Whisk in beaten egg whites. Return to freezer for 1 hour or until firm. If consistency is too hard, ripen in the refrigerator to soften.

Serves 4 to 6

Orange-Melon Sherbet

Tip
Use the pulp from Melon
Mania (see recipe, page 203)
or from any fruit juice recipe
containing melon.

● 9- by 5-inch (2 L) metal loaf pan

2 cups	melon pulp	500 mL
2 ½ cups	freshly squeezed orange juice	625 mL
2 tbsp	grated orange zest	25 mL
1	lemon, juiced	1
½ cup	granulated sugar	125 mL
1 cup	water	250 mL
2	egg whites	2

1. In loaf pan combine pulp, orange juice, orange zest, lemon juice, sugar and water. Freeze for 1 to 2 hours or until a mushy consistency is reached.

2. Beat egg whites in a bowl until stiff but not dry. Remove sherbet from freezer and beat with a fork for 20 seconds. Whisk in beaten egg whites. Return to freezer for 1 hour or until firm. If consistency is too hard, ripen in the refrigerator to soften.

Frozen Yogurts

In these desserts, natural yogurt replaces the heavy cream of ice creams, mousses and parfaits. You may substitute soft tofu for yogurt. Homemade frozen yogurt is truly healthier than the sweeter ices and fat-laden desserts made with 18% to 36% butterfat creams. It is superior to some commercial frozen yogurts, which may contain much more sugar and chemical additives.

Serves 4 to 6		

Banana-Orange Yogurt

- 9- by 5-inch (2 L) metal loaf pan

2 cups	pulp from C-Blend juice (see recipe, page 166)	500 mL
1 cup	natural yogurt	250 mL
1	ripe banana, mashed	1
2 tbsp	liquid honey	25 mL

1. In loaf pan combine pulp, yogurt, banana and honey. Freeze for 1 to 2 hours or until firm. If consistency is too hard, ripen in the refrigerator to soften.

Serves 4 to 6		

Frozen Strawberry Yogurt

- 9- by 5-inch (2 L) metal loaf pan

2 cups	natural yogurt	500 mL
2 cups	sliced strawberries or pulp from any juice containing strawberries	500 mL
½ cup	beet juice	125 mL
3 tbsp	liquid honey	45 mL

1. In loaf pan combine yogurt, strawberries, beet juice and honey. Freeze for 1 to 2 hours or until firm. If consistency is too hard, ripen in the refrigerator to soften.

Fruit Pulp Frozen Yogurt

Serves 4 to 6

If desired, add up to 2 tbsp (25 mL) chopped fresh sage, thyme, basil, tarragon, mint, lemon balm or hyssop.

• 9- by 5-inch (2 L) metal loaf pan

2 cups	fruit pulp or sweet vegetable pulp	500 mL
1 cup	natural yogurt	250 mL
3 tbsp	liquid honey, optional	45 mL
1 tbsp	freshly squeezed lemon juice	15 mL

1. In loaf pan combine pulp, yogurt, honey, if using, and lemon juice. Freeze for 1 to 2 hours or until firm. If consistency is too hard, ripen in the refrigerator to soften.

Instant Frozen Yogurt

Serves 4 to 6

To make instant frozen yogurt you will need a Vita-Mix machine. Pineapple Citrus juice and pulp (see recipe, page 174) works well for this recipe and requires no sweetening.

2 cups	chilled or frozen fruit pulp (see left)	500 mL
1 cup	natural yogurt	250 mL
1/2 cup	fruit juice	125 mL
2 tbsp	liquid honey, optional	25 mL
3 cups	ice cubes	750 mL

1. Combine pulp, yogurt, juice, honey, if using, and ice cubes in bowl of Vita-Mix and secure lid. Process, starting at variable speed #1, increasing speed to #10 and to High. Use the tamper while machine is processing. The process takes only 30 to 60 seconds. Serve immediately.

Ice Pops

Kids love ice pops. If started young enough, they will also love frozen fruit juices or a mixture of pulp and juice with no sweetener at all. To wean older children off commercial Popsicles, make this recipe with 2 to 3 tbsp (25 to 45 mL) liquid honey and gradually reduce it.

Use juice or a 1:2 ratio of pulp to juice. Always process pulp in the blender before using in ice pops. Carrot, fennel and beet juice can be mixed with sweeter fruit juices. If herbs are recommended for a particular condition, a tea may be made, strained and blended with fruit juice and frozen to make it easier for a child to take.

To freeze ice pops: Pour ¼ cup (50 mL) juice into waxed paper cups, freeze for 1 hour or until firm enough to hold stick. Insert wooden stick in middle and return to freezer for 1 hour or until hard. Re-useable plastic containers are available for making these refreshing treats at home.

Makes 12 ice pops

Berry Pops

● 12 waxed paper cups and 12 wooden sticks

2 cups	raspberry, strawberry or cherry juice	500 mL
½ cup	freshly squeezed orange juice	125 mL
½ cup	beet juice	125 mL
2 tbsp	liquid honey, optional	25 mL

1. In a medium bowl, combine raspberry juice, orange juice, beet juice and honey, if using. Pour ¼ cup (50 mL) juice into each waxed paper cup. Freeze for 1 hour or until firm enough to hold a stick. Insert wooden stick in middle and return to freezer for 1 hour or until hard.

Orange Icesicles

● 12 waxed paper cups and 12 wooden sticks

2 cups	freshly squeezed orange juice	500 mL
1 cup	carrot juice	250 mL
2 tbsp	liquid honey, optional	25 mL
2 tbsp	grated orange zest	25 mL

1. In a medium bowl, combine orange juice, carrot juice, honey, if using, and zest. Pour $\frac{1}{4}$ cup (50 mL) juice into each waxed paper cup. Freeze for 1 hour or until firm enough to hold a stick. Insert wooden stick in middle and return to freezer for 1 hour or until hard.

Appendix A
Food Allergies

Certain foods can trigger or aggravate conditions such as asthma, chronic fatigue syndrome, depression, chronic digestive problems, eczema, headaches, hives, irritable bowel syndrome, migraines, rheumatoid arthritis and ulcerative colitis in adults, and ear infections and epilepsy in children.

Symptoms of food allergies and intolerances can include chronic infections or inflammations, diarrhea, fatigue, anxiety, depression, joint pain, skin rashes, dark circles or puffiness under the eyes, itchy nose or throat, water retention, and swollen glands.

In the classic allergic reaction, a trigger (such as nuts) is mistakenly identified as an "enemy" by the immune system, which sets out to get rid of the offending toxin.

Food intolerances or sensitivities differ from "classic" allergies in that reactions do not happen immediately. As a result, allergy tests often cannot detect food intolerances. If you suspect that a food may be causing a chronic problem, the most effective method of identifying the culprit is to use an elimination diet.

Factors in food allergies include digestive system problems and lowered immune system functioning. While eliminating suspected foods from the diet, work to improve immunity (see Immune Deficiency, page 59) and digestion (see Indigestion, page 62). A key factor in digestion is liver functioning (see Liver Problems, page 71). Regular daily exercise and stress-reduction activities, such as meditation and yoga, improve immunity.

The most common foods that provoke chronic conditions are dairy products, wheat, corn, caffeine, yeast and citrus fruits. Other common food problems occur with processed and refined foods, food additives and preservatives, eggs, strawberries, pork, tomatoes, peanuts and chocolate. In irritable bowel syndrome, potatoes and onions are also common triggers. Dairy products are the most common trigger for children's chronic ear infections.

Foods that are especially helpful in reducing allergic reactions are:
- plenty of antioxidant fruit and vegetables
- yogurt with live bacterial cultures to re-establish helpful digestive bacteria
- flavonoids in the skins of fruits and vegetables, especially citrus
- essential fatty acids in oily fish (herring, salmon, sardines, mackerel), fish oils, flax seeds and evening primrose oil are anti-inflammatory and reduce the severity of allergies
- vitamin C decreases allergic reactions. Broccoli, lemon juice and rosehip tea are sources that are unlikely to cause allergic reactions.

The Elimination Diet

Preparation
Before starting on an elimination diet, consult with your health-care practitioner to eliminate the possibility of serious disease causing your symptoms. If disease is not evident, ask for (and follow) your health-care practitioner's advice about trying the elimination diet.

Choosing foods to eliminate
Start with the Guidelines to Eating Well (see page 12). This will eliminate refined and processed food, which will improve immunity and digestion. Avoid food additives and preservatives, which are common food allergens. If you regularly drink coffee or alcohol and are eliminating them, you may experience headache. To avoid this side affect, cut down on these gradually.

You can choose to eliminate one food at a time, or multiple foods. It is important that you maintain a wide variety of different types of food in your diet. Choose to eliminate the most common food allergens from the list on page 359. Do not add foods to which you have known allergies.

Steps in the Elimination Diet
1. Start a daily "diet diary," noting all the foods you eat each day and the symptoms you experience.
2. Eliminate one food item from your diet for a period of 1 week. Start with a food that most commonly causes symptoms, especially one that you eat regularly. The food must be completely eliminated. If you are eliminating eggs, avoid cakes, salad dressings and any other food that may contain eggs. If eliminating dairy products, check the ingredients of all foods for lactose, lactic acid and whey. Margarine commonly contains these ingredients.
3. If you have fewer symptoms while eliminating the chosen food or foods, proceed to step 4 to check each food you have eliminated. If there is no improvement in your symptoms, go back to the Guidelines to Good Health diet while you choose another food to eliminate.
4. Add the food item back into your diet, by eating 2 servings a day for the next 3 days. If you experience any symptoms, stop eating the food immediately and avoid it for 6 months while you work on improving your immunity, digestion and liver functioning.

Reintroducing foods that cause adverse reactions
After eliminating the food from the diet for a period of 6 months, the food can often be slowly reintroduced to the diet without adverse effects.

Appendix C
Herbs to Avoid in Pregnancy

Avoid medicinal doses of all herbs while pregnant unless you have full knowledge of the actions of the herb or recipe specific advice from a midwife. Following are some of the most common herbs to avoid during pregnancy.

Alder buckthorn *Rhamnus frangula*
Aloe *Aloe vera* (use externally only)
Angelica *Angelica archangelica*
Arbor vita *Thuja occidentalis*
Autumn crocus *Colchicum autumnale*
Barberry *Berberis vulgaris*
Bethroot Trillium (all species)
Black cohosh *Cimicifuga racemosa* (except as advised by midwife)
Blood root *Sanguinaria canadensis*
Blue cohosh *Caulophyllum thalacthroides* (except as advised by midwife)
Bogbean *Menyanthes trifoliata*
Broom *Sarothamnus scoparius*
Bryony *Bryonia dioica*
Buchu *Barosma betulina*
Calamus *Acorus calamus*
Cascara sagrada *Rhamnus purshiana*
Cayenne *Capsicum minimum* (use sparingly)
Celandine *Chelidonium majus*
Coffee *Coffea arabia*
Coltsfoot *Tussilago farfara*
Comfrey *Symphytum officinale*
Cotton root *Gossypium herbaceum*
Dong quai *Angelica sinensis*
Elecampane *Inula helenium*
Essential oils (except floral oils, use sparingly)
Fenugreek *Trigonella foenum-graecum*
Feverfew *Tanacetum parthenium*
Gentian *Gentiana lutea*
Ginger *Zingiber officinale* (use sparingly)
Ginkgo *Ginkgo biloba*
Ginseng *Panax ginseng, Panax quinquefolium, Eleutherococcus senticosus*

Goldenseal *Hydrastis canadensis*
Hops *Humulus lupulus*
Horehound *Marrubium vulgare*
Horseradish *Amoracia lapathifolia*
Hyssop *Hyssopus officinalis*
Jamaican dogwood *Piscidia erythrina*
Jimsonweed *Datura stramonium*
Juniper *Juniperus communis*
Licorice *Glycyrrhiza glabra*
Lobelia *Lobelia inflata*
Lomatium *Lomatium dissectum*
Ma huang (Ephedra) *Ephedra sinensis*
Male fern *Dryopteris felix-mas*
Mandrake *Podophyllum peltatum*
Mistletoe *Viscum album*
Mugwort *Artemesia vulgare*
Nutmeg *Myristica officinalis* (use sparingly)
Oregon/Mountain grape *Berberis aquafolia*
Osha root *Ligusticum porterii*
Parsley *Petroselinum crispum* (use sparingly)
Pennyroyal *Mentha pulegium*
Peruvian bark *Cinchona* spp.
Pleurisy root *Aesclepius tuberosa*
Poke root *Phytolacca decandra*
Poppy *Papiver somniferum*
Purging buckthorn *Rhamnus cathartica*
Rue *Ruta graveolens*
Sage *Salvia officinalis*
Saw palmetto *Serenoa serrulata*
Senna *Cassia senna*
Snake root *Polygala senega*
Southernwood *Artemesia arboratum*
Tansy *Tanacetum vulgare*
Thuja *Thuja occidentalis*
Thyme *Thymus vulgaris*
Turkey rhubarb root *Rheum palmatum*
Vervain *Verbena officinalis*
Wild indigo *Baptisia tinctoria*
Wormwood *Artemesia absinthum*
Yarrow *Achillea millefolium*
Yellow jasmine *Gelsemium sempervirens*
Yellow dock *Rumex crispus*

Glossary

Adaptogen. A substance that builds resistance to stress by balancing the functions of the glands and immune response, thus strengthening the immune system, nervous system, and glandular system. Adaptogens promote overall vitality. *Examples:* astragalus and ginseng.

Alterative. A substance that gradually changes a condition by restoring health.

Analgesic. A substance that relieves pain by acting as a nervine, antiseptic or counterirritant. *Examples:* German chamomile, meadowsweet, nutmeg and willow.

Anodyne. Herbs that relieve pain. *Example:* clove.

Antibiotic. Meaning "against life", antibiotics are substances that work to destroy infectious agents, including bacteria and fungi, without endangering the patient's health. *Examples:* garlic, green tea, lavender, sage and thyme.

Anti-inflammatory. Controlling or reducing swelling, redness, pain and heat, which is a reaction of the body to injury or infection. *Examples:* German chamomile and St. John's wort.

Antioxidant. A compound that protects cells by preventing polyunsaturated fatty acids (PUFAs) in cell membranes from oxidizing, or breaking down. They do this by neutralizing free radicals. Vitamins C, E and beta carotene are antioxidant nutrients and foods high in them will have antioxidant properties. *Examples:* alfalfa, beet tops, dandelion leaves, parsley, garlic, thyme and watercress.

Antiseptic. Herbs used to prevent or counteract the growth of disease germs in order to prevent infection. *Examples:* cabbage, calendula, German chamomile, clove, garlic, honey, nutmeg, onion, parsley, peppermint, rosemary, salt, thyme, turmeric and vinegar.

Antispasmodic. Relieving muscle spasm or cramp, including colic. *Examples:* German chamomile, ginger, licorice and peppermint.

Astringent. Drying and contracting substances that aid in reducing secretions. *Examples:* cinnamon, lemon, sage and thyme.

Beta carotene. The natural coloring agent (carotenoids) that gives fruits and vegetables (such as carrots) their deep orange colour. It converts in the body to vitamin A. Benefits of eating foods high in beta carotene include cancer prevention, lowering the risk of heart disease, increased immunity, lower risk of cataracts and better mental functioning. *Examples:* squash, carrots, yams, sweet potatoes, pumpkins and red peppers.

Bitters. See pages 217–18.

Carbohydrates. An important group of plant foods that are composed of carbon, hydrogen and oxygen. A carbohydrate is a simple sugar or a substance formed by combination of simple sugars. The chief sources of carbohydrates in a whole foods diet are grains, vegetables and fruits. Other sources include sugars, natural sweeteners and syrups.

Carminative. Herbs that relax the stomach muscles and are taken to relieve gas and gripe. *Examples:* allspice, cloves, caraway, dill, fennel, garlic, ginger, parsley, peppermint, sage and thyme.

Cathartic. Herbs that have a laxative effort. *Examples:* dandelion, licorice and parsley.

Cholagogue. Promotes the secretion of bile, assisting digestion and bowel elimination. *Examples:* dandelion root, licorice, yellow dock.

Decoction. A solution obtained by using the woody parts of plants (roots, seeds, bark) and boiling them in water for 10 to 20 minutes.

Demulcent. Soothing substances taken internally to protect damaged tissue. *Examples:* barley, cucumber, honey, marshmallow and fenugreek.

Depurative. Herbs taken to cleanse the blood. *Examples:* burdock, dandelion root, garlic, onion stinging nettles and yellow dock.

Diaphoretic. Herbs used to induce sweating. *Examples:* cayenne, German chamomile, cinnamon, ginger and horseradish.

Digestive. Substances that aid digestion. See Indigestion, page 62 and section on aperitifs and digestives, pages 206–16.

Diuretic. Herbs that increase the flow of urine. Should be used for the short term only. *Examples:* cucumber, burdock, dandelion leaf and root, fennel seed, lemon, linden, parsley and pumpkin seed.

Dysmenorrhea. Condition of menstruation accompanied by cramping pains that may be incapacitating in their intensity.

Ellagic acid. A natural plant phenol thought to have powerful anticancer/anti-aging properties. Research indicates that it blocks cells' receptor sites from taking up chemically induced carcinogens.

Elixir. A tonic that invigorates or strengthens the body by stimulating or restoring health.

Emetic. A substance taken to provoke vomiting to expel poisons. *Examples:* salt, nutmeg and mustard.

Emmenagogue. Herbs that promote menstruation. *Examples:* calendula and German chamomile.

Enzymes. The elements found in food that act as the catalyst for chemical reactions within the body, allowing efficient digestion and absorption of food, and enabling the metabolic processes that support tissue growth, high levels of energy and promote good health. Enzymes are destroyed by heat but juicing leaves them intact and readily absorbed.

Essential fatty acids (EFA's). Fat is an essential part of a healthy diet — about 20 fatty acids are used by the human body to maintain normal function. Fats are necessary to maintain healthy skin and hair, transport the fat-soluble vitamins (A, D, E and K), and to signal the feeling of fullness after meals. The three fatty acids considered to be most important — essential — are omega-6 linoleic, omega-3 linolenic and gamma linolenic acids. Evidence suggests that increasing the proportion of these fatty acids in the diet may increase immunity and reduce the risks of heart disease, high blood pressure and arthritis. The best vegetable source of omega-3 EFA in the diet is flax seed. Other sources of EFAs are hemp seeds, nuts, seeds, olives, avocados and cold-water fish.

Expectorant. Herbs that help to relieve mucus congestion from colds. *Examples:* coltsfoot, elder, garlic, ginger, hyssop, mullein and thyme.

Febriguge. Herbs that help reduce fever. *Examples:* German chamomile, sage and yarrow.

Fiber. indigestible carbohydrate. Fiber helps protect against intestinal problems and bowel disorders. *Best sources:* raw fruit and vegetables, seeds and whole grains.

Types of fiber include pectin, which reduces the risk of heart disease (by lowering cholesterol) and helps eliminate toxins. It is found mainly in fruits such as apples, berries, citrus fruit, vegetables and dried peas. Cellulose prevents varicose veins, constipation, colitis and plays a role in deflecting colon cancer. Because cellulose is found in the outer layer of fruit and vegetables, it is important to buy only organic produce and leave the peel on.

The hemicellulose in fruits, vegetables and grains aids in weight loss, prevents constipation, lowers risk of colon cancer and helps in removing cancer-forming toxins from the intestinal tract. Lignin is a fiber known to lower cholesterol, prevent gallstone formation, and help diabetics. It is found only in fruits, vegetables and Brazil nuts.

When juicing, the pulp or fiber is separated from the pure raw juice and is usually discarded. That is why it is important to include fresh raw fruits and vegetables or pulped drinks for a healthy diet.

Free Radicals. Highly unstable compounds that attack cell membranes and cause cell breakdown, aging and a predisposition to some diseases. Free radicals come from environment causes such as exposure to radiation, UV light, smoking, ozone and certain medications. Free radicals are also formed in the body by enzymes and during energy metabolism. See also Antioxidant, page 362.

Flatulence. The gas caused by poor digestion. See Carminative, page 362.

Food combining. See page 15.

Hepatic. Herbs that strengthen, tone and stimulate secretive functions of the liver. *Examples:* dandelion, lemon balm, milk thistle, rosemary and turmeric.

Hypotensive. Herbs used to lower blood pressure. *Examples:* garlic, hawthorn, linden flower and yarrow.

Isoflavones. Isoflavones are phytoestrogens, the plant versions of the human hormone estrogen. Found in nuts, soybeans and legumes, isoflavones help to prevent several cancers, including pancreatic cancer and cancer of the colon, breast and prostate, by preserving vitamin C in the body and acting as antioxidants.

Lactose intolerance. Deficiency of the enzyme lactase, which breaks down lactose, a sugar contained in milk from humans and animals. Without sufficient lactase, the sugar ferments in the large intestine causing bloating, diarrhea, abdominal pain and gas.

Laxative. Herbs that stimulate bowel movement should to be used for short term only. *Examples:* dandelion root, licorice root, rhubarb and yellow dock.

Macrobiotic diet. Eating whole food that is seasonal, and produced locally. Whole grains, vegetables, fruit (except tropical fruit), legumes and beans, small amounts of fish or organic meat, sea herbs and nuts and seeds are foods that are appropriate for North Americans.

Milk allergy. Many individuals, especially babies and young children, have allergic reactions to the protein in milk. Reactions include wheezing, eczema, rash, mucous build-up and asthma-like symptoms.

Mucilage. A thick, sticky glue-like substance, found in high concentrations in some herbs, that contains and helps spread the active ingredients of herbs, while soothing inflamed surfaces. *Examples:* comfrey root, marshmallow root and slippery elm root.

Nervine. Herbs used to ease anxiety and stress, and nourish the nerves, by strengthening nerve fibers. *Examples:* German chamomile, lemon balm, oats, skullcap, St. John's wort, thyme, valerian and vervain.

Non-reactive cooking utensils. The acids in foods can react with certain materials and promote the oxidation of some nutrients, as well as discolor the material itself. Non-reactive materials suitable for brewing teas include glass, enamel-coated cast iron or enamel-coated stainless steel. While cast iron pans are recommended for cooking (a meal cooked in unglazed cast iron can provide 20% of the recommended daily iron intake), and stainless steel is a non-reactive cooking material, neither is recommended for brewing or steeping teas.

Organosulfides. Compounds that have been shown to reduce blood pressure, lower cholesterol levels, and reduce blood clotting. *Examples:* garlic and onions.

Phytochemicals. Chemicals from a plant. Phyto, from the Greek, means "to bring forth", and is used as a prefix to designate "from a plant."

Protein. The dietary building block of body tissues. Protein is necessary for healthy growth and repair of cells, for reproduction and for protection against infection. Protein consists of 22 different amino acids, (called "essential amino acids") 8 of which are especially important because they can not be manufactured by the body.

A food that contains all 8 essential amino acids is said to be a complete protein. Protein from animal products — meat, fish, poultry, dairy products — is complete. The only accepted plant source of complete protein is soybeans and soy products, but research is establishing new theories that the protein content of legumes may be complete enough to replace animal protein.

A food that contains some, but not all 8, essential amino acids is called an incomplete protein source. Nuts and seeds, legumes and cereals and grains are plant products that provide us with incomplete protein. If your meals include foods from two complementary incomplete protein sources, your body will combine the incomplete proteins in the right proportions to make a complete protein. For example, many cultures have a tradition of using legumes and whole grains in dishes. Scientifically, this combination provides a good amino-acid (complete protein) balance in the diet because legumes are low in methionine and high in lysine, while whole grains are high in methionine and low in lysine. When eaten together, the body combines them to make complete protein. Nuts and seeds must be paired with dairy or soy protein in order to provide complete protein.

Purgative. Substances that promote bowel movement and increased intestinal peristalsis. *Example:* yellow dock.

Rhizome. Underground stem, usually thick and fleshy. *Examples:* ginger and turmeric.

Ripen. When applied to frozen desserts, means to allow to soften in the refrigerator.

Rubefacient. Herbs that, when applied to the skin, stimulate circulation in that area, bringing a good supply of blood to the skin, and increasing heat in the tissues. *Examples:* cayenne, garlic, ginger, horseradish, mustard seed, oils of rosemary, peppermint, thyme and wintergreen.

Sedative. Herbs that have a powerful quieting effect on the nervous system to relieve tension and induce sleep. *Examples:* German chamomile, lettuce, linden, lavender and valerian.

Stimulant. Herbs that have the effect of focusing the mind and increasing activity. *Examples:* basil, cayenne, cinnamon, peppermint and rosemary.

Styptic. Herbs causing capillaries to contract and thereby stop superficial bleeding. *Examples:* calendula and cayenne.

Tannin. A chemical component in herbs that causes astringency (see Astringent, page 362) and helps staunch internal bleeding. *Examples:* coffee, tea, vervain and witch hazel.

Therapeutic dose. Amount recommended by herbalist for healing certain ailments, usually higher and for longer periods of time than herbs used in cooking (which maintain health). Standardized amounts of specific herbs are used.

Tea. Strictly speaking, tea is defined as a solution made by pouring boiling water on the dried, fermented leaves and stems of a tea plant (green or black tea). In a broader sense, tea can be any solution made by pouring boiling water on a plant's leaves, petals or stems.

Tincture. A liquid herbal extract made by soaking a herb(s) in a solvent (usually alcohol) to extract the plant's medicinal components. Some herbalists maintain tinctures are the most effective way to take herbs because they contain a wide range of the plants chemical constituents and are easily absorbed.

Tisane. The "official" term used for steeping fresh or dried herbs in boiling water. The term is interchangeable with "tea" when herbs are used.

Tonic. See page 267.

Vasodilator. A herb that relaxes blood vessels, providing the benefits of increased circulation to the arms, hands, legs, feet and brain. *Examples:* peppermint and sage.

Volatile oil. Essential components found in the aerial parts of herbs. Often extracted to make "essential oils," volatile oils are antiseptic, easily assimilated and very effective in stimulating the body parts to which they are applied.

Vulnerary. A herbal remedy that helps to heal external wounds and reduce inflammation. *Examples:* aloe vera, calendula, comfrey, marshmallow root and slippery elm bark powder.

Wildcrafting. The practice of gathering herbs from the wild. Many plants today are endangered because of excessive wildcrafting. To avoid contributing to this problem, buy herbs that are organically cultivated.

Library and Archives Canada Cataloguing in Publication

Crocker, Pat
    The juicing bible / Pat Crocker. — 2nd ed.

Includes index.
ISBN 978-0-7788-0181-8

1. Fruit juices. 2. Vegetable juices. I. Title.

TX840.J84C76 2008   641.8'75   C2007-907101-5

Bibliography

Bartram's Encyclopedia of Herbal Medicine. Thomas Bartram. Dorset: Grace Publishers, 1995.

The Complete Book of Ayurvedic Home Remedies. Vasant Lad. New York: Three Rivers Press, 1998.

The Complete Woman's Herbal. Anne McIntyre. New York: Henry Holt and Company, 1995.

Encyclopedia of Natural Medicine. Michael Murray, N.D. and Joseph Pizzorno, N.D. Rocklin, CA: Prima Publishing, 1991.

A Field Guide to Medicinal Plants. Stephen Foster and James A. Duke. New York: Houghton-Mifflin Company, 1990.

Food: Your Miracle Medicine. Jean Carper. New York: Harper Collins Publishers, Inc., 1993.

The Green Pharmacy. James Duke, Ph.D. Emmaus, PA: Rodale Press, 1997.

The Healing Herbs Cookbook. Pat Crocker. Toronto: Robert Rose, 1996.

Healing Plants: A Medicinal Guide to Native North American Plants and Herbs. Ana Nez Heatherley. Toronto: HarperCollins Publishers, 1998.

Healing Wise. Susun Weed. Woodstock, NY: Ash Tree Publishing, 1989.

Healing with Herbal Juices. Siegfried Gursche. Vancouver: Alive Books, 1993.

Healing with Whole Foods: Oriental Traditions and Modern Nutrition. Paul Pitchford. Berkeley: North Atlantic Books, 1993.

Herbal Remedies for Women. Amanda McQuade Crawford. Rocklin, CA: Prima Publishing, 1997.

Herbal Tonics. Daniel B. Mowrey, Ph.D. New Canaan, CT: Keats Publishing, 1993.

Identifying and Harvesting Edible and Medicinal Plants. Steve Brill with Evelyn Dean. New York: Hearst Books, 1994.

The Lactose-Free Family Cookbook. Jan Main. Toronto: Macmillan Canada, 1996.

Meals That Heal. Lisa Turner. Rochester, VT: Healing Arts Press, 1996.

The Multiple Sclerosis Diet Book. Dr. Roy Swank. New York: Bantam Doubleday Dell Publishing Group, 1977.

The Natural Pregnancy Book. Aviva Jill Romm. Freedom, CA: The Crossing Press, 1997.

The New Holistic Herbal. David Hoffman. Rockport, MA: Element Books, 1992.

Nutritional Healing. Denise Mortimer. Boston: Element Books, 1998.

Nutritional Influences on Illness. Melvyn Werbach, M.D. Tarzana, CA: Third Line Press, 1996.

Rodale's Basic Natural Foods Cookbook. Charles Gerras, Editor. Emmaus, PA: Rodale Press, 1984.

The Vegetarian Cook's Bible. Pat Crocker. Toronto: Robert Rose, 2007.

Sources

Herb and Organic Associations/ Organizations/Information

American Botanical Council
P.O. Box 144345, Austin Texas, 78714-4345
Tel (512)926 4900
www.herbalgram.org

Canadian Herb Society
5251 Oak Street
Vancouver BC Canada V6M 4H1
A network of herb enthusiasts

Canadian Organic Growers (COG)
Box 6408, Station J
Ottawa, ON Canada K2A 3Y6
Tel (613)231 9047 www.cog.ca Canada's
national information network for organic
farmers, gardeners and consumers.

Herb Society of America
9019 Chardon Road, Kirtland, OH 44094
Tel (440)256-0514 Fax (440)256-0541
www.herbsociety.org
A well organized group of herb enthusiasts
with 6 Districts and many active local units.

International Herb Association
910 Charles Street
Fredericksburg, VA 22401
Tel (540)368-0590 Fax (540)370-0015
www.iherb.org
A professional organization of herb growers
and business owners.

Ontarbio
RR#1 Durham, Ontario N0G 1R0
Tel (519) 369 5316
www.ontarbio.com
An organic farmers' co-operative

Organic Consumers' Association
6101 Cliff Estate Road
Little Marais MN 55614
Tel (218)226-4164 Fax (218)226-4157
www.organicconsumers.org
Excellent tips, information on a wide range of
food issues

Organic Trade Association (OTA)
P.O. Box 547 Greenfield, MA 01302-0547
Tel (413)774-7511 Fax (413)774-6432
www.ota.com
Promotes awareness and understanding of
organic production, as well as providing a
unified voice for the industry.

Organic Herbs: Plants, Dried Herbs, Tinctures

www.chineseherbsdirect.com
Chinese herbs in bulk

www.wisewomanherbals.com
Formulas and tinctures

www.gaiagarden.com
dried herbs, teas, essential oils, tinctures

Four Elements Herbals
E. 8984 Weinke Road
North Freedom, WI, 53951
Tel (608)522-4492
natures@chorus.net
www.fourelementsherbals.com
Certified organic herb farm. Tinctures
(including Immune Blend, Chi Charge,
Sleep Support, Nerve Support and Liver-
Kidney Blend), Flower Essences, teas and
cosmetics. Wholesale and mail order
available. Catalogue.

Frontier Natural Products Co-operative
2990 Wilderness Place, Suite 200
Boulder, CO 80301
Tel (303)449-8137 Fax (303)449-8139
www.frontiercoop.com
Supplier of bulk herbs.

Richters Herbs
357 Highway 47
Goodwood, ON Canada L0C 1A0
Tel (905)640-6677 Fax (905)640-6641
orderdesk@richters.com
www.richters.com
Herb specialists with more than
800 varieties, selling herbs since 1969. Mail
order seeds, plants, books. Free, full-color
catalogue. Free seminars and herbal events.

Index